Robert Geffner, PhD, ABPN
Kristina Crumpton Franey, PsyD
Teri Geffner Arnold, MSSW
Robert Falconer, MA
Editors

Identifying and Treating Youth Who Sexually Offend: Current Approaches, Techniques, and Research

Identifying and Treating Youth Who Sexually Offend: Current Approaches, Techniques, and Research has been co-published simultaneously as *Journal of Child Sexual Abuse*, Volume 13, Numbers 3/4 2004.

*Pre-publication
REVIEWS,
COMMENTARIES,
EVALUATIONS . . .*

"**A**ny professional working with sexualized adolescents, either as a direct service provider or a supervisor of programs will find this collection A MOST EXCELLENT AND USEFUL RESOURCE FOR EVERYDAY PRACTICE."

David Bolton, MEd, LPC
Executive Director
Triad Behavioral Resources, PLLC
Greensboro, North Carolina

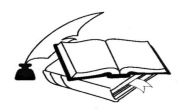

D1595603

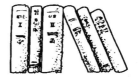

HMTP

The Haworth Maltreatment & Trauma Press®
An Imprint of The Haworth Press, Inc.

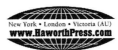

New York • London • Victoria (AU)
www.HaworthPress.com

2004

Identifying and Treating Youth Who Sexually Offend: Current Approaches, Techniques, and Research

Identifying and Treating Youth Who Sexually Offend: Current Approaches, Techniques, and Research has been co-published simultaneously as *Journal of Child Sexual Abuse,* Volume 13, Numbers 3/4 2004.

The *Journal of Child Sexual Abuse*™ Monographic "Separates"

Below is a list of " separates," which in serials librarianship means a special issue simultaneously pub - lished as a special journal issue or double-issue *and* as a "separate" hardbound monograph. (This is a format which we also call a "DocuSerial.")

"Separates" are published because specialized libraries or professionals may wish to purchase a specific thematic issue by itself in a format which can be separately cataloged and shelved, as opposed to purchasing the journal on an on-going basis. Faculty members may also more easily consider a "separate" for classroom adoption.

"Separates" are carefully classified separately with the major book jobbers so that the journal tie-in can be noted on new book order slips to avoid duplicate purchasing.

You may wish to visit Haworth's website at . . .

http://www.HaworthPress.com

. . . to search our online catalog for complete tables of contents of these separates and related publications.

You may also call 1-800-HAWORTH (outside US/Canada: 607-722-5857), or Fax 1-800-895-0582 (outside US/Canada: 607-771-0012), or e-mail at:

docdelivery@haworthpress.com

Identifying and Treating Youth Who Sexually Offend: Current Approaches, Techniques, and Research, edited by Robert Geffner, PhD, ABPN, Krisitina Crumpton Franey, PsyD, Teri Geffner Arnold, MMSW, and Robert Falconer, MA (Vol. 13, No. 3/4, 2004). *"Any professional working with sexualized adolescents, either as a direct service provider or a supervisor of programs will find this collection A MOST EXCELLENT AND USEFUL RESOURCE FOR EVERYDAY PRACTICE." (David Bolton, MEd, LPC, Executive Director, Triad Behavioral Resources, PLLC, Greensboro, North Carolina).*

Identifying and Treating Sex Offenders: Current Approaches, Research, and Techniques, edited by Robert Geffner, PhD, Kristina Crumpton Franey, PsyD, Terri Geffner Arnold, MSSW, and Robert Falconer, MA (Vol. 12, No. 3/4, 2003). *Address the assessment and treatment issues when working with adult sex offenders, exploring current issues, research, and theory behind sex offending, as well as the implications for new policies.*

Misinformation Concerning Child Sexual Abuse and Adult Survivors, edited by Charles L. Whitfield, MD, FASAM, Joyanna Silberg, PhD, and Paul J. Fink, MD (Vol. 9, No. 3/4, 2001). *"A THOROUGH, INTELLECTUALLY STIMULATING, AND COMPELLING PRIMER. . . . This collection of scholarly articles represents a comprehensive view of the issues. This is a must for everyone's bookshelf." (Ann Wolbert Burgess, RN, DNSc, CS, Professor of Psychiatric Nursing, School of Nursing, Boston College)*

Identifying and Treating Youth Who Sexually Offend: Current Approaches, Techniques, and Research

Robert Geffner, PhD, ABPN
Kristina Crumpton Franey, PsyD
Teri Geffner Arnold, MSSW
Robert Falconer, MA
Editors

Identifying and Treating Youth Who Sexually Offend: Current Approaches, Techniques, and Research has been co-published simultaneously as *Journal of Child Sexual Abuse,* Volume 13, Numbers 3/4 2004.

HMTP

The Haworth Maltreatment & Trauma Press®
An Imprint of The Haworth Press, Inc.

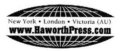

New York • London • Victoria (AU)
www.HaworthPress.com

Published by

The Haworth Maltreatment & Trauma Press, 10 Alice Street, Binghamton, NY 13904-1580 USA

The Haworth Maltreatment & Trauma Press is an imprint of The Haworth Press, Inc., 10 Alice Street, Binghamton, NY 13904-1580 USA.

Identifying and Treating Youth Who Sexually Offend: Current Techniques, Approaches, and Research has been co-published simultaneously as *Journal of Child Sexual Abuse*, Volume 13, Numbers 3/4 2004.

The development, preparation, and publication of this work has been undertaken with great care. However, the publisher, employees, editors, and agents of The Haworth Press and all imprints of The Haworth Press, Inc., including The Haworth Medical Press® and The Pharmaceutical Products Press®, are not responsible for any errors contained herein or for consequences that may ensue from use of materials or information contained in this work. Opinions expressed by the author(s) are not necessarily those of The Haworth Press, Inc.

Cover design by Kerry E. Mack

Library of Congress Cataloging-in-Publication Data

Identifying and treating youth who sexually offend : current approaches, techniques, and research / Robert Geffner, editor . . . [et al.]

     p. cm.

     "Co-published simultaneously as Journal of child sexual abuse, volume 13, numbers 3/4 2004."
Includes bibliographical references and index.

     ISBN 0-7890-2786-0 (hard cover : alk. paper)–ISBN 0-7890-2787-9 (soft cover : alk. paper)

     1. Teenage sex offenders. 2. Geffner, Robert. II. Journal of child sexual abuse.

RJ506.S48I346 2005

618.92′8583–dc22   2005001316

Indexing, Abstracting & Website/Internet Coverage

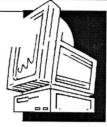

This section provides you with a list of major indexing & abstracting services and other tools for bibliographic access. That is to say, each service began covering this periodical during the year noted in the right column. Most Websites which are listed below have indicated that they will either post, disseminate, compile, archive, cite or alert their own Website users with research-based content from this work. (This list is as current as the copyright date of this publication.)

Abstracting, Website/Indexing Coverage . . . . Year When Coverage Began

- *Academic Search Elite (EBSCO)* **1996**

- *Academic Search Premier (EBSCO)*
  <http://www.epnet.com/academic/acasearchprem.asp> **1996**

- *Applied Social Sciences Index & Abstracts (ASSIA)*
  (Online: ASSI via Data-Star) (CDRom: ASSIA Plus)
  <http://www.csa.com> **1992**

- *Behavioral Medicine Abstracts (Annals of Behavioral Medicine)* . . . **1992**

- *Business Source Corporate: coverage of nearly 3,350 quality*
  magazines and journals; designed to meet the diverse information
  needs of corporations, EBSCO Publishing
  <http://www.epnet.com/corporate/bsourcecorp.asp> **1996**

- *CareData: the database supporting social care management*
  and practice <http://www.elsc.org.uk/caredata/caredata.htm> . . . **2001**

- *Child Development Abstracts & Bibliography (in print & online)*
  <http://www.ukans.edu> **1994**

- *CINAHL (Cumulative Index to Nursing & Allied Health*
  Literature), in print, EBSCO, and SilverPlatter, Data-Star,
  and PaperChase. (Support materials include Subject Heading List,
  Database Search Guide, and instructional video)
  <http://www.cinahl.com> **1992**

(continued)

(continued)

(continued)

(continued)

Special Bibliographic Notes related to special journal issues (separates) and indexing/abstracting:

- indexing/abstracting services in this list will also cover material in any "separate" that is co-published simultaneously with Haworth's special thematic journal issue or DocuSerial. Indexing/abstracting usually covers material at the article/chapter level.
- monographic co-editions are intended for either non-subscribers or libraries which intend to purchase a second copy for their circulating collections.
- monographic co-editions are reported to all jobbers/wholesalers/approval plans. The source journal is listed as the "series" to assist the prevention of duplicate purchasing in the same manner utilized for books-in-series.
- to facilitate user/access services all indexing/abstracting services are encouraged to utilize the co-indexing entry note indicated at the bottom of the first page of each article/chapter/contribution.
- this is intended to assist a library user of any reference tool (whether print, electronic, online, or CD-ROM) to locate the monographic version if the library has purchased this version but not a subscription to the source journal.
- individual articles/chapters in any Haworth publication are also available through the Haworth Document Delivery Service (HDDS).

Identifying and Treating Youth Who Sexually Offend: Current Approaches, Techniques, and Research

CONTENTS

RECIDIVISM, RESILIENCE,
AND TREATMENT EFFECTIVENESS
FOR YOUTH WHO SEXUALLY OFFEND

ABOUT THE EDITORS

Robert Geffner, PhD, ABPN, is the Founder and President of the Family Violence and Sexual Assault Institute located in San Diego, CA. Dr. Geffner is a Clinical Research Professor of Psychology at the California School of Professional Psychology, Alliant International University in San Diego, and is also a Licensed Psychologist and a Licensed Marriage and Family Therapist in California and in Texas. He was the clinical director of a large private practice mental health clinic in East Texas for over 15 years; one of his roles was the supervision of the sex offender assessment and treatment programs. Dr. Geffner is the Editor-in-Chief of Haworth's Maltreatment and Trauma Press, which includes being the Editor of the *Journal of Child Sexual Abuse* and *Journal of Aggression, Maltreatment & Trauma,* and co-editor of *Journal of Emotional Abuse,* all internationally disseminated. He also is Senior Editor of the Maltreatment, Trauma, and Interpersonal Aggression book program for The Haworth Press, Inc. He has a Diplomate in Clinical Neuropsychology from the American Board of Professional Neuropsychology. He served as an adjunct faculty member for the National Judicial College for 10 years, and was a former Professor of Psychology at the University of Texas at Tyler for 16 years. Dr. Geffner has published extensively and given presentations and workshops world-wide in the areas of family violence, sexual assault, child abuse, family and child psychology, child custody issues, forensic psychology, neuropsychology, and diagnostic assessment. He has served on several national and state committees dealing with various aspects of family psychology, family violence, child abuse, and family law. In addition, he has served as a consultant for various agencies and centers of the federal government, including the Department of Health and Human Services, National Center for Child Abuse and Neglect, Department of Defense and different branches of the military.

Kristina Crumpton Franey, PsyD, received her doctorate in Psychology from the California School of Professional Psychology at Alliant International University in San Diego, CA, with specialized training in child and adolescent psychology. Her research has focused on the experiences of adolescent sexual offenders who have re-entered society following treatment. Dr. Franey is currently working with juvenile sex offenders at the Sexual Treatment and Recovery Program in San Diego, and is working with Forensic Psych Consultants in San Diego, CA. She has worked with the Family Violence and Sexual Assault Institute (FVSAI) since 1998, and co-edited *The Cost of Child Maltreatment: Who Pays? We All Do*, published in 2001 by FVSAI.

Teri Geffner Arnold, MSSW, received her Bachelor of Arts in Psychology from the University of Texas at Austin, and her Master of Science in Social Work, also at UT Austin. Currently, she is a victims advocate at the Williamson Crisis Center in Austin, Texas. Since 2001, Ms. Geffner Arnold has been an assistant editor with the Family Violence & Sexual Assault Institute (FVSAI) for the *Journal of Child Sexual Abuse,* the *Journal of Emotional Abuse*, and the *Family Violence & Sexual Assault Bulletin.* She has provided editing assistance on three prior books and treatment manuals for the FVSAI in the past five years. She was a co-editor of a recent book, entitled *Identifying and Treating Sex Offenders.* Her primary interest lies in clinical practice with both adults and children.

Robert Falconer, MA, is currently the executive director of the Institute for Trauma Oriented Psychotherapy. He has been involved in the child maltreatment arena for over a decade, has been the President of a foundation, and has supported numerous intervention and educational projects concerning child sexual abuse. He has previously co-edited three books in this field: *Trauma, Amnesia, & the Denial of Abuse*, *Identifying and Treating Sex Offenders*, and *The Cost of Child Maltreatment: Who Pays? We All Do*, published as joint projects by FVSAI and the Institute for Trauma Oriented Psychotherapy.

About the Contributors

Josephine Bonomo, MS, is a licensed marriage and family therapist and doctoral candidate at Purdue University currently doing research at the Center for Adolescent and Family Studies at Indiana University. She has worked with a wide array of clients including abused and neglected children and juvenile delinquents and their families. She is a national consultant and trainer in the implementation of Functional Family Therapy (FFT) across the country. Her research interests include process and outcome research in the treatment of juvenile delinquency and the application of FFT in treatment of juvenile sex offenders.

Robert Brager, PhD, is Associate Professor at CSPP-AIU. Over the past ten years, Dr. Brager has provided clinical services to Juvenile Sex Offenders. He maintains an independent practice in San Diego, CA.

Marci Mandel Brewer, LCSW, is currently the Clinical Supervisor of Juvenile Programming at the Resource Center for High Risk Youth, an outpatient sexual offense-specific treatment facility in Denver, Colorado. She conducts a private clinical practice and has over 13 years of experience working with a variety of clientele in such settings as the county department of human services, outpatient, day treatment, after-school programming, and residential agencies. Ms. Brewer offers particular expertise in the field of sexual abuse and trauma recovery, and she has presented at many trainings and conferences statewide.

Jill Efta-Breitbach, PsyD, is a Captain in the U.S. Army, currently stationed at Fort Bragg, NC. She is a member of the American Psychological Association, the Silver Cadeceus Society, and the Association for the Treatment of Sexual Abusers. She works in the areas of trauma, resilience, and assessment and is currently involved in research projects examining the biological, psychological, and social effects of PTSD/ASD in combat soldiers returning from deployments.

Clark Clipson, PhD, is an assessment psychologist in private practice, specializing in forensic and neuropsychological evaluations. He is also an adjunct faculty member at the California School of Professional Psychology in San Diego, where he taught professional ethics for ten years.

Kurt A. Freeman, PhD, is Assistant Professor in the Department of Pediatrics, Child Development and Rehabilitation Center, Oregon Health & Science University. His clinical and research interests focus primarily on the assessment and treatment of common and severe behavior problems in children and adolescents. In addition to conducting his own research, Dr. Freeman serves on the editorial boards of *Aggression & Violent Behavior: A Review Journal, Behavior Modification,* and *Journal of Developmental and Physical Disabilities.*

Raymond Knight, PhD, earned his doctorate from the University of Minnesota, and then joined the faculty of Brandeis University, where he is now Gryzmish Professor of Human Relations. He has developed and validated taxonomic models for rapists and child molesters, has completed a 25-year follow-up of sex offenders released from the Massachusetts Treatment Center, and has created a computerized inventory to evaluate juvenile and adult sexual offenders. In addition to publishing 38 journal articles or book chapters on sexual aggression and over 40 papers on various other areas of psycho pathology, he has been President of the Society for Research in Psychopathology and is currently President of the Association for the Treatment of Sexual Aggression.

David J. Kolko, PhD, is Professor of Psychiatry, Psychology, and Pediatrics at the University of Pittsburgh School of Medicine. At Western Psychiatric Institute and Clinic, he directs the Services for Adolescent and Family Enrichment (SAFE) Program that conducts treatment and research with sexually abusive youth referred by the Juvenile Court. He is also a consultant for the Pittsburgh Child Advocacy Center at Children's Hospital of Pittsburgh. A sample of Dr. Kolko's clinical-research activities and articles may be found online at *<http://www.pitt.edu/~kolko>.*

Ian Lambie, PhD, is Senior Lecturer in clinical psychology at the University of Auckland, New Zealand and Clinical Consultant and Clinical Psychologist for SAFE Adolescent Programme. He has 14 years clinical experience in the field of adolescent sexual offenders. His clinical and research interests are youth forensic psychology and in particular adolescent sexual offending, arson, and the relationship between trauma and violence.

Robert E. Longo, MRC, LPC, is Corporate Director of Special Programming and Clinical Training at New Hope Treatment Centers in North Charleston, SC.

John McCarthy, MSW, is the Director of the SAFE Programme and has 14 years clinical experience with both adult and adolescent sexual offenders. SAFE is New Zealand's largest community program specializing in treating children with sexualized behavior problems and adolescent and adult sexual offenders. John has a particular interest in treating Internet offenders.

David McCormick, MEd, received his BA in General Experimental Psychology from the University of Oklahoma in 1988 and his Master's degree in Community Counseling from the University of Oklahoma in 1991. He has worked with juvenile offenders for over 10 years and was Senior Therapist at St. Michael's Juvenile offender program. He has participated in a variety of research projects during both his graduate and undergraduate work yielding publications in the field of health psychology. He currently resides in Juneau, AK where he provides therapy services in the field of chemical dependency at Juneau Recovery Hospital.

Shannon K. McGovern, MA, is a doctoral student in clinical psychology at the Graduate School of Psychology, Fuller Theological Seminary. Her clinical and research interests include violence prevention among adolescents and the treatment of juvenile offenders.

Talley Moore, PhD, completed her undergraduate studies at the College of Santa Fe, New Mexico. She continued her education, earning a Masters Degree in Forensic Psychology at John Jay College of Criminal Justice in New York City. Dr. Moore earned her PhD at the California School of Professional Psychology at Alliant International University in San Diego, CA. Her doctoral research focused on a comparison study of sexually victimized and non-sexually victimized juvenile sexual offenders. Dr. Moore is currently employed at Forensic Psych Consultants in San Diego, CA specializing in the assessment and treatment of persons with a history of abusive behaviors.

David Nahum, EdD, is a licensed psychologist and approved juvenile treatment provider and evaluator through the Colorado Sex Offender Management Board (SOMB). He has supervised and developed both outpatient and residential sexual offense-specific treatment programs. Dr. Nahum maintains a private practice in child/adolescent psychology south of Denver, has presented at numerous local conferences, and is busy in the development of novel theoretical models to accelerate the therapy process for high-risk youth.

Colleen Noel, MSW, LSW, is Treatment Clinician with the SAFE Program in Pittsburgh, PA. Colleen has a Master's degree from the School of Social Work at the University of Pittsburgh. Her main interests are family therapy, family involvement and the juvenile sex offender, the impact of the juvenile justice system on families, creative therapy with children and adolescents, and program evaluation.

Kathryn E. Otis, MA, is a doctoral student in clinical psychology at the Graduate School of Psychology, Fuller Theological Seminary. Her current research interests center around the relationship of personality with therapists' choice of therapeutic orientation. She works with the persistently mentally ill and juvenile offenders.

Evelyn L. Poey, MA, earned her Master's degree in Psychology from Fuller Theological Seminary and is currently completing her PhD in clinical psychology. She works as a psychological assistant treating adolescents, children, and adults.

David S. Prescott, LICSW, oversees the treatment of sexually abusive adolescents in a residential treatment center in Bennington, VT. He has written a number of articles, consulted to a wide variety of agencies, and has presented workshops on residential treatment and risk assessment at the local, national, and international level. He is currently the editor of the Forum, a newsletter published by the Association for the Treatment of Sexual Abusers (ATSA), and serves on that organization's Executive Board of Directors.

Lucinda A. Rasmussen, PhD, is Associate Professor at San Diego State University School of Social Work and a therapist at Sharper Future–San Diego. She has over 15 years clinical experience treating sexually abused children, children with sexual behavior problems, adolescent sexual offenders, and adult sexual offenders.

Sue Righthand, PhD, obtained her BA in Sociology from Beloit College in 1975, her MS in criminal justice in 1977 from Northeastern University, and her PhD in clinical psychology from the University of Wyoming in 1985. Dr. Righthand provides consultation and training, and has an independent clinical and forensic practice in Rockland, Maine. Dr. Righthand also has an adjunct faculty position in the University of Maine's Department of Psychology.

Judith E. Sims-Knight, PhD, is Chancellor Professor of Psychology at the University of Massachusetts, Dartmouth where she has taught for 25 years. She earned her BA at Brown University, her MA at City University of New York, and her PhD at the University of Minnesota. Since that time she has published on a wide range of topics, including sexual aggression, cognitive development, instructional psychology, and infancy.

Gretchen Thomas, MSW, LSW, is Treatment Clinician with the SAFE Program in Pittsburgh, Pennsylvania. Gretchen has a Master's degree from Columbia University's School of Social work. Her professional experiences and interests are focused on sexuality, specifically deviant sexual interests and behaviors, sexual minorities, STD transmission, and HIV/AIDS.

Eunice Torres, MS, is Assessment Clinician with the SAFE Program in Pittsburgh, Pennsylvania. Eunice has a Master's degree in Child Development and Family Studies and a Certificate in Child Welfare Interdisciplinary Studies from the School of Social Work at the University of Pittsburgh. She is a PhD candidate in the Developmental Psychology Program at the University of Pittsburgh. Her main interests involve assessment of juvenile sex offenders and their families, family treatment, behavioral disorders, and ecological theory.

Donald Viglione, PhD, is Professor and Director of the Clinical PhD program at the California School of Professional Psychology-Alliant International University in San Diego. He has conducted research on the Rorshach and other assessment instruments for more than twenty years. He is Diplomat of the American Board of Assessment Psychology and a Fellow of the Society for Personality Assessment. His recent book is entitled *Rorschach Coding Solutions: A Reference Guide for the Comprehensive System.* In his consultation practice he evaluates sexual offenders and performs other forensic, clinical, and psycho-educational evaluations.

C. Eugene Walker, PhD, President of Psychological Consultants, Inc., is Professor Emeritus at the University of Oklahoma Medical School. While at the University of Oklahoma, he was instrumental in establishing and doing research on treatment programs for adolescent and juvenile sex offenders. He is currently program consultant to St. Michael Hospital in Oklahoma City, OK for a twenty-bed inpatient unit devoted to treatment of male adolescent sex offenders.

Donald F. Walker, MA, is currently a doctoral candidate in the Graduate School of Psychology at Fuller Theological Seminary. His research interests include treatment with adolescent sexual offenders, violence prevention among adolescents, and the integration of spirituality in therapy.

Peter Wayson, PhD, attended college in the Midwest prior to attending graduate school in California. He received his PhD in 1983 from CSPP-San Diego. He currently serves as an adjunct faculty member at CSPP and is in private practice. He also currently serves as a consultant at the LGBT Center in San Diego.

Carlann Welch, PsyD, obtained her BS in nursing from the University of Massachusetts in 1978, her MS in psychiatric nursing from Boston College in 1981, and her PsyD in clinical psychology from Antioch/New England in 1994. Dr. Welch has an independent practice conducting juvenile forensic evaluations and a clinical practice in Intensive Short-Term Dynamic Psychotherapy. Her practice is located in Portland, ME.

Scott Zankman, MA, is a certified sex offender treatment provider in Washington State. He has worked in varying contexts with adolescent sex offenders since 1990; the last 8 years have been in private practice. He has been a Functional Family Therapy (FFT) therapist since 1999, and he has used the FFT model with juvenile sex offenders since 2001. In 2002, Scott began his work as a national supervisor of FFT, working with agencies across the country to implement the model. Scott is a clinical member of ATSA and works in the Seattle area.

Introduction:
Assessment and Treatment
of Youth Who Sexually Offend:
An Overview

Talley Moore
Kristina Crumpton Franey
Robert Geffner

SUMMARY. This introductory article provides an overview of the significant issues involved when dealing with youth who sexually offend, sometimes referred to as juvenile sex offenders or sexually reactive children or adolescents. There is not an accepted term or definition that is widely used to describe or refer to this population, and the precise prevalence or incidence rates are not known. Statistics are presented from various national studies, but methodological problems in the research are also noted. The authors briefly discuss the current research concerning youth who sexually offend, present some of the important issues in this area of research and practice, and list various types of sexual victimization that have been included when dealing with youth who sexually offend. The article then introduces the current volume, describing the articles and con-

Address correspondence to: Robert Geffner, PhD, FVSAI, 6160 Cornerstone Court East, San Diego, CA 92121.

[Haworth co-indexing entry note]: "Introduction: Assessment and Treatment of Youth Who Sexually Offend: An Overview." Moore, Talley, Kristina Crumpton Franey, and Robert Geffner. Co-published simultaneously in *Journal of Child Sexual Abuse* (The Haworth Maltreatment and Trauma Press, an imprint of The Haworth Press, Inc.) Vol. 13, No. 3/4, 2004, pp. 1-13; and: *Identifying and Treating Youth Who Sexually Offend: Current Approaches, Techniques, and Research* (ed: Robert Geffner et al.) The Haworth Maltreatment and Trauma Press, an imprint of The Haworth Press, Inc., 2004, pp. 1-13. Single or multiple copies of this article are available for a fee from The Haworth Document Delivery Service [1-800-HAWORTH, 9:00 a.m. - 5:00 p.m. (EST). E-mail address: docdelivery@haworthpress.com].

tent. Identifying and treating youth who sexually offend is in its infancy in many ways. It is hoped that this volume will provide important information to help those in research and practice better understand the issues and dynamics of this population. *[Article copies available for a fee from The Haworth Document Delivery Service: 1-800-HAWORTH. E-mail address: <docdelivery@haworthpress.com> Website: <http://www.HaworthPress.com> © 2004 by The Haworth Press, Inc. All rights reserved.]*

KEYWORDS. Sexually reactive children, juvenile sex offenders, child sexual abuse, forensic psychology, crime statistics

Historically, the phenomenon of juvenile sexual offending has been generally ignored, as society assumed that adult males perpetrated all sexual assaults (Becker & Hunter, 1997). As society moved away from a "boys will be boys" attitude and began to realize that youth do indeed commit sexual crimes, act out sexually, and sexually offend, researchers began to explore this phenomenon. Yet, the study of youth who sexually offend is still a fairly new field. For instance, prior to 1970, only nine major articles were published on the juvenile sexual offender. By 1993, however, over 100 major articles had been published (Barbaree, Hudson, & Seto, 1993), and the number continues to grow. Likewise, the number of treatment programs targeting this population has increased (Kahn & Chambers, 1991). According to a survey by the Safer Society Foundation, there are 249 community-based programs and 115 residential programs in the United States that specialize in treating youth who sexually offend (Burton & Smith-Darden, 2000), and more than 1,000 treatment programs worldwide (Ryan, 2000).

Research among this population has faced many challenges. Among them is the difficulty with definitions related to this group. For instance, some researchers prefer the legal term of "juvenile sex offender," labeling the population based on their crime. This emulates the adult offender model. However, given the ramifications of the term "sex offender" in today's society (e.g., civil commitment laws, forced registration), some researchers are hesitant to utilize this term with young people. Many of these researchers prefer the label "adolescents with sexually abusive behaviors." This term focuses more on the behavior rather than labeling a youth as a sex offender. It speaks to the rehabilitative property of young people. Finally, there are researchers and clinicians who prefer the term "sexually reactive youth." This refers to children and adolescents who offend as a way to reenact their own sexual abuse. It focuses on the youths' abuse history rather than on their offensive behavior. Yet, this term does not address those youth without a history of their own abuse who offend against others. Thus, this term is very limited. More recently, some have suggested the term "youth who sexually offend," since it appears to have fewer negative connotations while still dealing with the main issues. Thus, the title of this volume and many of the articles utilize this terminology.

Another difficulty with the research concerning youth who sexually offend includes dividing participants into subgroups. Some researchers classify youth according to their abuse histories, criminal histories, or the type of offense they have committed (e.g., rape versus molestation, age of the victim, age difference between victim and offender, gender of the victim, relationship to victim, etc.). Often times these variables can overlap, causing problems in research design. Nonetheless, research has pressed forward.

As the field continues to grow, we are beginning to understand the depth and breadth of the problem. Youth who sexually offend present a serious, ongoing problem, with high costs for the victim, families, the offender him/herself, and society at large. American society and the criminal justice system look to the mental health professions for interventions and solutions to the problem of youth-perpetrated sexual offending (Becker & Murphy, 1998; Winick, 1998; Zonana, Abel, Bradford, Hoge, & Metzner, 1998).

NATIONAL CRIME STATISTICS

Juveniles who sexually offend are responsible for a significant number of sexual assaults and child molestations perpetrated in the United States each year. In 2001 alone, more than 15,500 adolescent males and females were charged with one or more sexual offenses (Maguire & Pastore, 2002). Although over 7,600 of the adolescents arrested in 2001 were between 15 and 18 years of age, more than 7,300 were between the ages of 10 and 14, with an additional 462 under the age of 10 (Maguire & Pastore, 2002). Adolescent males are believed responsible for one in every five sexual assaults (e.g., forcible rape) of a male or female 12 years of age and older in the United States each year, while adolescent females accounted for 1 in every 16 arrests for sexual assault in 2001 (Maguire & Pastore, 2002). For victims under the age of 12, adolescent males are believed responsible for one in every two incidents of male child sexual victimization and one in three incidents of female child sexual victimization (Ryan, 1999; Zonana et al., 1998)

Whereas the literature and statistics on adolescent males who sexually offend indicate the severity of their crimes, little has been studied about the females who sexually offend. In a 1983 study, Brown, Flanagan, and McLeod (1984) determined that only 7% of all sexual offenses and 2% of all rapes are committed by adolescent females. Generally speaking, studies on juvenile sex offenders usually cite what percentage of their population is female, but then continue to discuss the males who sexually offend in their population, or combine the two genders when reporting statistics on the population being studied (Barbaree et al., 1993). Given the lower base rate of occurrence, it is difficult to research just females who sexually offend, which in turn leaves the literature lacking in information regarding this subpopulation.

In general, arrest rates for sexual offenses have declined over the last decade (Federal Bureau of Investigation [FBI], 2002). Between 1993 and 2002, the number of arrests for forcible rape declined by more than 25% (FBI, 2002). However, arrests for juvenile sex offenders have not diminished at rates comparable to their adult counterparts. While the number of adult males arrested and charged with a sexual offense other than forcible rape (e.g., exhibitionism, child molestation, sodomy) decreased by more than 17%, adolescent males charged with a similar sexual offense declined by less than 9% (FBI, 2002). While any number of factors or theories may account for differences in decline of arrest rates for sexual offenders over the last decade, including the current social-political hard-line approach to adolescent-perpetrated crime (Becker & Murphy, 1998; Steinberg & Scott, 2003), national crime statistics clearly support the severe and chronic nature of youth-perpetrated sexual crime.

Problems with national crime statistics. Unfortunately, national crime statistics significantly misrepresent the magnitude of youth-perpetrated sexual crime. National crime data are based almost exclusively on arrest rates obtained from reporting agencies and therefore do not include: (a) youth-perpetrated sexual crimes that are never reported to a legal agency, (b) incidents when the youth perpetrators are never identified, (c) cases where the youth offender is apprehended but not charged with a sexual offense, (d) incidents when charges were dropped as part of a plea agreement to enter treatment, or (e) cases where the juvenile sex offender was adjudicated as an adult (Maguire & Pastore, 2002; Weinrott, 1996). Clearly, the problem of youth-perpetrated sexual offending is much greater than national crime statistics indicate.

Crime victim reports. National crime data generated from victim reports indicates that the problem of the young sexual offender is much greater than the image depicted from national arrest rates. Statistical data obtained from the National Crime Victims Survey proffers that 200,000 to 450,000 adolescents perpetrate a sexual act(s) involving the use of force in the United States every year (U.S. Department of Justice [DOJ], 2003). Unfortunately, crime victim reports also under-represent the magnitude of the problem of youth-perpetrated sexual crime, because the majority of sexual crime is never reported.

UNDERREPORTING OF SEXUAL CRIME

Victim. Retrospective research indicates that an estimated three out of four incidents of sexual assault and child sexual molestations are never reported to a legal agency (FBI, 2002; Stevenson, 1999; U. S. Department of Justice, 2002). Holmes and Slap (1998) reviewed more than 169 empirically based studies published between 1985 and 1997 and concluded that three out of every four adolescent (71%) and adult (77%) males sexually victimized prior to age 12 never reported their abuse experience(s) to parents, friends, physician, or a reporting agency.

Type of sexual victimization. In addition, the type of sexual offense has been found to contribute to underreporting of sexual crime. When an incident of sexual victimization is reported, often only the most severe forms of hands-on assault (e.g., fondling, oral copulation, penetration) reach the attention of a legal agency (Becker & Murphy, 1998; Ryan & Lane, 1997). However, the general consensus is that the range of sexual offenses perpetrated by an adolescent male "is enormous . . . (and) hands-off offenses such as peeping, flashing, and obscene communications often precede hands-on offenses and continue between the hands-on assaults" (Ryan & Lane, 1997, p. 8).

Ryan and Lane (1997) reviewed the legal and clinical records of more than 1,500 male juveniles who sexually offended in an attempt to gain a better understanding of the magnitude and scope of adolescent-perpetrated sexual crime. The authors concluded that by the time an offender first encountered the criminal justice system ($M = 14$ years of age), he had averaged seven (range 0-30) prior hands-off and hands-on sexual offenses, for which he was neither caught nor reported. Wieckowski, Hartsoe, Mayer, and Shortz (1998) reported similar findings in that, within their sample of juveniles who sexually offended, 30 offenders had committed a median 69.5 sexual offenses, the majority of which were hands-on offenses, highlighting the prodigious nature of adolescent sexual offending.

Summary. Although national crime statistics, crime victim reports, offender records, and self-report must be viewed with caution, these sources of data converge, indicating youth-perpetrated sexual crime is a serious and on-going problem in the United States. Youth who sexually offend profoundly impact the lives of a substantial number of men, women, and children each year. For every reported sexual offense, large time and financial demands are placed on the criminal justice system, which must investigate, apprehend, and adjudicate the youth offender. Upon conviction, the youth is often court mandated into state or county funded juvenile detention centers, residential care, and/or day- or outpatient-treatment facilities. Upon release, the criminal justice system must subsequently monitor and track a number of juveniles' return to their communities (Becker & Murphy, 1998; Freeman-Longo, 2000; Winick, 1998).

In tandem, mental health professionals are expected to provide well informed, empirically based services to the courts regarding assessment, adjudication, and release of youth who sexually offend back into the community. Further, mental health professionals are expected to develop and provide well informed, empirically based interventions and treatment for both the victim and the offender (Becker & Murphy, 1998; Marshall, 1997; Winick, 1998). Clearly, the problem of youth-perpetrated sexual offending provides an ongoing impetus for research addressing the etiology, developmental pathway, and salient personality characteristics of these offenders.

Adolescent Sexual Offender Research

A great deal of empirical and clinical research has focused on identifying psychological, behavioral, and environmental factors that predispose an adolescent to sexually offend (Becker & Murphy, 1998; Holmes & Slap, 1998; Zonana et al., 1998). As a result, a long list of personality characteristics, family dynamics, demographic factors, life experiences, delinquent behaviors, and offense characteristics associated with adolescent sexual offending has been generated in the research literature (Becker, 1998; Lee, Jackson, Pattison, & Ward, 2002; Zonana et al., 1998). Further, statistical and clinical trends have been observed regarding offender and offense characteristics, resulting in the development of a large number of adolescent sex offender typologies and classification systems (Araji, 1997; Becker, 1998; Gray, Pithers, Busconi, & Houchens, 1999; Hunter, Figueredo, Malamuth, & Becker, 2003; Knight & Prentky, 1993; Worling, 2001).

However, a majority of factors statistically associated with adolescent sexual offending fail to consistently discriminate youth who sexually offend from each other, from non-sexually offending delinquents, or general population controls upon replication of the study (Becker, 1998; Marshall, 1997). Classification systems and offender typologies often share a similar outcome when utilized in subsequent research, failing to consistently distinguish between offenders and non-sexually offending controls. Weinrott (1996) concluded after his review of three decades of juvenile sex offender research:

> There is great variation in victim characteristics, degree of force, chronicity, variety of sexual outlets (e.g., other paraphilias), arousal patterns, and motivation/intent. Other factors thought to be relevant . . . intelligence, social competence, cultural values, attachment bonds, personal victimization, substance abuse, presence of Conduct Disorder, observation of sexual vio-

lence, and use of pornography . . . often fail to discriminate [youth who sexually offend] from either non-sexual delinquents or normal adolescents. Others [factors] do not appear correlated with treatment amenability, recidivism, or other criteria. (p. 20)

Therefore, while much more is known regarding the juvenile offender, no empirically validated psychological or behavioral profile has emerged. After decades of research, "the only . . . definitive conclusion that can be drawn to date is that . . . [adolescent] sex offenders are a very heterogeneous group" (Zolondek, Abel, Northey, & Jordan, 2001, p. 1). Chronic heterogeneity impedes identification of the etiology and developmental pathway(s) of sexual offending, impacting the development of empirically driven theoretical models guiding intervention and treatment (Becker, 1998). It is clear that research in this field has far to go. Yet a review of what is known is crucial for those who work with these young offenders on a daily basis.

PURPOSE AND DESCRIPTION OF THIS VOLUME

Youth who sexually offend profoundly impact the lives of a significant number of men, women, and children each year. Society in general and the criminal justice system in particular demand answers and solutions to the problem of youth-perpetrated sexual offending. Focusing on salient offender characteristics may be key to understanding why some youth sexually offend and may provide a springboard towards identifying appropriate intervention and treatment. It is hoped that this volume will assist those who are working with youth who sexually offend, by discussing up-to-date research topics as well as providing theory, techniques, and guidelines for assessment and treatment of this challenging population.

In the first section of this volume, a theoretical overview is presented related to youth who sexually offend. The first article, "Characteristics of Youth Who Sexually Offend" by Sue Righthand and Carlann Welch, provides an overview of the characteristics of youths who have committed sex offenses. The article discusses factors such as abuse history, family environment, social skills, cognitive functioning, sexual experiences, and mental health of these youth. This comprehensive overview provides readers with an understanding of the factors believed to be related to sex offending among youth as well as an up-to-date review of current theory.

Once this foundation has been laid, the volume then explores a specific theory regarding the antecedents that lead to juvenile male sex offending. For instance, in "Testing an Etiological Model for Male Juvenile Sexual Offending Against Females," Raymond A. Knight and Judith E. Sims-Knight test an etiological model that is frequently applied to adult sex offenders. They begin by exploring the current research on the origin of sexual aggression against women and the identified contributing factors, such as early abuse, personality/behavioral traits, and attitudinal/cognitive variables. They then discuss an etiological model of sexual coercion against women that they have developed and tested on adult samples from both the community and sexual offenders. Finally they go on to test this model on a juvenile sexual offender sample in an effort to determine whether one unified theory can account for sexual offending in both adult and juvenile populations.

The volume then begins to tackle the challenges one faces when conducting assessments of sexually abusive youth. Assessment can be focused on the youth's abilities and characteristics or on the ongoing risk for re-offense. These juveniles have usually been accused of or have admitted to a sexual crime considered to be heinous by society at large. The shame and fear associated with their crimes makes assessing these offenders that much more difficult. By understanding the challenges one faces when meeting with these youth, from choosing assessment tools to utilizing interviewing techniques aimed at decreasing denial, the clinician is much more equipped to handle this daunting task.

First, Lucinda A. Rasmussen addresses the issue of distinguishing subtypes among this population. In her article, "Differentiating Youth Who Sexually Abuse: Applying a Multidimensional Framework When Assessing and Treating Subtypes," Rasmussen begins by reviewing the known research regarding typologies of youth who sexually offend. Based on the research, she then describes and compares five clinical typologies and two empirical typologies. She continues by discussing how the empirical typologies can be incorporated into a multidimensional assessment framework based on the Trauma Outcome Process model. She concludes by giving examples of how this model can be utilized in clinical practice.

Next, in "Emerging Strategies for Risk Assessment of Sexually Abusive Youth: Theory, Controversy, and Practice," David S. Prescott attempts to assist clinicians who are called upon to predict risk of re-offense among youth who sexually offend. As he notes, clinicians and other professionals are frequently called upon to offer judgments regarding risk for sexual re-offense. He asserts that there are currently no empirically validated methods for accurately classifying risk among this population. Therefore, those faced with this task must first evaluate the research on the assessment of risk and recidivism before choosing their methodology. To assist clinicians in this daunting task, Prescott reviews five methods of risk assessment and four scales, and he provides readers with directions on how to obtain the measures. The measures include the Juvenile Sex Offender Assessment Protocol (JSOAP), the Protective Factors Scale (PFS), and Estimate of Risk of Adolescent Sex Offender Recidivism (ERASOR).

The section concludes by addressing the "nuts and bolts" of the interviewing and clinical assessment phase of treatment. Ian Lambie and John McCarthy, in their article, "Interviewing Strategies with Sexually Abusive Youth," discuss the challenges often faced by a clinician when attempting to obtain information through a clinical interview. Juveniles who have sexually offended often harbor strong feelings of shame, guilt, mistrust, and embarrassment about their behaviors and crimes. Asking any juvenile about his or her sexual practices is likely to result in minimal information and denial at best. Yet, as Lambie and McCarthy point out, the clinical interview is an integral but often overlooked part of juvenile offender assessment and treatment.

The authors discuss methods for interviewing clients in a way that elicits accurate information as well as facilitates the development of a therapeutic relationship, when applicable. They assert that this relationship will be the foundation upon which effective therapy can be undertaken. The authors describe interviewing strategies, the process of change, the stages of change model, as well as motivational interviewing with sexually abusive youth and their families. Moreover, they go on to highlight the importance of the client-therapist relationship in providing effective therapeutic interventions.

In the next section, the authors provide guidelines and strategies for treating juveniles who sexually offend. The articles cover individual, group, and family treatment modalities. The first article, "Treatment of Juveniles Who Sexually Offend: An Overview," by Jill Efta-Breitbach and Kurt A. Freeman gives an introductory overview of types of treatments generally used with youth who sexually offend. This review includes an overview of treatment goals, common cognitive-behavioral techniques, psycho-educational techniques, and the different modalities, such as family, individual, and group treatment.

We then move on to discussing a rationale for including parents of youth who sexually offend in treatment. In their article "Working with Parents to Reduce Juvenile Sex Offender Recidivism," Scott Zankman and Josephine Bonomo address the importance of including family therapy with treatment of this population. As the authors point out, since living with the family poses a potential risk factor for the juvenile, integrating relapse prevention into daily family life can contribute to the success or failure of the juvenile in the community. The authors address ways to include parents in relapse prevention planning as well as discussing treatment providers' misconceptions about family therapy with juvenile sex offenders. They conclude by providing their rationale for including parents in treatment, as well as reviewing research regarding different parenting styles.

Specific treatment models are then presented in the article, "Cognitive-Behavioral Treatment for Adolescents Who Sexually Offend and Their Families." David J. Kolko, Colleen Noel, Gretchen Thomas, and Eunice Torres describe an outpatient treatment program for adolescent sexual abusers. Individualized treatment in their program is based on a comprehensive clinical assessment with the youth and guardian, for which examples are provided. They then describe several treatment strategies directed to various individual or family clinical targets, including psychological dysfunctions, sexual deviance and sexuality, adolescent development and adaptive skills, parent and family relationships. A key component of their program is the integration of mental health and probationary services as part of juvenile court services for a balanced approach to the community management and treatment of the low-risk, primarily first-time, adolescent sexual offender.

Next, in "An Integrated Experiential Approach to Treating Young People Who Sexually Abuse," Robert E. Longo endorses the use of an integrated (holistic) experiential approach to treating youth who sexually offend. He provides a description of this model, with its emphasis on the importance of the therapeutic relationship. He provides readers with sample exercises to be implemented into treatment. Longo recommends this model as an alternative to some of the more commonly used treatments. He continues by discussing the pros and cons of many current treatment modalities.

Supplementing Longo's article is the one by David Nahum and Marci Mandel Brewer entitled, "Multi-Family Group Therapy for Sexually Abusive Youth." This treatment approach involves having several families meet at one time in a group environment. The authors point out that Multi-Family Group Therapy (MFGT) has only more recently been used with sexually abusive youth. They contend that MFGT is a powerful clinical intervention that has unique advantages, including economic benefits, family-to-family support and mentoring, community-based resourcefulness, and accelerated catalyzing of emotions. The authors provide direction to other clinicians on how to establish a MFGT format for treatment as well as discussing the goals, curriculum, facilitation priorities, and strategies of the groups.

The last article in this section, "Current Practices in Residential Treatment for Adolescent Sex Offenders: A Survey," by C. Eugene Walker and David McCormick, reviews the most common type of treatment offered to youth who sexually offend. Utilizing a survey, the authors contacted sex offender treatment facilities to determine their policies and practices regarding treatment. They inquired as to the major aspects of residential programs, including number of beds, average daily census, and number of males and females in treatment. They continue by reviewing testing and assessment procedures utilized as well as therapeutic approaches used, number and types of individual and group treatment sessions per week, qualifications of therapists, and average length of treatment. The authors also look at the participants in the programs, addressing the most frequent diagnoses and characteristics. Finally, the authors review follow-up research on treatment effectiveness.

The final section of this volume explores what happens to youth who sexually offend after they leave treatment. First, Jill Efta-Breitbach and Kurt A. Freeman provide a review of the literature regarding recidivism rates among juveniles who sexually offend. In their article, "Recidivism and Resilience in Juvenile Sexual Offenders: An Analysis of the Literature," the authors discuss factors that have been found to influence recidivism rates among this population. Included in this discussion are variables such as abuse, family dysfunction, peer group, deviant arousal, and mental stability. They then discuss positive factors that have been associated with resiliency (i.e., factors that help such offenders succeed after treatment). These factors include self-esteem, locus of control, spirituality, family environment, and socioeconomic status.

Next, Donald F. Walker, Shannon K. McGovern, Evelyn L. Poey, and Kathryn E. Otis address the issue of treatment outcome studies. In their article, "Treatment Effectiveness for Male Adolescent Sexual Offenders: A Meta-Analysis and Review," the authors evaluate the effectiveness of treatment of 644 juvenile sex offenders through the meta-analysis of 10 studies. The authors report that the results were encouraging, suggesting that treatments for male adolescent sexual offenders appear effective. They provide a descriptive review of the 10 studies and indicate that studies utilizing cognitive behavioral therapy approaches were the most effective.

Building upon this theme is the final article, entitled, "An Investigation of Successfully Treated Adolescent Sex Offenders," by Kristina Crumpton Franey, Donald J. Viglione, Peter Wayson, Clark Clipson, and Rob Brager. Here the authors qualitatively explore the life experiences of a sample of successfully treated adolescents who sexually offend. Through qualitative interviews with seven participants who graduated from treatment and did not re-offend after being released, the authors utilize the youth as "teachers." The juveniles explain in their own words how it felt to be labeled a sex offender, aspects of treatment they felt were helpful, and components of the treatment program they would change. In addition, they discuss challenges they faced after returning to society. The article concludes with a discussion regarding what other treatment programs can learn from these successfully treated youth.

Youth who sexually offend continue to pose a problem for society at large. Although they may also be victims themselves, the youth create a new generation of victims. The research on this population is still in its infancy. There are numerous controversies in trying to identify and treat youth who sexually offend, including the labels and definitions being used, whether a clinical versus criminal justice approach should be used, the types and effectiveness of interventions, and the policies that should be implemented.

Thirty years of research have provided clinicians with descriptors of youth who sexually offend and have begun to indicate types of treatment that may be effective with this population. It is hoped that this volume will assist clinicians, researchers, and others who choose to work with this population to better understand the issues and controversies, and to be able to improve their intervention and prevention programs. Although the work is challenging, the prevention of future victims makes the work worth the efforts.

REFERENCES

Araji, S. (1997). *Sexually aggressive children: Coming to understand them*. Newbury Park, CA: Sage Publications.

Barbaree, H. E., Hudson, S., & Seto, M. C. (1993). Sexual assault in society: The role of the juvenile offender. In H. E. Barbaree, W. L. Marshall, & S. Hudson (Eds.), *The juvenile sex offender* (pp. 1-24). New York: Guilford Press.

Becker, J. V., & Hunter, J. (1997). Understanding and treating child and adolescent sexual offenders. *Advances in Clinical Child Psychology, 19*, 177-197.

Becker, J. V., & Murphy, W. D. (1998). What we know and do not know about assessing and treating sex offenders. *Psychology, Public Policy, and Law, 4*(1/2), 116-137.

Brown, J., Flanagan, T. J., & McLeod, M. (1984). *Sourcebook of criminal justice statistics–1983*. Washington DC: Bureau of Justice Statistics.

Burton, D., & Smith-Darden, J. (2000). North American survey of sexual abuser treatment and models summary data. Brandon, VT: The Safer Society Foundation Inc.

Federal Bureau of Investigation (2002). *Uniform Crime Reports* [Online]. Retrieved April 21, 2004 from: http://www.fbi.gov/ucr/ucr.htm

Freeman-Longo, R. E. (2000). *Revisiting Megan's law and sex offender registration: Prevention or problem?* [Online]. Retrieved April 21, 2004 from: http://www.appa-net.org/revisitingmegan.pdf

Gray, A., Pithers, W. D., Busconi, A., & Houchens, P. (1999). Developmental and etiological characteristics of children with sexual behavior problems: Treatment implications. *Child Abuse & Neglect, 23*(6), 601-621.

Holmes, W. C., & Slap, G. B. (1998). Sexual abuse of boys: Definition, prevalence, correlates, sequelae, and management. *Journal of the American Medical Association, 280*(21), 1855-1862.

Hunter, J. A., Figueredo, A. J., Malamuth, N. M., & Becker, J. V. (2003). Juvenile sex offenders: Toward the development of a typology. *Sexual Abuse: Journal of Research & Treatment, 15*, 27-48.

Kahn, T., & Chambers, H. (1991). Assessing reoffense risk with juvenile sexual offenders. *Child Welfare, LXX*(3), 333-345.

Knight, R. A., & Prentky, R. A. (1993). Exploring characteristics for classifying juvenile sex offenders. In H. E. Barbaree, W. L. Marshall, & S. Hudson (Eds.), *The juvenile sex offender* (pp. 45-83). New York: The Guilford Press.

Lee, J. K. P., Jackson, H. J., Pattison, P., & Ward, T. (2002). Developmental risks factors for sexual offending. *Child Abuse & Neglect, 26*, 73-92.

Maguire, K., & Pastore, A. L. (Eds.) (2002). *Sourcebook of criminal justice statistics* [Online]. Retrieved April 21, 2004 from: http://www.albany.edu/sourcebook/

Marshall, W. L. (1997). Pedophilia: Psychopathology and theory. In D. R. L. W. O'Donohue (Ed.), *Sexual deviance: Theory, assessment, and treatment* (pp. 152-173). New York: Guilford Press.

Ryan, G. (1999). Treatment of sexually abusive youth. *Journal of Interpersonal Violence, 14*(4), 422-436.

Ryan, G. D. (2000). *Fact sheet recidivism and treatment effectiveness of youth who sexually abuse.* Denver, CO: National Adolescent Perpetrator Network.

Ryan, G. D., & Lane, S. L. (Ed.). (1997). *Juvenile sexual offending: Causes, consequences, and correction.* San Francisco: Jossey-Bass Inc.

Steinberg, L., & Scott, E. S. (2003). Less guilty by reason of adolescence. *American Psychologist, 58*(12), 1009-1017.

Stevenson, J. (1999). The treatment of the long-term sequelae of child abuse. *Journal of Child Psychology & Psychiatry & Allied Disciplines, 40*(1), 89-111.

U.S. Department of Justice. (2002). *Bureau of Justice Statistics* [Online]. Retrieved April 21, 2004 from: http://www.usdoj/gov

U.S. Department of Justice. (2003). *Bureau of Justice Statistics* [Online]. Retrieved April 22, 2004 from: http://www.ojp.usdoj/gov/bjs

Weinrott, M. R. (1996). *Juvenile sexual aggression: A critical review* [Center Paper 005-F-1450]. Boulder, CO: Center for the Study and Prevention of Violence, Institute for Behavioral Sciences, Center for the Study and Prevention of Violence.

Wieckowski, E., Hartsoe, P., Mayer, A., & Shortz, J. (1998). Deviant sexual behavior in children and young adolescents: Frequency and patterns. *Sexual Abuse: Journal of Research & Treatment, 10*(4), 293-303.

Winick, B. J. (1998). Sex offender law in the 1990s: A therapeutic jurisprudence analysis. *Psychology, Public Policy, and Law, 4*(1/2), 505-570.

Worling, J. R. (2001). Personality-based typology of adolescent male sexual offenders: Differences in recidivism rates, victim-selection characteristics, and personal victimization histories. *Sexual Abuse: A Journal of Research and Treatment, 12*(3), 149-166.

Zolondek, S., Abel, G., Northey, W., & Jordan, A. D. (2001). The self-reported behaviors of juvenile sexual offenders. *Journal of Interpersonal Violence, 16*(1), 73-85.

Zonana, H., Abel, G., Bradford, J., Hoge, S., & Metzner. J. (1998). *Task force report on sexually dangerous offenders.* Washington DC: American Psychological Association.

YOUTH WHO SEXUALLY OFFEND: THEORETICAL ISSUES

Characteristics of Youth Who Sexually Offend

Sue Righthand
Carlann Welch

SUMMARY. Sexual abuse by juveniles is widely recognized as a significant problem. As communities have become more aware of juvenile sex offending they have responded with increasingly severe responses. This is despite recidivism data suggesting that a relatively small group of juveniles commit repeat sexual offenses after there has been an official response to their sexual offending. Research has shown that juveniles who commit sexual offenses are a heterogeneous mix, varying according to a wide range of variables. This article provides an overview of the characteristics of youths who have committed sex offenses. Factors that

---

Address correspondence to: Sue Righthand, PhD, P.O. Box 1047, Rockland, ME 04841 (E-mail: rtnds@aol.com).

[Haworth co-indexing entry note]: "Characteristics of Youth Who Sexually Offend." Righthand, Sue, and Carlann Welch . Co-published simultaneously in *Journal of Child Sexual Abuse* (The Haworth Maltreatment and Trauma Press, an imprint of The Haworth Press, Inc.) Vol. 13, No. 3/4, 2004, pp. 15-32; and: *Identifying and Treating Youth Who Sexually Offend: Current Approaches, Techniques, and Research* (ed: Robert Geffner et al.) The Haworth Maltreatment and Trauma Press, an imprint of The Haworth Press, Inc., 2004, pp. 15-32. Single or multiple copies of this article are available for a fee from The Haworth Document Delivery Service [1-800-HAWORTH, 9:00 a.m. - 5:00 p.m. (EST). E-mail address: docdelivery@haworthpress.com].

Digital Object Identifier: 10.1300/J070v13n03_02

will be discussed include types of offending behaviors, family environment, histories of child maltreatment, social skills and interpersonal relationships, sexual knowledge and experiences, academic and cognitive functioning, and mental health. *[Article copies available for a fee from The Haworth Document Delivery Service: 1-800-HAWORTH. E-mail address: <docdelivery@haworthpress.com> Website: <http://www.HaworthPress.com>*

KEYWORDS. Juvenile sex offending, juvenile sex offenders, characteristics, juveniles, sexual abuse

Sexual abuse by juveniles is widely recognized as a significant problem. Federal Bureau of Investigation Uniform Crime data (2001) indicate that in 2000, 16% of arrests for forcible rape and 19% of arrests for all other sex offenses involved youths under 18 years old: Juveniles who commit sex offenses have abused significant numbers of people (Araji, 1997; Weinrott, 1996).

Official records such as arrest records underestimate the scope of the problem, because juvenile sex offenders who become known to the system may represent only a subset of juveniles who have committed such offenses. For example, Knight and Prentky (1993) found that only 37% of the adult sex offenders in their sample had official records documenting juvenile sex offending histories. In contrast, when these subjects completed a computer-generated questionnaire, and were assured that their responses would remain confidential, 55% acknowledged engaging in sexually abusive behavior as juveniles.

Juvenile sex offending involves a wide range of sexual misconduct including non-contact sexual behaviors (such as exhibitionism and voyeurism) and penetrative acts. Research has shown that the sexual behavior problems exhibited by these juveniles are "not simply isolated incidents involving normally developing adolescents" (Fehrenbach, Smith, Monastersky, & Deisher, 1986, p. 231).

As communities have become more aware of juvenile sex offending, they have responded with legislation for stiffer sentences, sex offender registration, community notification, and even sexual predator laws concerning juvenile offenders (Zimring, in press). These severe responses are in spite of recidivism data suggesting that a relatively small group of juveniles commit repeat sexual offenses after there has been an official response to their sexual offending, and that most of those who recidivate appear to do so with nonsexual crimes (Righthand & Welch, 2001).

The costs of sex offending are substantial for victims and society as well as for youths who offend and their families. In addition to the human costs in terms of emotional and physical anguish and suffering, staggering financial costs are incurred as a result of child welfare and criminal justice system involvement, therapeutic intervention, and so forth (Prentky & Burgess, 1990). To minimize these costs, timely and appropriate interventions are needed.

Historically, approaches and interventions with youths who commit sexual offenses have been based upon those utilized with adult offenders, often without sufficient consideration of relevant developmental issues and needs. There are important differences between juvenile and adult sex offenders (Association for the Treatment of Sexual Abusers, 1997; Becker, 1998; Bonner, 1997). Yet, only recently have a growing number of professionals pointed to the research literature to emphasize that the notion of "once a sex offender, always a sex offender" has not been empirically supported, particularly when it comes to juveniles.

In fact, the appropriateness and ethics of the term "juvenile sex offender" have been called into question (Bonner, 1997). Language describing these young people as children or teenagers who have been sexually abusive (rather than as juvenile sex offenders) holds them accountable for their behavior yet does not suggest that they are and always will be disreputable sex offenders. Because most papers and studies in the literature have used the term "juvenile sex offenders," this term will be used, at times, in this article. However, language that emphasizes behavior rather than the person may help avoid self-fulfilling prophecies that can contribute to offending behavior by promoting the belief that a person can never be more than his or her past. When the past includes sex offending, this can be a hopeless and esteem-deflating perspective.

Juveniles who have committed sex offenses are a heterogeneous mix (Bourke & Donohue, 1996; Knight & Prentky, 1993). They vary according to victim and offense characteristics. They also differ on a wide range of other variables, including types of offending behaviors, family environment, histories of child maltreatment, social skills and interpersonal relationships, sexual knowledge and experiences, academic and cognitive functioning, and mental health (Knight & Prentky, 1993; Weinrott, 1996).

In spite of the apparent heterogeneity of juveniles who sexually offend, findings from the few existing studies that compared juveniles who committed sex offenses with those who committed other types of offenses frequently have not revealed significant differences between samples (Becker & Hunter,

1997). This finding suggests that a substantial number of youths who commit sex offenses do not differ significantly from other juvenile offenders, although subgroups may differ.

OFFENDING BEHAVIORS

Sexually abusive behaviors and offense characteristics. The sexually abusive behavior these youths engage in range from non-contact offenses to penetrative acts. Studies have found that more than half of the abusive acts may involve oral-genital contact or attempted or actual vaginal or anal penetration (Righthand, Hennings, & Wigley, 1989; Righthand, Welch, Carpenter, Young, & Scoular, 2001). Other offense characteristics are presented in Table 1.

Nonsexual criminal behavior. Juvenile sex offenders frequently engage in nonsexual criminal and antisocial behavior (Fehrenbach et al., 1986; Righthand et al., 2001; Ryan, Miyoshi, Metzner, Krugman, & Fryer, 1996). Such behavior may in fact be quite typical of these youths, suggesting that sexual offending may be one facet of an overall pattern of delinquent behavior. In spite of many similarities between youths who commit sex offenses and those who commit other types of offenses, some unique characteristics have been reported. These have included an overall negative attitude regarding most types of delinquent behavior and a disengagement from family interactions (Miner & Crimmins, 1995), as well as increased rates of child sexual abuse victimization, major mental health difficulties, sexual identity problems, and fewer appropriate peer relationships (Milloy, 1994). Milloy also found that compared to youths who committed other types of offenses, those who sexually offended tended to have more adequate academic performance, fewer prior offenses and convictions, and less substance abuse. Findings from the 3-year follow-up period indicated that none of the sex offenders were convicted of a new sex offense and their overall recidivism rate was lower than that of other offenders. In addition, when the youths who had sexually offended did reoffend, their crimes tended to be nonsexual and nonviolent (Milloy, 1994). Milloy concluded, "These findings suggest that when a longitudinal perspective is used, sex offending among juveniles appears to be but one piece of a pattern of generalized delinquency" (p. 9) (for further comparison between the profiles of juvenile sex offenders and juvenile nonsexual offenders, see Zankman & Bonomo, this issue).

TABLE 1. Sex Offense Characteristics

Domain	Characteristics
Victim Characteristics	Female children targeted most frequently[b,c,d,f,g,h,i,j]
	Male victims represent up to 25% of some samples[g,j,k]
Relationship Characteristics	Victims are more often substantially younger than the offender, rather than peer age[b,c,d,f,g,h,i,j,k]
	Victims are usually relatives or acquaintances; rarely are they strangers[b,g,h,f,j,k]
	Babysitting frequently provides the opportunity to offend[c,j]
Use of Aggression	Although less physically violent than adults, compliance may be secured via intimidation, threats of violence, physical force, or extreme violence[b,e]
	Approximately 40% of the youths from a sample of 91 displayed expressive aggression in their sex offense(s)[f]
	Youths who victimized peers or adults tended to use more force, vs. those who victimized younger children[a]
Triggers	Some of the "triggers" that have been described as related to sex offending include anger, boredom, and family problems[i]

Note. [a]Becker, 1998; [b]Davis & Leitenberg, 1987; [c]Fehrenbach, Smith, Monastersy, & Deisher, 1986; [d]Hunter & Figueredo, 1999; [e]Knight & Prentky, 1993; [f]Miner, Siekert, & Ackland, 1997; [g]Rasmussen, 1999; [h]Righthand, Hennings, & Wigley, 1989; [i]Ryan, Miyoshi, Metzner, Krugman, & Fryer, 1996; [j]Smith & Monastersky, 1986; [k]Wieckowski, Hartsoe, Mayer, & Shortz, 1998.

CHILD MALTREATMENT HISTORIES

Childhood experiences of sexual abuse have been associated with juvenile sex offending (Burton, 2000; Fehrenbach et al., 1986; Kahn & Chambers, 1991; Kobayashi, Sales, Becker, Figueredo, & Kaplan, 1995). Rates of juvenile sex offenders who have experienced sexual abuse as children reportedly range from 40 to 80% (Becker & Hunter, 1997). Yet, such abusive experiences have not consistently been found to differ significantly from those of other juvenile offenders (e.g., Spaccarelli, Bowden, Coatsworth, & Kim, 1997) and have been associated with other forms of offending (Smith & Monastersky, 1986).

Not surprisingly, childhood experiences of being physically abused, being neglected, and witnessing family violence have been independently associated with sexual violence in juvenile offenders (Kobayashi et al., 1995; Righthand et al., 2001; Ryan et al., 1996). Proportions of juvenile sex offenders who have experienced physical abuse as children reportedly range from 25 to 50% (Becker & Hunter, 1997). A study comparing juvenile sex offenders with juveniles who have committed nonsexual offenses found that the sex offenders had higher rates of childhood physical abuse (Ford & Linney, 1995). When juvenile sex offenders were compared only with juveniles who had committed nonsexual violent offenses, however, this result was not replicated (Lewis, Shanok, & Pincus as cited in Knight & Prentky, 1993). This latter finding suggests that a history of physical abuse is correlated with some type of violent behavior but not necessarily with sexually violent behavior.

The role of child maltreatment in the etiology of sex offending appears to be quite complex (Prentky, Harris, Frizzell, & Righthand, 2000). For example, Hunter and Figueredo (as cited in Becker & Hunter, 1997) found that compared to other youths, those who sexually offended were younger at the time of victimization, had higher rates of abusive incidents, longer periods between abuse and disclosure, and a lower level of perceived family support following the disclosure of the abuse. Similarly, Burton, Miller, and Shill (2002) found that compared to juveniles who committed other offenses, those that sexually offended had closer relationships with their perpetrators, were more likely to have a male perpetrator, had longer durations of victimization, and experienced more force and penetration. Other studies have found that more serious childhood experiences of sexual abuse (e.g., penetration) were associated with persisting sexual offending from childhood into adolescence (Burton, 2000) and greater numbers of sex offense victims (Righthand, Knight, & Prentky, 2002).

Similarly, Cooper, Murphy, and Haynes (1996) compared juvenile sex offenders who had been sexually or physically abused with those who had not. They found that the abused juveniles began their sex offending 1.6 years earlier than the non-abused group, had twice the number of victims, were more likely to have both female and male victims, and were less likely to limit their offending to family members. The finding that offenders with histories of maltreatment often begin offending at earlier ages than offenders who were not maltreated is consistent with other research (Knight & Prentky, 1993; for further discussion on the role of abuse in the etiology of juvenile sexual offending, see Knight & Sims-Knight, this issue).

FAMILY FACTORS

Studies vary in regards to the number of youths whose families experience significant difficulties such as separations, significant stress, or family dysfunction, with residential samples reflecting higher rates of difficulties. Factors such as family instability, substance abuse, psychopathology, criminality, and violence have been found to be prevalent in some samples (Bagley & Shewchuk-Dann, 1991; Miner, Siekert, & Ackland, 1997; Morenz & Becker, 1995). Studies vary as to the percentages of these juveniles who are from intact families (Fehrenbach et al., 1986; Kahn & Chambers, 1991). However, even when families are intact, some parents have been described as disengaged and physically and/or emotionally inaccessible and distant from their children (Miner & Crimmins, 1995; Smith & Israel, 1987).

In addition, Kimball and Guarino-Ghezzi (1996) have found high rates of ongoing family conflict among juveniles who sexually abused younger children and little support for treatment among parents of those who sexually assaulted peers. Together, these various studies suggest that many youths who have sexually offended have been exposed to significant forms of psychopathology and family dysfunction and may have been cut off from possible sources of emotional support. As a consequence of such difficulties, these youths may experience ongoing stress and may be less able to form positive attachments and relationships (for discussion on attachment disorders, see Longo, this issue).

SOCIAL SKILLS AND RELATIONSHIPS

Research repeatedly documents that juveniles with sexual behavior problems have significant deficits in social competence (Becker, 1990; Knight & Prentky, 1993). Inadequate social skills, shyness, poor peer relationships, and social isolation are some of the difficulties identified in these juveniles (Carpenter, Peed, & Eastman, 1995; Fehrenbach et al., 1986; Righthand et al., 2001). Miner and Crimmins (1995) found that juveniles who have sexually offended had fewer peer attachments and felt less positive attachments to their schools compared with other delinquent juveniles and non-delinquent juveniles. In fact, the authors stated that this and other research point to the primacy of isolation and poor social adjustment as distinguishing characteristics of adolescent sex offenders. This indicates that interventions that maximize the ability to build respectful, prosocial, interpersonal attachments potentially will reduce the propensity to engage in sexually abusive and aggressive behaviors.

SEXUAL KNOWLEDGE AND EXPERIENCES

Sexual histories and beliefs. Research suggests that adolescents who commit sex offenses generally have had previous consenting sexual experiences (e.g., Ryan et al., 1996). Research also suggests that sometimes their experiences have exceeded the experience of control juveniles who have not committed sex offenses (McCord, McCord, & Venden as cited in Knight & Prentky, 1993). A study of 1,600 juvenile sex offenders described by 90 independent contributors from 30 states (Ryan et al., 1996) found that only about one-third of the juveniles perceived sex as a way to demonstrate love or caring for another person; others perceived sex as a way to feel power and control (23.5%), to dissipate anger (9.4%), or to hurt, degrade, or punish (8.4%).

Pornography. Investigations into the role of pornography in juvenile sex offending are limited in number. One study (Ford & Linney, 1995) found higher rates of exposure to hardcore, sexually explicit magazines among youths who sexually offended compared with youths who committed other offenses. The juvenile sex offenders also had been exposed at younger ages ranging from 5 to 8. Wieckowski, Hartsoe, Mayer, and Shortz (1998) also found that exposure to pornographic material at a young age was common among youths who sexually offended. Additionally, high rates of exposure to pornography have been found in girls who have committed sex offenses (Mathews, Hunter, & Vuz, 1997).

Deviant sexual arousal. Deviant sexual arousal is strongly associated with sexually coercive behavior in adults (e.g., Hanson & Bussière, 1998). Knight and Prentky (1993) found that adult sex offenders who began offending as juveniles did not differ from those who began as adults in terms of preoccupation with sexual fantasies, problems with sexuality, or sexually deviant conduct. Controlled studies of deviant sexual arousal in juvenile sex offenders are lacking in number, although some related research has been reported (e.g., Kahn & Chambers, 1991; Schram, Milloy, & Rowe, 1991; Worling & Curren, 2000). These studies found deviant sexual arousal was related to increased rates of sexual reoffending (for discussion of deviant sexual arousal as a factor in recidivism, see Efta-Breitbach & Freeman, this issue). The studies, however, relied on self-report and clinical judgments to determine the existence of deviant arousal, rather than on more objective means such as phallometric assessment.

In their review of the role of deviant sexual arousal in juvenile sex offending, Hunter and Becker (1994) noted the limited research in this area and encouraged further investigations. They stressed that deviant arousal may be more of a factor for sex offenders who target children (particularly those who target boys). They emphasized that the sexual interest and arousal patterns of juveniles are more changeable than those of adult sex offenders and cautioned against applying to juveniles what is known about deviant arousal in adults.

ACADEMIC AND COGNITIVE FUNCTIONS

Academic performance. Studies typically report that as a group, juveniles who sexually offended experienced school and academic difficulties (Fehrenbach et al., 1986; Kahn & Chambers, 1991; Miner et al., 1997; Righthand et al., 2001). Reported difficulties include disruptive behavior, truancy, academic problems, learning disabilities, and placement in special classes. Academic functioning is not determined solely by intellectual or neurological functioning. Parental level of education and support, truancy, and other variables are important. Some juveniles who have sexually offended, however, do well in school. For example, O'Brien (as cited in Ferrara & McDonald, 1996) found that 32% of the offenders in his sample were described as above average in their academic performance.

Intellectual and cognitive impairments. Research that focuses on the intellectual and cognitive functioning of juveniles who have committed sex offenses is limited. Ferrara and McDonald (1996) noted that research on juvenile delinquents has demonstrated two areas of impairment: (a) difficulties with executive functions, such as planning, abstraction, inhibition of inappropriate impulses, and cognitive flexibility, and (b) difficulties with receptive and expressive language. As noted above, some juveniles who sexually offend do not differ from juveniles who commit other types of offenses. Similarly, some juvenile sex offenders experience cognitive deficits similar to those identified in other groups of juvenile offenders. Based on their review of the literature, Ferrara and McDonald concluded that between one-quarter and one-third of juvenile sex offenders might have some form of neurological impairment. They noted, "Furthermore, it is likely that the neurologically impaired juvenile sex offender who goes undetected will not attain the [optimal] benefit from treatment due to problems in concentration, comprehension, and memory" (p. 13).

Cognitive distortions and attributions. Knight and Prentky (1993) pointed out that some factors observed in abused children may have relevance for juvenile sex offenders who have been maltreated. For example, they noted that abused children exhibit less empathy than non-abused children, have trouble recognizing appropriate emotions in others, and have difficulty taking another person's perspective. This observation is consistent with research indicating that cognitive distortions, such as blaming the victim, were associated with increased rates of sexual offending among juveniles that committed sex offenses (Kahn & Chambers, 1991; Schram et al., 1991).

MENTAL HEALTH ISSUES

Symptoms and disorders. Studies vary in regards to the number of youths that experience significant mental health difficulties, with residential samples evidencing higher rates. Conduct disorder diagnoses and antisocial behavior have frequently been observed in populations of juveniles who have sexually offended (Kavoussi, Kaplan, & Becker, 1988; Miner et al., 1997; Righthand et al., 2001). In addition, mental health difficulties as reflected in higher rates of depression and anxiety have been found to be greater than in comparison samples (Bagley & Shewchuk-Dann, 1991). Becker, Kaplan, Tenke, and Tartaglini (1991) also found that juveniles with histories of childhood physical abuse or sexual abuse had higher rates of depressive symptoms. They pointed out that their findings illustrate the importance of evaluating whether juvenile sex offenders are experiencing symptoms of depression, especially if they have been victimized themselves.

Substance abuse. Studies vary widely on the importance of substance abuse as a factor in sex offending. Lightfoot and Barbaree (1993) reported that rates at which juvenile sex offenders were found to be under the influence of drugs or alcohol at the time they committed their offenses ranged from 3.4 to 72%. Although substance abuse has been identified as a problem for many juveniles who have sexually offended (Kahn & Chambers, 1991; Miner et al., 1997), the role of substance abuse in sex offending remains unclear, and for some juveniles, substance abuse may not be related to sex offending. However, substance abuse can have a disinhibiting effect. Thus, problems such as poor impulse control, problem-solving difficulties, and poor social skills can be exacerbated by even small amounts of substance abuse, and consequently, may increase the risk of sex offending. Therefore, even infrequent users may benefit from substance abuse treatment efforts that are part of a comprehensive treatment program. More chronic users may require more intensive substance abuse treatment interventions, possibly prior to treatment related to sex offending (Lightfoot & Barbaree, 1993).

PERSONALITY TYPES AND CLASSIFICATIONS

A variety of personality characteristics have been identified among juveniles who have sexually offended, yet few studies have attempted to classify these juveniles according to the characteristics. Similarities and differences have been found (e.g., Hunter, Figueredo, Malamuth, & Becker, 2003; Smith, Monastersky, & Deisher, 1987; Worling, 2001). Because information about different types of juveniles is of great importance for determining and applying appropriate treatment strategies, further research in this area is needed.

GIRLS WHO HAVE COMMITTED SEX OFFENSES

Incidence. Studies and literature reviews have estimated the incidence of juvenile sex offending by girls to be between 2 and 11% (Lane & Lobanov-Rostovsky, 1997; Righthand et al., 1989; Righthand & Welch, 2001; Righthand et al., 2001). Incidence reports on juvenile sex offenders may underestimate the extent of the problem for girls even more than for boys. For example, sex offending in childcare situations may be less likely to be detected, because young victims may not have the language skills, abilities, or knowledge-base that can facilitate disclosures of sexually abusive behaviors.

Characteristics. More thorough reviews of the limited literature pertaining to girls who have sexually offended are available from other sources (e.g., Bumby & Bumby, 1997; Righthand & Welch, 2001). Most studies are limited by small sample sizes, but have findings that are relatively consistent. Ray and English (1995) found that compared with boys, girls tend to select younger victims, use less force, are less frequently involved in the criminal justice system, and are more frequently referred for assessment and treatment. Like boys, girls engage in a variety of types of offenses, including penetration (Fehrenbach & Monastersky, 1988; Mathews et al., 1997; Righthand et al., 2001), although penetrative acts occur less often (Ray & English, 1995). Childcare situations frequently provide the opportunity for abusive behaviors (Bumby & Bumby, 1997; Fehrenbach & Monastersky, 1988).

Although boys who sexually offend often have high rates of child maltreatment histories, girls typically evidence higher rates and more severe histories (Bumby & Bumby, 1997; Kubik, Hecker, & Righthand, 2003; Ray & English, 1995). In addition to having high rates of abuse and trauma, in one of the largest studies to date, Mathews and associates (1997) found that the girls typically came from families evidencing high levels of family dysfunction and an absence of parental support. Their family environments were described as usually appearing detrimental for the development of healthy attachments and a positive sense of self.

Like boys who commit sexual offenses, girls who sexually offend often engage in other forms of delinquent behaviors and evidence a range of behavior problems including sexually promiscuous behaviors. Peer relationship problems and school difficulties have been found to be common (Righthand et al., 2001). Girls typically have had high rates of previous involvement in mental health systems (Bumby & Bumby, 1997; Hunter, Lexier, Goodwin, Browne, &

Dennis, 1993). Mathews and colleagues (1997) found that although a small subgroup of girls evidenced little psychopathology and limited offending behaviors, around half of the sample appeared to have moderate to severe psychopathology. Problems included behaviors associated with conduct disorders, impulsivity, substance abuse, suicidal behaviors, and unprotected sex. A subgroup of the girls also evidenced deviant sexual arousal patterns, post-traumatic stress disorder, depression, and anxiety. In sum, the authors surmised:

> Biological and socialization factors create a higher threshold for the externalization of experienced developmental trauma in females than males. In this regard, it may be that females are generally less likely than males to manifest the effects of maltreatment in the form of interpersonal aggression of violence and that females who develop such patterns of behavior are generally those who have experienced remarkable high levels of such developmental trauma in the absence of environmental support for recovery and the presence of healthy female role models. (p. 194)

DEVELOPMENTALLY DISABLED JUVENILES WHO HAVE COMMITTED SEXUAL OFFENSES

In one of the few studies focusing on adolescent sex offenders with mental retardation, Gilby, Wolf, and Goldberg (1989) compared sexual behavior problems in a sample of intellectually normal youths (defined by the author as borderline intellectual functioning or higher) and youths with mental retardation (including mild and moderate mental retardation). The authors found that the frequency of sexual behavior problems of the groups did not differ significantly according to their levels of intellectual functioning. They noted that, for both groups, the closer the adolescent was observed (e.g., within a residential setting), the greater the number of sexual behavior problems recorded. This finding was especially true for the mentally retarded inpatient group. The authors suggested that reports of a greater-than-expected number of sexual problems among persons with mental retardation might be related to the increased levels of supervision these individuals receive.

Gilby and colleagues (1997) did find increased levels of inappropriate, non-assaultive sexual behavior (e.g., exhibitionism and public masturbation) among the adolescents with mental retardation and more indiscriminate sexual behavior. Although the rate of sexual assault did not vary between the intellectually normal and mentally retarded groups, there were fewer "consented to" sexual activities among the mentally retarded outpatient group. The authors suggested that this difference could reflect a lack of opportunity.

Interventions with juveniles with intellectual and cognitive disabilities must be appropriate for their special needs and learning styles. For example, due to differences in information processing styles and/or as a result of negative experiences in educational settings, these youths may prefer to avoid therapeutic situations that resemble their negative experiences, such as psychoeducational programs and other cognitive-behavioral methods (Langevin, Marentette, & Rosati, 1996).

A review of the literature (Stermac & Sheridan, 1993) regarding treatment of "developmentally disabled" adult and adolescent sex offenders revealed a "dearth of work in this area" (p. 237). Most studies have focused on adults and have stressed behaviorally oriented interventions. Strategies that enhance learning and generalizing skills, such as clear and concrete information or instruction, opportunities to rehearse new skills, and strategies to facilitate the development and use of new skills in a variety of settings are recommended. Modified relapse prevention strategies have been found to be effective with some cognitively impaired sex offenders. Yet, as Stermac and Sheridan pointed out, relapse prevention emphasizes self-management and therefore may not be appropriate for all intellectually or cognitively impaired sex offenders. Ferrara and McDonald (1996) provide an in-depth discussion of specialized interventions with juveniles who have cognitive and neurological challenges.

RISK FOR REOFFENDING

In a recent commentary, Chaffin and Bonner (1998) pointed out that there are no true experimental studies comparing untreated and treated juvenile sex offenders and no prospective studies evaluating risk factors or the natural course of sexual offending. Becker (1988) suggested that adolescent sex offenders were probably more likely to sexually reoffend if one or more of the following factors were present: (a) the initial offending was pleasurable, (b) consequences for the offenses were minimal, (c) the deviant sexual behavior was reinforced through masturbation or fantasy, and/or (d) the offender had social skills deficits. These factors appear to have good face validity but require additional evaluation (for an in-depth discussion of factors related to reoffense, see Efta-Breitbach & Freeman, this issue).

Relatively few studies have investigated the factors associated with the risk of repeat or persistent sexual offending. Most findings have not been replicated and some are contradictory. Methodological problems such as small sample sizes further limit this research. This is not to say that these findings should be ignored. Empirically supported as well as other theoretically sound factors may be important for reducing reoffending, however, pending further research caution is necessary and these limitations must be kept in mind.

CONCLUSIONS

The findings of this literature review indicate that juveniles who have committed sex offenses are heterogeneous. Like other juveniles, they are in the process of growing up. Yet, as this review demonstrates, they present with an array of social, emotional, and behavioral problems and may present with special risks related to their abusive behaviors.

Research also indicates that known rates of sexual recidivism are quite low, suggesting that a substantial proportion of these juveniles desist from committing sex offenses following the initial disclosed offense and intervention. The higher rates of nonsexual recidivism, and the relatively low rates of sexual reoffending, suggest that there are subgroups that commit additional offenses, primarily nonsexual offenses, and that a relatively small group goes on to commit additional sexual offenses or both sexual and nonsexual crimes.

Finally, it should be remembered that the goal when working with juveniles who have committed sex offenses is to help them stop their abusive behaviors. To label them "juvenile sex offenders" at a time when they are developing their identity may have deleterious effects. There is no evidence pertaining to these juveniles that suggests "once a sex offender always a sex offender." Chaffin and Bonner (1998) pointed out in an editorial, "Don't Shoot, We're Your Children: Have We Gone Too Far in Our Response to Adolescent Sexual Abusers and Children with Sexual Behavior Problems?"

It is important to remember that youths who commit sex offenses are children and adolescents first; they are young people who have committed offenses, but they are more than their crimes. They require individualized and developmentally appropriate interventions as well as our attention and concern.

REFERENCES

Araji, S. (1997). *Sexually aggressive children: Coming to understand them.* Thousand Oaks, CA: Sage Publications.

Association for the Treatment of Sexual Abusers. (1997). *Position on the effective legal management of juvenile sexual offenders.* Beaverton, OR: Author.

Bagley, C., & Shewchuk-Dann, D. (1991). Characteristics of 60 children and adolescents who have a history of sexual assault against others: Evidence from a controlled study. *Journal of Child and Youth Care: Special Issue*, 43-52.

Becker, J. V. (1988). The effect of child sexual abuse on adolescent sexual offenders. In G.E. Wyatt, & G.J. Powell (Eds.), *Lasting effects of child sexual abuse* (pp. 193-207). Beverly Hills: Sage Publications.

Becker, J. V. (1990). Treating adolescent sexual offenders. *Professional Psychology: Research and Practice, 21*(5), 362-365.

Becker, J. V. (1998). What we know about the characteristics and treatment of adolescents who have committed sexual offenses. *Child Maltreatment, 3*(4), 317-329.

Becker, J. V., & Hunter, J. A. (1997). Understanding and treating child and adolescent sexual offenders. In T. H. Ollendick, & R. J. Prinz (Eds.), *Advances in clinical child psychology: Vol. 19* (pp. 177-197). New York: Plenum Press.

Becker, J. V., Kaplan, M. S., Tenke, C.E., & Tartaglini, A. (1991). The incidence of depressive symptomatology in juvenile sex offenders with a history of abuse. *Child Abuse & Neglect, 15*(4), 531-536.

Bonner, B. (1997, October). *Child, adolescent, and adult sex offenders: Similarities and differences.* Paper presented at the meeting of the Association for the Treatment of Sexual Abusers, Arlington, VA.

Bourke, M. L., & Donohue, B. (1996). Assessment and treatment of juvenile sex offenders: An empirical review. *Journal of Child Sexual Abuse, 5*(1), 47-70.

Bumby, K. M., & Bumby, N. H. (1997). Adolescent female sexual offenders. In B. K. Schwartz, & H. K. Cellini (Eds.), *The sex offender: New insights, treatment innovations, and legal developments, Vol. 2* (pp. 10.1-10.16). Kingston, NJ: Civic Research Institute.

Burton, D. L. (2000). Were adolescent sexual offenders children with sexual behavior problems? *Sexual Abuse: A Journal of Research & Treatment, 12*(1), 37-48.

Burton, D. L., Miller, D. L., & Shill, C.T. (2002). A social learning theory comparison of the sexual victimization of adolescent sexual offenders and nonsexual offending male delinquents. *Child Abuse & Neglect, 26*, 893-907.

Carpenter, D.R., Peed, S.F., & Eastman, B. (1995). Personality characteristics of adolescent sexual offenders: A pilot study. *Sexual Abuse: A Journal of Research and Treatment, 7*(3), 195-203.

Chaffin, M., & Bonner, B. (1998). Don't shoot, we're your children: Have we gone too far in our response to adolescent sexual abusers and children with sexual behavior problems? *Child Maltreatment, 3*(4), 314-316.

Cooper, C.L., Murphy, W.D., & Haynes, M.R. (1996). Characteristics of abused and non-abused adolescent sex offenders. *Sexual Abuse: A Journal of Research and Treatment, 8*(2), 105-120.

Davis, G. E., & Leitenberg, H. (1987). Adolescent sex offenders. *Psychological Bulletin, 101*(3), 417-427.

Efta-Breitbach, J., & Freeman, K.A. (2004). Recidivism and resilience in youth who sexually offend: An analysis of the literature. *Journal of Child Sexual Abuse, 13*(3/4), pp. 257-294.

Federal Bureau of Investigation. (2001). *Crime in the United States 2000.* Washington, DC: U.S. Department of Justice.

Fehrenbach, P. A., & Monastersky, C. (1988). Characteristics of female adolescent sexual offenders. *American Journal of Orthopsychiatry, 58*(1), 148-151.

Fehrenbach, P. A., Smith, W., Monastersky, C., & Deisher, R. W. (1986). Adolescent sexual offenders: Offender and offense characteristics. *American Journal of Orthopsychiatry, 56*(2), 225-233.

Ferrara, M. L., & McDonald, S. (1996). *Treatment of the juvenile sex offender: Neurological and psychiatric impairments.* Northvale, NJ: Jason Aronson.

Ford, M.E., & Linney, J.A. (1995). Comparative analysis of juvenile sexual offenders, violent nonsexual offenders, and status offenders. *Journal of Interpersonal Violence, 10*(1), 56-70.

Gilby, R., Wolf, L., & Goldberg, B. (1989). Mentally retarded adolescent sex offenders: A survey and pilot study. *Canadian Journal of Psychiatry, 34*, 542-548.

Hanson, R. K., & Bussière, M. T. (1998). Predicting relapse: A meta-analysis of sexual offender recidivism studies. *Journal of Consulting and Clinical Psychology, 66*(2), 348-362.

Hunter, Jr., J. A., & Becker, J. V. (1994). The role of deviant sexual arousal in juvenile sexual offending: Etiology, evaluation, and treatment. *Criminal Justice and Behavior, 21*(1), 132-149.

Hunter, Jr. J. A., & Figueredo, A. J. (1999). Factors associated with treatment compliance in a population of juvenile sexual offenders. *Sexual Abuse: A Journal of Research and Treatment, 11*(1), 49-67.

Hunter, J. A., Figueredo, A.J., Malamuth, N.M., & Becker, J.V. (2003). Juvenile sex offenders: Toward the development of a typology. *Sexual Abuse: A Journal of Research and Treatment, 15*(1), 27-48.

Hunter, Jr., J. A., Lexier, L. J., Goodwin, D.W., Browne, P.A., & Dennis, C. (1993). Psychosexual, attitudinal, and developmental characteristics of juvenile female sexual perpetrators in a residential treatment setting. *Journal of Child & Family Studies, 2*(4), 317-326.

Kahn, T. J., & Chambers, H. J. (1991). Assessing reoffense risk with juvenile sexual offenders. *Child Welfare, LXX*(3), 333-345.

Kavoussi, R. J., Kaplan, M., & Becker, J. V. (1988). Psychiatric diagnoses in adolescent sex offenders. *Journal of the American Academy of Child and Adolescent Psychiatry, 27*(2), 241-243.

Kimball, L M., & Guarino-Ghezzi, S. (1996). *Sex offender treatment: An assessment of sex offender treatment within the Massachusetts department of youth services* (Juvenile Justice Series Report: No. 10). Boston: Northeastern University, Privatized Research Management Initiative.

Knight, R. A., & Prentky, R. A. (1993). Exploring characteristics for classifying juvenile sex offenders. In H. E. Barbaree, W. L. Marshall, & S. M. Hudson (Eds.), *The juvenile sex offender* (pp. 45-83). New York: Guilford Press.

Knight, R.A., & Sims-Knight, J.E. (2004). Testing an etiological model for male juvenile sexual offending against females. *Journal of Child Sexual Abuse, 13*(3/4), pp. 33-56.

Kobayashi, J., Sales, B. D., Becker, J. V., Figueredo, A. J., & Kaplan, M. S. (1995). Perceived parental deviance, parent-child bonding, child abuse, and child sexual aggression. *Sexual Abuse: A Journal of Research and Treatment, 7*(1), 25-43.

Kubik, E. K., Hecker, J. E., & Righthand, S. (2002). Adolescent females who have sexually offended: A comparison with adolescent males who have sexually offended. *Journal of Child Sexual Abuse, 11*(3), 63-83.

Lane, S., & Lobanov-Rostovsky, C. (1997). Special populations: Children, families, the developmentally disabled, and violent youth. In G.D. Ryan, & S. L. Lane (Eds.), *Juvenile sexual offending: Causes, consequences, and correction* (pp. 322-359). San Francisco: Jossey-Bass Publishers.

Langevin, R., Marentette, D., & Rosati, B. (1996). Why therapy fails with some sex offenders: Learning difficulties examined empirically. In E. Coleman, M. Dwyer, & N. J. Pallone (Eds.), *Sex offender treatment: Biological dysfunction, intrapsychic conflict, interpersonal violence* (pp. 143-155). Binghamton, NY: The Haworth Press, Inc.

Lightfoot, L.O., & Barbaree, H. E. (1993). The relationship between substance use and abuse and sexual offending in adolescents. In H. E. Barbaree, W. L. Marshall, & S. M. Hudson (Eds.), *The juvenile sex offender* (pp. 203-224). New York: Guilford Press.

Longo, R.E. (2004). An integrated experiential approach to treating young people who sexually abuse. *Journal of Child Sexual Abuse, 13*(3/4), pp. 193-213.

Mathews, R., Hunter, Jr., J. A., & Vuz, J. (1997). Juvenile female sexual offenders: Clinical characteristics and treatment issues. *Sexual Abuse: A Journal of Research and Treatment, 9*(3), 187-200.

Milloy, C. D. (1994). *A comparative study of juvenile sex offenders and non-sex offenders.* Olympia, WA: Washington State Institute for Public Policy.

Miner, M. H., & Crimmins, C. L. S. (1995). Adolescent sex offenders: Issues of etiology and risk factors. In B. K. Schwartz, & H. K. Cellini (Eds.), *The sex offender: Vol. 1. Corrections, treatment, and legal practice* (pp. 9.1-9.15). Kingston, NJ: Civic Research Institute.

Miner, M. H., Siekert, G. P., & Ackland, M.A. (1997). *Evaluation: Juvenile sex offender treatment program, Minnesota Correctional Facility–Sauk Centre* (Final report–Biennium 1995-1997). Minneapolis, MN: University of Minnesota, Department of Family Practice and Community Health, Program in Human Sexuality.

Morenz, B., & Becker, J.V. (1995). The treatment of youthful sexual offenders. *Applied & Preventive Psychology, 4,* 247-256.

Prentky, R., & Burgess, A. W. (1990). Rehabilitation of child molesters: A cost-benefit analysis. *American Journal of Orthopsychiatry, 60*(1), 108-117.

Prentky, R., Harris, B., Frizzell, K., & Righthand, S. (2000). An actuarial procedure for assessing risk in juvenile sex offenders. *Sexual Abuse: A Journal of Research and Treatment, 12*(2), 71-93.

Rasmussen, L.A. (1999). Factors related to recidivism among juvenile sexual offenders. *Sexual Abuse: A Journal of Research and Treatment, 11*(1), 69-85.

Ray, J. A., & English, D. J. (1995). Comparison of female and male children with sexual behavior problems. *Journal of Youth and Adolescence, 24*(4), 439-451.

Righthand, S., Hennings, R., & Wigley, P. (1989). *Young sex offenders in Maine.* Portland, ME: University of Southern Maine, Public Policy and Management Program, Human Services Development Institute.

Righthand, S., Knight, R., & Prentky, R. (2002, October). *A path analytic investigation of proximal antecedents of J-SOAP risk domains.* Paper presented at the Association for the Treatment of Sexual Abusers' 21st Annual Research and Treatment Conference, Montreal, Quebec, Canada.

Righthand, S., & Welch, C. (2001). *Youths who have sexually offended: A review of the professional literature.* Washington, DC: Office of Juvenile Justice and Delinquency Prevention.

Righthand, S., Welch, C., Carpenter, E. M., Young, G. S., & Scoular, R. J. (2001). *Sex offending by Maine youth: Their offenses and characteristics (Part 1 & Part II).* Augusta, ME: Department of Corrections and Department of Human Services.

Ryan, G., Miyoshi, T. J., Metzner, J. L., Krugman, R. D., & Fryer, G. E. (1996). Trends in a national sample of sexually abusive youths. *Journal of the American Academy of Child and Adolescent Psychiatry, 35*(1), 17-25.

Schram, D. D., Milloy, C. D., & Rowe, W. E. (1991). *Juvenile sex offenders: A follow up study of reoffense behavior.* Olympia, WA: Washington State Institute for Public Policy, Urban Policy Research and Cambie Group International.

Smith, H., & Israel, E. (1987). Sibling incest: A study of dynamics of 25 cases. *Child Abuse and Neglect, 11,* 101-108.

Smith, W. R., & Monastersky, C. (1986). Assessing juvenile sexual offenders' risk for reoffending. *Criminal Justice and Behavior, 13*(2), 115-140.

Smith, W. R., Monastersky, C., & Deisher, R.M. (1987). MMPI-based personality types among juvenile sexual offenders. *Journal of Clinical Psychology, 43,* 422-430.

Spaccarelli, S., Bowden, B., Coatsworth, J. D., & Kim, S. (1997). Psychosocial correlates of male sexual aggression in a chronic delinquent sample. *Criminal Justice and Behavior, 24*(1), 71-95.

Stermac, L., & Sheridan, L. (1993). The developmentally disabled adolescent sex offender. In H. E. Barbaree, W. L. Marshall, & S. M. Hudson (Eds.), *The juvenile sex offender* (pp. 235-242). New York: Guilford Press.

Weinrott, M. (1996). *Juvenile sexual aggression: A critical review.* Boulder, CO: University of Colorado, Institute for Behavioral Sciences, Center for the Study and Prevention of Violence.

Wieckowski, E., Hartsoe, P., Mayer, A., & Shortz, J. (1998). Deviant sexual behavior in children and young adolescents: Frequency and patterns. *Sexual Abuse: A Journal of Research and Treatment, 10*(4), 293-304.

Worling, J.R. (2001). Personality-based typology of adolescent male sexual offenders: Differences in recidivism rates, victim-selection characteristics, and personal victimization histories. *Sexual Abuse: A Journal of Research & Treatment, 13*(3), 149-166.

Worling, J.R., & Curren, T. (2000). Adolescent sexual offender recidivism: Success of specialized treatment and implications for risk prediction. *Child Abuse & Neglect, 24,* 965-982.

Zankman, S., & Bonomo, J. (2004). Working with parents to reduce juvenile sex offender recidivism. *Journal of Child Sexual Abuse, 13*(3/4), pp.139-156.

Zimring, F. (in press). *The changing legal world of adolescent sexuality.* Berkeley, CA: University of California. Manuscript in preparation.

Testing an Etiological Model for Male Juvenile Sexual Offending Against Females

Raymond A. Knight
Judith E. Sims-Knight

SUMMARY. Research on the origin of sexual aggression has identified several important contributing factors: (a) early abuse (physical and sexual), (b) personality/behavioral traits (callousness and unemotionality, antisocial behavior/impulsivity, and hypersexuality), and (c) attitudinal/cognitive variables (negative masculinity, hostility toward women, misogynistic fantasies). We developed and tested an etiological model of sexual coercion on adult samples of sexual offenders and community controls. The model proposes three major causal pathways to sexual coercion. Using data gathered from a computerized interview, we employed this same model to predict sexually coercive behavior in a sample of 218 juvenile sexual offenders. The cross- sample consistency of the model provides support for a unified theory of sexual aggression against women. *[Article copies available for a fee from The Haworth Document Delivery Service: 1-800-HAWORTH. E-mail address: <docdelivery@ haworthpress.com> Website: <http://www.HaworthPress.com> © 2004 by The Haworth Press, Inc. All rights reserved.]*

Address correspondence to: Raymond A. Knight, PhD, Department of Psychology, MS 062, Brandeis University, Waltham, MA 02454-9110 (E-mail: knight2@brandeis. edu).

[Haworth co-indexing entry note]: "Testing an Etiological Model for Male Juvenile Sexual Offending Against Females." Knight, Raymond A., and Judith E. Sims-Knight. Co-published simultaneously in *Journal of Child Sexual Abuse* (The Haworth Maltreatment and Trauma Press, an imprint of The Haworth Press, Inc.) Vol. 13, No. 3/4, 2004, pp. 33-55; and: *Identifying and Treating Youth Who Sexually Offend: Current Approaches, Techniques, and Research* (ed: Robert Geffner et al.) The Haworth Maltreatment and Trauma Press, an imprint of The Haworth Press, Inc., 2004, pp. 33-55. Single or multiple copies of this article are available for a fee from The Haworth Document Delivery Service [1-800-HAWORTH, 9:00 a.m. - 5:00 p.m. (EST). E-mail address: docdelivery@haworthpress.com].

KEYWORDS. Juvenile sexual offenders, rape, causal analysis, sexual coercion, path analysis, sex offenders, child abuse, psychopathy

Juvenile sexual offending is a serious societal problem that elicits concern from community, clinical, legal, and research quarters (Barbaree, Hudson, & Seto, 1993). It is estimated that juveniles account for 30% to 60% of cases of child molestation and 20% to 30% of the rapes reported each year in the United States (Brown, Flanagan, & McLeod, 1984; Fehrenbach, Smith, Monastersky, & Deishner, 1986). The widespread concern about sexual aggression has been reflected in the numerous recent legislative initiatives directed at reducing the incidence of sexual coercion, such as sexual predator laws, required community notification about high-risk offenders, and mandated treatment of offenders (Grubin & Prentky, 1993; Prentky, 1996).

Such legislative attention has been directed at juveniles without questioning the appropriateness of applying adult models to juveniles. Clearly, decisions about which adult initiatives to apply to juveniles should be informed by data. Unfortunately, our knowledge of juvenile sexual offenders has not matched the seriousness of the problem they pose (Becker, Harris, & Sales, 1993). Much of the existing research is riddled with methodological flaws (Becker & Hunter, 1997; Knight & Prentky, 1993) and has been largely descriptive.

Although questions about the etiology and the course of sexually aggressive behavior in adolescents are crucial, there are few research studies specifically addressing these issues. The gaps in our knowledge constitute a formidable roadblock to any attempts at adapting a public health model of sexual aggression (McMahon & Puett, 1999; Mercy, 1999; Wurtele, 1999). The practical implementation of a primary prevention perspective requires well-founded models of etiology and course to guide its policies and interventions. A few hypotheses about important etiological factors contributing to juvenile sexual aggression have been proposed (e.g., Becker, 1988; Caputo, Frick, & Brodsky, 1999), but these have not been tested empirically.

Fortunately, data from a variety of sources indicate that there are empirically validated guidelines available to orient our speculations about the etiology of juvenile sexual aggression. In their review, Loeber and Stouthamer-Loeber (1998) concluded that the aggression literature with both adolescents and adults supports the hypothesis that a single theory may be able to account for the diversity in findings across different antisocial behaviors and aggressive outcomes. They argued further that incorporating into such a general theory factors unique to a particular domain of aggression could enhance the understanding of specific types of antisocial outcomes and behaviors. We have been able to confirm this claim in several recent studies (Johnson & Knight, 2000; Knight & Sims-Knight, 2003).

Combining elements from studies of non-criminal aggressors (Malamuth, 1998) with our own work on criminal sexual aggressors, we developed and successfully tested on both adult community males and adult sexual offenders an etiological model of sexual coercion (Knight & Sims-Knight, 1999; 2003). It is the intent of the present article to describe the components of this model, to examine the relevance of these components to juvenile offenders, and to test the validity of a version of this model on a sample of juvenile sexual offenders.

THE ETIOLOGICAL MODEL

Our model of the origins of sexual aggression (see Figure 1) proposes that early abuse experiences (physical/verbal and sexual) plus personality predispositions combine to produce three latent traits that predict sexual aggression: (a) arrogant, deceitful personality/emotional detachment, (b) impulsivity/antisocial behaviors, and (c) sexual preoccupation/hypersexuality.

Physical/Verbal Abuse

Physical/verbal abuse was found to have two roles in our two samples of adults (sexual offenders and community males) (Knight & Sims-Knight, 2003). First, it increased the likelihood of arrogant/deceitful personality/emotional detachment (Callous/Unemotional trait in Figure 1), the first of Hare's two factors on the Psychopathy Checklist (PCL-R) (see Hare et al., 1990; Harpur, Hakstian, & Hare 1988; Harpur, Hare, & Hakstian, 1989). Second, it served as a model of aggression, thus increasing the likelihood of the manifestation of aggressive behavior and antisocial, impulsive acting out, similar to Factor 2 of the PCL-R. Behavioral genetic research suggests that this second factor has high heritability (Depue, 1996; Edelbrock, Rende, Plomin, & Thompson, 1995; Krueger, 2000; Mason & Frick, 1994; but see Livesley, 1998, for contrary evidence), but it is also purported to be influenced by physical/verbal abuse (e.g., Bennett et al., 2002).

Research with children suggests that physical/verbal abuse has similar effects. It is correlated with personality disorders (Goldman, D'Angelo, DeMaso, & Mezzacappa, 1992) and dissociation (Chu, & Dill, 1990; Sandberg & Lynn, 1992). It has been found to covary with sexual coercion in adolescence (Awad & Saunders, 1991; Boone-Hamilton, 1991; Fehrenbach et al., 1986), and juvenile sex offenders have been found to have experienced more abuse than other delinquent groups (Ford &

FIGURE 1. Adjusted three component structural model predicting sexual coercion against women, tested in a sample of 275 adult male sexual offenders.

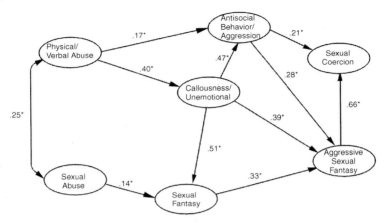

Note. *Standardized beta is significant at least p < .05.

Linney, 1995; for additional review of the literature on physical abuse as a factor in juvenile sexual offending, see Righthand & Welch, this issue).

Sexual Abuse

In both samples of adults, sexual abuse led to sexual preoccupation and compulsivity, which in turn increased the risk of aggressive sexual fantasies (Knight & Sims-Knight, 2003). Research with children corroborates the importance of sexual abuse, but does not allow specification of the mechanisms through which it might work. Although it is clear that only a proportion of males who are sexually abused become sexually abusive (Friedrich & Chaffin, 2000; Widom, 1996; Williams, 1995), and not all juvenile and adult sexual offenders have experienced sexual abuse as children or adolescents, there is nonetheless considerable evidence that sexual abuse is a risk factor in sexually coercive behavior. A high proportion of juvenile sexual offenders were also themselves victims of sexual abuse; estimates range from 19% to 81% (Becker, Kaplan, Cunningham-Rathner, & Kavoussi, 1986; Fehrenbach et al., 1986; Friedrich & Luecke, 1988; Longo, 1982). These incidences exceed estimates of sexual abuse in the general male population, and they are higher than the incidences of such abuse among juvenile offenders who have been accused of non-sexual offenses (Burton, Miller, & Shill, 2002) or of non-contact sexual offenses (Fehrenbach et al., 1986).

There are some indications that sexual abuse plays a more critical role in juvenile than adult sexual coercion. Knight and Prentky (1993) found that among sexual offenders, those who had begun their sexually coercive behavior in adolescence could be distinguished from offenders who began their offending as adults by the higher frequency and level of the childhood sexual abuse they experienced. There is also evidence that the sexually abusive history of juveniles predicts the nature of their predatory acts (Burton, 2001; DiCenso, 1992; for additional review of the literature on sexual abuse as a factor in juvenile sexual offending, see Righthand & Welch, this issue).

Psychopathy

Factor analytic studies of Hare's Psychopathy Checklist (PCL-R) (Hare et al., 1990) have revealed two correlated dimensions, labeled Predatory Personality (or Arrogant and Deceitful Personality/Emotional Detachment) and Antisocial Behavior (Cooke & Michie, 2001; Patrick, Bradley, & Lang, 1993). In their review of the correlative work on these two dimensions, Patrick and Zempolich (1998) argued that whereas the Predatory Personality factor has been related to low anxiety, low fear reactivity, high social dominance, and narcissism, the Antisocial factor has been related to impulsivity, sensation seeking, alcohol and drug abuse, and the frequency of criminal offending.

If these factors are indeed related to different underlying mechanisms, each could play a unique role in sexual aggression. Arrogant, Deceitful Personality/Emotional Detachment and Antisocial Behavior/Impulsivity appear to play differential roles both in psychopathy and as predictors of sexual coercion in both criminal and non-criminal samples (Malamuth, Linz, Heavey, Barnes, & Acker, 1995; Prentky, Knight, Lee, & Cerce, 1995; Quinsey, Harris, Rice, & Cormier, 1998). This suggests that these factors may relate to basic processes that underlie all aggressive behavior, and psychopathy may simply represent the extreme end of both dimensions (Loeber & Stouthamer-Loeber, 1998).

Arrogant and deceitful personality/emotional detachment. In our adult samples, this trait predicted sexual fantasy and antisocial behavior/aggression (Knight & Sims-Knight, 2003). Although this factor has received little attention in the literature on juvenile sexual offenders, what research does exist suggests that this personality/affective factor is an important predictor in this population. Caputo et al. (1999) found that, consistent with the adult literature, juvenile sexual offenders had more callous and unemotional traits than other offenders. Moreover, among children with significant conduct disorder problems, those who also exhibited callous and unemotional traits had more severe behavioral problems than those with only conduct disorders (Christian, Frick, Hill, Tyler, & Frazer, 1997; Frick, 1998; Lynam, 1998).

Antisocial behavior/impulsivity. Consistent with earlier research (Knight, 1999; Langton, 2002; Prentky et al., 1995; Quinsey et al., 1998), our research with adults found that antisocial behavior/impulsivity predicted sexual coercion, both directly and indirectly through aggressive sexual fantasy (Knight & Sims-Knight, 2003). A history of antisocial behavior is also common in juvenile sexual offending, as is reflected in the criminal records of these adolescents (e.g., Awad & Saunders, 1991; Becker et al., 1986). Knight and Prentky (1993) found that sexual offenders who had begun their sexually coercive behavior in adolescence exhibited significantly more antisocial behavior as juveniles than offenders who began their offending as adults. In our direct comparison of juvenile and adult sexual offenders (Knight, in press) we found that the reported frequency and degree of juvenile antisocial behavior were significantly higher for incarcerated juvenile sexual offenders than they were in a sample of incarcerated adult sexual offenders.

Sexual Drive and Sexual Promiscuity

The notion that some aspects of sexual drive or sexual appetitive behavior may be a critical component of sexual aggression has found considerable empirical support (Ellis, 1993; Malamuth, Heavey, & Linz, 1993). We found that sexual drive and preoccupation discriminated sexually coercive males from non-coercives in both community and criminal samples (Knight & Prentky, in preparation). Regardless of criminal status, sexually coercive participants reported higher levels of sexual drive, higher frequency of sexual behavior, and greater sexual deviance than non-coercive participants. Moreover, in Hanson and Bussière's (1998) meta-analysis, sexual deviance and drive were important predictors of recidivism.

There is, however, considerable debate about what the core construct underlying this dimension is. Whereas for Ellis (1993) the core seems to be simply the strength of the sexual drive, Malamuth (1998) has postulated that the proclivity to engage in promiscuous/impersonal sex is the critical construct. He described the dimension of impersonal sex as similar to the concept of "sociosexuality," a hypothetical dimension of willingness to engage in sexual activity in the relative absence of attachment or emotional ties. In our studies, we found that sexual drive, preoccupation, and compulsivity were highly correlated with each other and in turn were correlated with pornography use, expressive aggression toward women, sadism, pervasive anger, and offense planning for both adult and juvenile sexual offenders (Knight, 1999; Knight & Cerce, 1999).

Our latent trait of sexual fantasy, accordingly, included sexual drive, sexual preoccupation, and sexual compulsivity. In adults it predicted aggressive sexual fantasy directly, and indirectly it increased the likelihood of sexually coercive behavior (Knight & Sims-Knight, 2003).

Sexualization appears to be at least as important in juvenile samples as in adult samples. In our direct comparison of juvenile and adult sexual offenders on the Multidimensional Assessment of Sex and Aggression (the MASA; a computerized inventory that assesses multiple domains relevant to sexual coercion) (Knight, in press), we found that juvenile offenders were equivalent to the adult offenders in their reported Sexual Drive and Preoccupation factors, and were significantly lower only on Sexual Compulsivity. Also, the reported frequencies of the factors Exhibitionism, Transvestitism, Voyeurism, and Atypical Paraphilia were significantly higher for incarcerated juvenile sexual offenders than for incarcerated adult sexual offenders. Moreover, there is some evidence that juvenile sexual offenders with deviant sexual interests are more likely to recidivate (Schram, Malloy, & Rowe, 1992; Worling & Curwen, 2000).

Conclusion

The data we reviewed supports the hypothesis that the components of our adult model, which has successfully predicted sexually coercive behavior in both sexual offender and community adult samples (Knight & Sims-Knight, 2003), are equally important for juveniles. Consequently, in this present study we tested the utility of our latent trait model on juvenile sexual offenders, which is presented in Figure 1. Specifically, we predicted that there are three paths that antecede sexual coercion in juveniles. The first path leads from physical/verbal abuse through antisocial behavior/aggression to sexual coercion. The second path leads from physical/verbal abuse through callous/unemotional trait through aggressive sexual fantasy to sexual coercion. The third path leads from sexual abuse through sexual fantasy and through aggressive sexual fantasy to sexual coercion. It is important to remember that although structural equation models make claims about causal paths, they are in the end, always based on correlations and therefore cannot be considered definitive tests of causality.

METHOD

Participants

The 218 juveniles in the sample came from inpatient juvenile sexual offender treatment facilities in Maine, Massachusetts, Minnesota, and Virginia.

All participants had been adjudicated for sexual offenses involving sexual contact with a victim. The mean age of the sample was 15.97 years, and these offenders had been incarcerated an average of 3.06 times including the present offense. The sample was ethnically diverse, comprising 8.9% African American, 9.9% Asian, 28.3% Caucasian, 38.2% Hispanic, 3.7% Native American, and 11% other races.

PROCEDURE

Test Administration

These juveniles were administered one of the computerized versions of the MASA (3, 4, 5, or 6) in groups of 3 to 15 participants. Starting with Version 3 the MASA had been revised to have a 4th grade reading level and to use language understandable to juveniles. The juveniles were assured that all of their responses were completely confidential and that no information would be entered into their clinical files or reported to their counselors. A Certificate of Confidentiality protected this assurance.

The MASA. The MASA was originally developed to supplement our coding of archival records, which we had found significantly lacking in the area of sexual behavior, cognitions, and fantasies. As we expanded our subject pool, additional inadequacies in record sources at some institutions motivated us to expand the domains tested. In the first version of the MASA we assessed the following 10 domains: Social competence, juvenile and adult antisocial behavior, sexualization, paraphilias, pornography exposure, offense planning, sadism, expressive aggression, and pervasive anger. We factor analyzed the items in each of these domains. The resulting factors have been replicated on new samples, and the factor scores show both high internal consistency and test-retest reliability (Knight & Cerce, 1999). The versions of the MASA used in the present study added sexual abuse, physical abuse, emotional detachment, and arrogant and deceitful personality to the 10 original domains. The MASA has been revised six times and is now only administered in a computerized format. It has been administered to over 2,200 males and 200 females.

RESULTS

In testing the model, for each of the latent traits we created observational measures (depicted in the rectangles in Figure 2) comparable to those measures we had used in our adult model. We tested their internal consistency, where appropriate, to provide an indication of whether these components cohered in juveniles the way that they did in adults. Of the 21 scales 15 were summative scales, appropriate for internal consistency analysis. Only 2 of these 15 scales had alphas that fell below .70, Sexual Compulsivity ($\alpha = .56$) and Sexual Drive ($\alpha = .58$). Of the remaining 13 summative scales, 6 had alphas between .70 and .79, and the remaining 7 were equal to or greater than .80. The 6 non-summative scales in the model were all early developmental scales, calculated either as a maximum, minimum, or count over a number of responses or response categories (e.g., physical abuse frequency) or as a complex algorithm over a number of responses (e.g., degree of penetration).

As we had done in generating the adult model, we did factor analyses of both the early developmental antecedents and the psychopathy-related scales. The former analysis yielded, as it did for the adults, two separate, theoretically clean factors, one for Physical/Verbal Abuse and the other for Sexual Abuse. In contrast with the adult analyses, the factor analysis of the components of psychopathy yielded three separate factors that corresponded more closely to Cooke and Michie's (2001) three-factor solution. Because the empathy, perspective taking, and guilt factor was completely independent of the callousness factor, we decided to exclude it from the analysis. This analysis also differed from the adult analysis in that a scale made up mostly of items from Monroe's (1978) Dyscontrol scale, a self-report measure of impulsivity, loaded highly on the CU factor, and significantly less on the Antisocial Behavior/Aggression factor. We left the scale on the CU factor.

Outcome measures were three sexual coercion scales against a woman or an age-appropriate female. Serious coercion involved attempted or completed intercourse. Moderate coercion involved oral sex or anal penetration. Mild coercion included touching, feeling, kissing, or petting. Mild coercion was included in the juvenile model, although it did not appear in the adult model, because of the significantly greater incidence of mild coercion in the offense histories of juveniles as compared to adult offenders (Miranda & Corcoran, 2000).

In all three scales the victim was defined as a woman or peer-aged girl, if she was less than 4 years younger, same age, or older than the offender at the time of the sexual assault. The dependent measure was the maximum number of the specific sexual acts against an age appropriate or older female, regardless of the method of coercion (plying with alcohol, manipulation against their will, verbal threats, or physical force). Sexually coercive acts against males and younger females were not counted in these measures of sexual coercion.

FIGURE 2. A priori three component theoretical structural model predicting sexual coercion against women, tested in a sample of 218 juvenile sexual offenders.

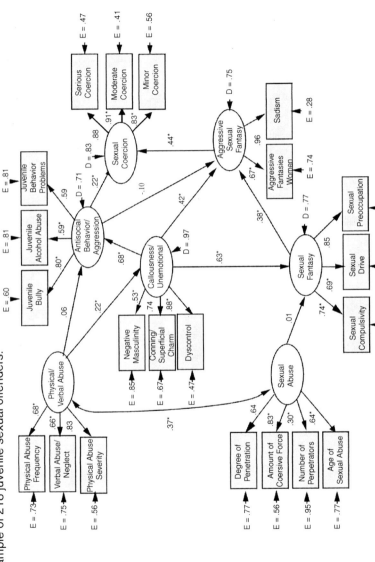

Note. *Standardized beta is significant at least p < .05.

42

THE JUVENILE STRUCTURAL EQUATION MODEL

We tested the three-path model presented in Figure 2 on this sample of juveniles using AMOS (Byrne, 2001). We also tested two alternative models that have been proposed in the literature. The first alternative model assessed the proposal that the sexual aggression in juveniles against women was primarily the result of childhood sexual abuse. The effect may be due either to a recapitulation of their own sexual victimization (Rogers & Terry, 1984) or to childhood victimization initiating an abusive cycle that is maintained and reinforced by sexually aggressive fantasies (Ryan, Lane, Davis, & Isaac, 1987). The second alternative model tested was Malamuth's (1998; Malamuth et al., 1993). He proposed that sexually coercive behavior against women was predicted by the confluence of negative masculinity and sexual promiscuity. The explanatory power of these three alternative models was compared.

Figure 2 presents the juveniles' standardized beta results for the three-path, a priori model developed on the adult offenders. In this figure rectangles represent the observable measurement scales, and ovals represent the latent traits. The E's for the observable scales are the residuals associated with the measurement of each variable, and the D's or disturbances are the residuals associated with the prediction of each trait (Byrne, 1994).

This model showed a reasonable fit to the data as indicated by a Comparative Fit Index (CFI) of .90 (Byrne, 1994, 2001) and a root mean square error of approximation (RMSEA) of .07 (a RMSEA below .08 indicates a reasonable fit; Brown & Cudeck, 1993). The alternative one-path model, which was allotted all of the proposed relations of the three-path model except the projections of CU and antisocial behavior to Sexual Fantasy, Aggressive Sexual Fantasy, or Sexual Coercion, did not fit to the data as well (CFI = .82, RMSEA = .09). Malamuth's two-path alternative, which required the restructuring of the model to closely match his model (Malamuth et al., 1993), fit even less well (CFI = .81, RMSEA = .10). It should be noted that this test of Malamuth's model used sexual preoccupation, compulsivity, and drive rather than sexual promiscuity.

Despite the reasonableness of the fit of the juvenile data, there are notable differences between the adult and the juvenile results. First, although 65% of the variance of both sexual coercion and aggressive sexual fantasy was accounted for in the model applied to adult sexual offenders, the comparable percents of variance accounted for in the juvenile sample were 37% and 44%, respectively $(1 - D^2)$. Second, three paths that were significant in the adults' solution failed to yield significant standardized betas in the juvenile data: Physical/Verbal Abuse to Antisocial Behavior/Aggression, Antisocial Behavior/Aggression to Aggressive Sexual Fantasy, and Sexual Abuse to Sexual Fantasy.

Modification indices suggested a significant direct effect of Sexual Abuse on Sexual Coercion ($\beta = .25$). Nonetheless, when a revised post hoc model was calculated with this new path added and non-significant paths eliminated, the CFI increased only slightly to .91. It is worth noting that in this post hoc model, the only significant path from Sexual Abuse projected directly to Sexual Coercion.

DISCUSSION

The most impressive finding in the testing of the three-path model was the consistency of the pattern in relations among traits in adult and juvenile sexual offender samples. The three paths in the model and their developmental antecedents appear to play an important role in the prediction of sexual coercion against women in both adolescents and adults. This same model also shows reasonable fit in college students, community non-offenders, and nonsexual criminal samples (Knight & Sims-Knight, 1999; 2003), which lends further support to the explanatory power of the model and indicates the potential for the unified theory of rape that was discussed in relation to the adult model.

It is important to emphasize that the three traits that define the three paths–sexual drive/preoccupation, antisocial behavior, and callousness/unemotionality–correspond to core theoretical processes identified in both the experimental and psychometric research on psychopathy and in the personality literature. In addition, it can be argued that these same three traits account for a considerable proportion of the variance of factors identified as predictors of general recidivism (Gendreau, Little, & Goggin, 1996) and more specifically of factors that predict recidivism for a sexual crime in adults (Barbaree, Seto, Langton, & Peacock, 2001; Hanson & Bussière, 1998; Langton, 2002). These variables play a prominent role in the risk assessment scales that have been fashioned to predict recidivism in adult sexual offenders (Hanson, 2000; Roberts, Doren, & Thorton, 2002). Similarly, for juveniles the first two factors for the JJPI Juvenile Sex Offender Assessment Protocol are sexual drive/sexual preoccupation and impulsive, antisocial behavior (Prentky, Harris, Frizzel, & Righthand, 2000).

These three components are also important in the treatment of both juvenile and adult sexual offenders. There is some evidence that aspects of both psychopathy and sexual maladjustment may be related to treatment compliance in juvenile sexual offenders (Hunter & Figueredo, 1999). These three components, or their related behavioral correlates, constitute key targets of therapeutic intervention for sexual aggression (e.g., Knight, 1999; Righthand & Welch, 2001). Thus, these three components appear to play a critical role in the etiology of sexual coercion and in the modulation of such behavior across the life span. Note that the notion of how many specific paths are involved in the model does not, as Malamuth (2003) suggests, rest on whether the relation of two components to sexual coercion is mediated through another construct (e.g., aggressive sexual fantasies), but on whether one can empirically identify core underlying processes to account for each causal component. Our review of the relevant literature suggests that the three components in our model covary with different underlying processes.

In both the adult and the juvenile models, early traumatic physical and sexual abuse play an important etiological role, increasing the likelihood of sexually coercive behavior either indirectly through the three intervening paths or directly. The significant role of physical abuse in predicting recidivism in adult offenders (Knight, 1999), when added to the etiological role of childhood maltreatment, mandates that such abuse and its sequelae be the target of therapeutic intervention (Barbaree, Marshall, & McCormick, 1998). The childhood abuse variables will also be important in identifying high-risk children and providing them with the opportunity of early intervention and possibly prevention.

Despite the considerable similarity of the juvenile and adult models, the differences in their solutions were noteworthy. First, although Physical Abuse in the juvenile sexual offenders predicted the CU trait, it did not predict Antisocial Behavior. Second, although Sexual Abuse directly predicted Sexual Coercion, it did not predict Sexual Fantasy or Aggressive Sexual Fantasy. Third, the proportion of variance accounted for, although substantial, was much smaller for the juveniles than for the adults.

Discussion of the possible reasons for the differences in the results between the juvenile and adult samples can be divided into two major categories. The first category focuses on issues related to the different developmental stages of the two populations. Three related, overlapping issues must be considered: (a) the developmental timeline for the coalescence of particular attitudes and behavioral traits, (b) the problem in adolescent samples of differentiating between those whose sexual transgressions are adolescence-limited, and those whose sexual coercion will be life course-persistent (terms borrowed from Moffitt's [1993] distinction in the adolescent aggression literature), and (c) the increased difficulty in juvenile samples relative to adult samples of differentiating between those whose sexual targets are age-appropriate females and those who are fixated on children as sexual objects. The second category considers moderating theoretical constructs that might account for the greater instability of the paths that were not found significant for the juvenile sample. We will consider each of these four explanations in turn.

Trait Development

It could be argued that in both the domains of sexual fantasy and the generation of the core personality characteristics that are represented in the callous, unemotional and antisocial behavior constructs, juveniles are in the process of development and trait consolidation. These constructs might not yet represent sufficiently cohesive targets for clear linkage to particular earlier experiences, but they may nonetheless still have sufficient power to predict sexual coercion. Other data (Frick, 1998; Lynam, 1998) suggest that in adolescence, callousness and emotional detachment are involved in a complex, interactive interplay with antisocial behavior and aggression. Although the patterning of the transactional sequence that determines whether and how these traits develop into the more stable and persistent behavioral and attitudinal adult characteristics remains controversial, the ultimate stable coping pattern rather than transitional turmoil may provide the better link to earlier traumatic experiences. This would explain why the abuse traits had fewer significant relations with the three mediating paths in the juvenile solution. It would also explain the lower proportion of variance explained.

The complete lack of a relation in the juvenile solution between Sexual Abuse and both Sexual Fantasy and Aggressive Sexual Fantasy was surprising, especially when viewed in light of the significant direct relation from Sexual Abuse to Sexual Coercion? ($\beta = .25$) found in the post hoc model. Such a direct path from Sexual Abuse to Sexual Coercion, not mediated by Sexual Fantasy, suggests that juveniles may imitate the abuse they suffered (Burton, 2001; DiCenso, 1992) rather than fantasizing about it. Sexual abuse and sexual fantasy appear to make independent contributions to sexually coercive behavior against women in adolescents.

Differentiating Persistent Traits from Transitional Noise

The transitional turmoil that characterizes the life course of some adolescents might turn up the volume on certain behavioral dispositions, and affect both the elevation of particular dimensions and the patterns of their relation to other dimensions. Such turmoil might contribute noise that masks the more cross-temporally stable signal patterns. Transition into adulthood allows a dampening of the transitory problems of adolescence and a sharper differentiation of core traits. This same process has been offered as one possible explanation for the higher percent of genetic variance attributed to adult than adolescent antisocial behavior (Raine, 1993). Such transitory problems might contribute to the loss of particular relations in the juvenile solution, especially those involving the antisocial behavior/aggression trait, which Knight (in press) found significantly higher in juvenile sexual offenders than in adult offenders.

In comparing juveniles to adult sexual offenders it is important to remain cognizant of two important factors. First, the recidivism rate among juveniles appears to be significantly lower than that of adults (Weinrott, 1996; for an in-depth discussion of recidivism in juvenile sexual offenders, see Efta-Breitbach & Freeman, this issue). Second, the majority of adults have begun their sexually coercive behavior as juveniles (Knight & Prentky, 1993). Comparable evidence for these two factors has been found for antisocial behavior (Robins & Radcliff, 1978) and for aggression (Loeber & Stouthamer-Loeber, 1998). Whatever models are created for juveniles and adults must ultimately account for these factors. The retrospective study of development is limited in its potential resolution of important issues. The ultimate explication of the differences between juvenile and adult sexual offenders will require a large-scale, detailed prospective study of juvenile offenders with adequate community controls.

Discriminating Among Different Types of Sexual Aggression

When one is predicting sexual coercion against women in samples of generic sexual offenders, one has a more difficult task than when predicting the same coercion among nonsexual offenders, whether they be college students, community samples, or nonsexual offending criminal samples. All participants in a sexual offender sample have been selected because of presumed involvement in some form of sexually coercive behavior, whether rape or child molestation. Thus, when the outcome sexual coercion measure attempts to predict sexually aggressive behavior against females, those who deny such acts are likely to have molested children. Consequently, any ambiguities in the offender's understanding of his acts, inaccuracies in the criteria for differentiating age-appropriate from inappropriate sexual acts, or other problems differentiating these two sexual offender groups will increase the error variance in the distal, outcome sexual coercion measure and reduce predictability.

The difficulty determining whether a young female victim constitutes an age appropriate sexual partner for a young adolescent or is rather a fixated child victim has created problems in attempts to test adult taxonomic models on juvenile samples (Knight & Prentky, 1993). Although the R^2 values in the juvenile solution of .37 and .44 for Sexual Coercion against woman and Aggressive Sexual Fantasies against women, respectively, are substantial, they are far below the comparable .65s in the adult model. The difficulty identifying true rapists in a juvenile sample may account for part of this drop in the percent of variance accounted for in these outcome traits.

In this context it is important to emphasize that the three-path model presented here is intended as a model for sexual coercion against women. Clearly, an alternative model must be created to account for sexual behavior focused on children. From the sparse literature that has attempted to differentiate rapists from child molesters within juvenile samples, it is clear and consistent with our model, that the juvenile rapists evidence more antisocial behavior (Richardson, Kelly, Bhate, & Graham, 1997) and a higher use of alcohol (Hsu & Starzynski, 1990). Moreover, they come from more disturbed families, and they have experienced more caregiver instability (Saunders, Awad, & White, 1986). They have committed more violent offenses than offenders against younger children, and they evidence a higher frequency of borderline intellectual functioning (Saunders et al., 1986). Many of these discriminating characteristics are captured in the present three-path model.

The fact that both the adult and the juvenile models are in essence discriminating between rapists and child molesters might also partially explain the weak role of Sexual Abuse in the model. There are some data that suggest that among both juveniles (Knight & Prentky, 1993; Richardson et al., 1997) and adults (Bard et al., 1987; Seghorn, Prentky, & Boucher, 1987), offenders with child victims rather than age-appropriate female victims are more likely to have experienced sexual abuse themselves. This would explain the relatively low predictive strength of such abuse in a model aimed at predicting coercion against women (for more information on differentiating subtypes of juvenile sexual offenders, see Rasmussen, this issue).

Alternative Theoretical Explanations of the Differences

The failures in the juvenile model of the Antisocial Behavior and the Sexual Fantasy traits to be linked to childhood maltreatments are, at first glance, surprising, because one might predict that the immediacy of early traumas would have a greater impact in adolescence. Both physical and sexual abuse did ultimately predict sexual coercion for adolescents, but the differences in their causal path trajectories warrant further consideration.

Both research on the relation between physical abuse and child aggression and our results with adults led us to expect that physical abuse would predict the Antisocial Behavior/Aggression trait, though not to the degree that it would predict CU. The non-significance of this path in the juveniles might be due to a number of factors. First, in the juvenile model the dyscontrol (impulsivity) scale loaded more highly on CU and therefore was not included as an observable measure of the Antisocial Behavior trait. Second, only the Juvenile Bully scale on the Antisocial Behavior trait really measured aggression per se, which is the most consistent consequence of physical abuse. Interestingly, Juvenile Bully had the highest zero order correlations with the observable scales measuring Physical/Verbal Abuse, and was significantly correlated with the Verbal Abuse, Neglect scale ($r(216) = .29, p < .001$). In addition, the relative weakness of the path Physical/Verbal Abuse to Antisocial Behavior compared to the path to CU is consistent with the adult model and with Dodge, Bates, Pettit, and Valente's (1995) conclusion that attributional biases (such as our negative masculinity scale) partially mediate the effect of early abuse on later conduct problems, as it did in the juvenile model.

CONCLUSIONS

The three-path model presented in this article has not only provided a good fit for data used to predict sexual coercion in both adult sexual offender and community samples, but it has also predicted sexual coercion among juvenile sexual offenders. In our review of the three latent traits defining the paths–sexual drive/preoccupation, antisocial behavior/impulsivity, and callous/unemotional trait–we have argued that they correspond to core theoretical processes identified in both the psychopathy and personality literature. We have argued further that these traits play a critical role across the life span for sexually coercive males, are critical in assessing risk of recidivism, and should be targets of therapeutic intervention.

As we indicated at the beginning of this article, identifying the developmental antecedents of sexual aggression not only informs treatment planning (i.e., tertiary intervention), but also will ultimately be the basis for identifying at-risk groups for primary and secondary interventions. Having a validated model of the etiology of sexual aggression is the cornerstone of any public health approach to sexual aggression and a necessary prerequisite for implementation of a primary prevention perspective.

Clearly, the model presented is only a preliminary structure. Throughout the article we have noted the problems and the inconsistencies that remain. Other developmental antecedents must be measured and explored. It must be determined whether the callous, arrogant, and deceitful personality and emotional detachment are better conceived as a single factor or two separate traits. The core processes underlying the traits in the model must be explored, and behavioral-based, psychometrically sound measures of these processes must be developed. There are many questions that remain unanswered, but the model provides a solid, empirically disconfirmable, beginning.

REFERENCES

Awad, G. A., & Saunders, E. B. (1991). Male adolescent sexual assaulters: Clinical observations. *Journal of Interpersonal Violence, 6,* 446-460.

Barbaree, H. E., Hudson, S. M., & Seto, M. C. (1993). Sexual assault in society: The role of the juvenile offender. In H. E. Barbaree, W. L. Marshall, & S. M. Hudson (Eds.), *The juvenile sex offender* (pp. 1-24). New York: Guilford Press.

Barbaree, H. E., Marshall, W. L., & McCormick, J. (1998). The development of deviant sexual behaviour among adolescents and its implications for prevention and treatment. *Irish Journal of Psychology, 19,* 1-31.

Barbaree, H. E., Seto, M., Langton, C. M., & Peacock, E. J. (2001). Evaluating the predictive accuracy of six risk assessment instruments for adult sex offenders. *Criminal Justice and Behavior, 28,* 490-521.

Bard, L. A., Carter, D. L., Cerce, D. D., Knight, R. A., Rosenberg, R., & Schneider, B. (1987). A descriptive study of rapists and child molesters: Developmental, clinical, and criminal characteristics. *Behavioral Sciences and the Law, 5,* 203-220.

Becker, J. V. (1988). The effects of child sexual abuse on adolescent sexual offenders. In G. E. Wyatt, & G. J. Powell (Eds.), *Lasting effects of child sexual abuse* (pp. 193-207). Newbury Park, CA: Sage Publications.

Becker, J. V., Harris, C. D., & Sales, B. D. (1993). Juveniles who commit sex offenses: A critical review of research in sexual aggression. In G. C. N. Hall, R. Hirschman, J. R. Graham, & M. S. Zaragoza (Eds.), *Sexual aggression: Issues in etiology and assessment, treatment, and policy* (pp. 215-228). Washington, DC: Taylor & Francis.

Becker, J. V., & Hunter, J. (1997). Understanding and treating child and adolescent sexual offenders. In T. H. Ollendick, & R. J. Prinz (Eds.), *Advances in clinical child psychology, volume 19* (pp. 177-197). New York: Plenum Press.

Becker, J. V., Kaplan, M. S., Cunningham-Rathner, J., & Kavoussi, R. J. (1986). Characteristics of adolescent incest sexual perpetrators: Preliminary findings. *Journal of Family Violence, 1,* 85-97.

Bennett, A. J., Lesch, K. P., Heils, A., Long, J. C., Lorenz, J. G., Shoaf, S. E., Champoux, M., Suomi, S. J., Linnoila, M. V., & Higley, J. D. (2002). Early experience and serotonin transporter gene variation interact to influence primate CNS function. *Molecular Psychiatry, 7,* 118-122.

Boone-Hamilton, B. (1991, April). *A family psychosocial assessment tool: Implications for treatment of the adolescent sex offender and the family.* Paper presented at the 62nd Annual Meeting of the Eastern Psychological Association, New York.

Brown, E. J., Flanagan, T. J., & McLeod, M. (Eds.). (1984). *Sourcebook of criminal justice statistics–1983.* Washington, DC: Bureau of Justice Statistics.

Brown, M. W., & Cudeck, R. (1993). Alternative ways of assessing model fit. In K. A. Bollen, & J. S. Long (Eds.), *Testing structural equation models* (pp. 445-455). Newbury Park, CA: Sage.

Burton, D. L. (2001). *The relationship between the sexual victimization of and the subsequent sexual abuse by male adolescents.* Manuscript submitted for publication.

Burton, D. L., Miller, D. L., & Shill, C. T. (2002). A social learning theory comparison of the sexual victimization of adolescent sexual offenders and non-sexual offending male delinquents. *Child Abuse and Neglect, 26,* 893-907.

Byrne, B. M. (1994). *Structural equation modeling with EQS and EQS/Windows: Basic concepts, applications, and programming.* Thousand Oaks, CA: Sage Publications.

Byrne, B. M. (2001). *Structural equation modeling with AMOS: Basic concepts, applications, and programming.* Mahwah, NJ: Lawrence Erlbaum.

Caputo, A. A., Frick, P. J., & Brodsky, S. L. (1999). Family violence and juvenile sex offending: The potential mediating role of psychopathic traits and negative attitudes toward women. *Criminal Justice and Behavior, 26,* 338-356.

Christian, R. E., Frick, P. J., Hill, N. L., Tyler, L., & Frazer, D. R. (1997). Psychopathy and conduct problems in children II: Implications for subtyping children with conduct problems. *Journal of the American Academy of Child and Adolescent Psychiatry, 36,* 233-241.

Chu, J. A., & Dill, D. L. (1990). Dissociative symptoms in relation to childhood physical and sexual abuse. *American Journal of Psychiatry, 147,* 887-892.

Cooke, D. J., & Michie, C. (2001). Refining the construct of psychopathy: Towards a hierarchical model. *Psychological Assessment, 13,* 171-188.

Depue, R. A. (1996). A neurobiological framework for the structure of personality and emotion: Implications for personality disorders. In J. F. Clarkin, & M. F. Lenzenweger (Eds.), *Major theories of personality disorder* (pp. 347-390). New York: Guilford Press.

DiCenso, C. (1992). The adolescent sexual offender: Victim and perpetrator. In E. Viano (Ed.), *Critical issues in victimology: International perspectives* (pp. 190-200). New York: Springer.

Dodge, K. A., Bates, J. E., Pettit, G. S., & Valente, E. (1995). Social information-processing patterns partially mediate the effect of early physical abuse on later conduct problems. *Journal of Abnormal Psychology, 104,* 632-643.

Edelbrock, C., Rende, R., Plomin, R., & Thompson, L. A. (1995). A twin study of competence and problem behavior in childhood and early adolescence. *Journal of Child Psychology & Psychiatry, 36,* 775-785.

Efta-Breitbach, J., & Freeman, K.A. (2004). Recidivism and resilience in youth who sexually offend: An analysis of the literature. *Journal of Child Sexual Abuse, 13*(3/4), 257-280.

Ellis, L. (1993). Rape as a biosocial phenomenon. In G. C. Nagayama Hall, R. Hirschman, J. R. Graham, & M. S. Zaragoza (Eds.), *Sexual aggression: Issues in etiology and assessment, treatment and policy* (pp. 17-41). Washington, DC: Hemisphere Publishing Corp.

Fehrenbach, P. A., Smith, W., Monastersky, C., & Deisher, R. W. (1986). Adolescent sexual offenders: Offender and offense characteristics. *American Journal of Orthopsychiatry, 56,* 225-233.

Ford, M. E., & Linney, J. A. (1995). Comparative analysis of juvenile sexual offenders, violent homosexual offenders, and status offenders. *Journal of Interpersonal Violence, 10,* 56-70.

Frick, P. J. (1998). Callous-unemotional traits and conduct problems: A two-factor model of psychopathy in children. In D. J. Cooke, R. D. Hare, & A. Forth (Eds.), *Psychopathy: Theory, research, and implications for society* (pp. 47-51). Cordresch, The Netherlands: Kluwer Press.

Friedrich W. N., & Chaffin, M. (2000, November). *Developmental-systemic perspectives on children with sexual behavior problems.* Paper presented at the 19th Annual Meeting of the Association for the Treatment of Sexual Abusers, San Diego, CA.

Friedrich, W. N., & Luecke, W. J. (1988). Young school-age sexually aggressive children. *Professional Psychology Research and Practice, 19,* 155-164.

Gendreau, P., Little, T., & Goggin, C. (1996). A meta-analysis of the predictors of adult offender recidivism: What works! *Criminology, 34,* 575-607.

Goldman, S. J., D'Angelo, E. J., DeMaso, D. R., & Mezzacappa, E. (1992). Physical and sexual abuse histories among children with borderline personality disorder. *American Journal of Psychiatry, 149,* 1723-1726.

Grubin, D., & Prentky, R. (1993). Sexual psychopathy laws. *Criminal Behaviour and Mental Health, 3,* 381-392.

Hanson, R. K. (2000). *Risk assessment.* Beaverton, OR: Association for the Treatment of Sexual Abusers.

Hanson, R. K., & Bussière, M. T. (1998). Predicting relapse: A meta-analysis of sexual offender recidivism studies. *Journal of Consulting and Clinical Psychology, 66,* 348-362.

Hare, R. D., Harpur, T. J., Hakstian, A. R., Forth, A. E., Hart, S. D., & Newman, J. P. (1990). The revised psychopathy checklist: Reliability and factor structure. *Psychological Assessment, 2,* 338-341.

Harpur, T. J., Hakstian, A., & Hare, R. D. (1988). Factor structure of the Psychopathy Checklist. *Journal of Consulting and Clinical Psychology, 56,* 741-747.

Harpur, T. J., Hare, R. D., & Hakstian, A. (1989). Two-factor conceptualization of psychopathy: Construct validity and assessment implications. *Psychological Assessment: A Journal of Consulting and Clinical Psychology, 1,* 6-17.

Hsu, L. K. G., & Starzynski, J. (1990). Adolescent rapists and adolescent child sexual assaulters. *International Journal of Offender Therapy and Comparative Criminology, 34,* 23-30.

Hunter, J. A., & Figueredo, A. J. (1999). Factors associated with treatment compliance in a population of juvenile sexual offenders. *Sexual Abuse: A Journal of Research and Treatment, 11,* 49-67.

Johnson, G. M., & Knight, R. A. (2000). Developmental antecedents of sexual coercion in juvenile sex offenders. *Sexual Abuse: A Journal of Research and Treatment, 12,* 165-178.

Knight, R. A. (1999). Validation of a typology for rapists. *Journal of Interpersonal Violence, 14,* 297-323.

Knight, R. A. (in press). Comparisons between juvenile and adult sexual offenders on the Multidimensional Assessment of Sex and Aggression. In G. O'Reilly, W. L. Marshall, A. Carr, & R. Beckett (Eds.), *Handbook of clinical interventions with young people who sexually abuse.* London: Brunner-Routledge Ltd.

Knight, R. A., & Cerce, D. D. (1999). Validation and revision of the Multidimensional Assessment of Sex and Aggression. *Psychologica Belgica, 39 (2/3),* 187-213.

Knight, R. A., & Prentky, R. A. (1993). Exploring the characteristics for classifying juvenile sexual offenders. In H. E. Barbaree, W. L. Marshall, & S. M. Hudson (Eds.), *The juvenile sex offender* (pp. 45-83). New York: Guilford Press.

Knight, R. A., & Prentky, R. A. (In preparation). *The role of sexual motivation in sexually coercive behavior.* Manuscript submitted for publication.

Knight, R. A., & Sims-Knight, J. E. (1999, November). *Family and early behavioral antecedents of sexual coercion.* Paper presented at the 14th Annual Meeting of the Society for Research in Psychopathology, Montreal, Canada.

Knight, R. A., & Sims-Knight, J. E. (2003). Developmental antecedents of sexual coercion against women: Testing of alternative hypotheses with structural equation modeling. In R. A. Prentky, E. S. Janus, & M. C. Seto (Eds.), *Sexually coercive behavior: Understanding and management* (pp. 72-85). New York: Annals of New York Academy of Sciences, Vol. 989.

Krueger, R. F. (2000). Phenotypic, genetic, and nonshared environmental parallels in the structure of personality: A view from the Multidimensional Personality Questionnaire. *Journal of Personality and Social Psychology, 79,* 1057-1067.

Langton, C. M. (2002). *Contrasting approaches to risk assessment with adult male sexual offenders: An evaluation of recidivism prediction schemes and the utility of supplementary clinical information for enhancing predictive accuracy.* Doctoral dissertation, University of Toronto.

Livesley, W. J. (1998). The phenotypic and genotypic structure of psychopathic traits. In, D. J. Cooke, A. Forth, & R. D. Hare (Eds.), *Psychopathy: Theory, research, and implications for society* (pp. 69-79), Dordtrecht, The Netherlands: Kluwer Academic Publishers.

Loeber, R., & Stouthamer-Loeber, M. (1998). Development of juvenile aggression and violence. *American Psychologist, 53,* 242-259.

Longo, R. F. (1982). Sexual learning and experience among adolescent sexual offenders. *International Journal of Offender Therapy and Comparative Criminology, 26,* 235-241.

Lynam, D. R. (1998). Early identification of the fledgling psychopath: Locating the psychopathic child in the current nomenclature. *Journal of Abnormal Psychology, 107,* 566-575.

Malamuth, N. M. (1998). An evolutionary-based model integrating research on the characteristics of sexually coercive men. In J. Adair, K. Dion, & D. Belanger, D. (Eds.), *Advances in psychological science, Vol. 1: Social, personal, and developmental aspects.* (pp. 151-184). Hove, England: Psychology Press/Erlbaum.

Malamuth, N. M. (2003). Integrating psychopathy in a hierarchical-mediational confluence model. In R. A. Prentky, E. S. Janus, & M. C. Seto (Eds.), *Sexually coercive behavior: Understanding and management* (pp. 33-58). New York: Annals of New York Academy of Sciences, Vol. 989.

Malamuth, N. M., Heavey, C. L., & Linz, D. (1993). Predicting men's antisocial behavior against women: The interaction model of sexual aggression. In G. C. Nagayama Hall, R. Hirschman, J. R. Graham, & M. S. Zaragoza (Eds.), *Sexual aggression: Issues in etiology and assessment, treatment and policy* (pp. 63-97). Washington, DC: Hemisphere Publishing Corp.

Malamuth, N. M., Linz, D., Heavey, C. L., Barnes, G., & Acker, M. (1995). Using the confluence model of sexual aggression to predict men's conflict with women: A 10-year follow-up study. *Journal of Personality and Social Psychology, 69,* 353-369.

Mason, D. A., & Frick, P. J. (1994). The heritability of antisocial behavior: A meta-analysis of twin and adoption studies. *Journal of Psychopathology & Behavioral Assessment, 16*, 301-323.

McMahon, P., & Puett, R. (1999). Child sexual abuse as a public health issue: Recommendations of an expert panel. *Sexual Abuse: A Journal of Research and Treatment, 11*, 257-266.

Mercy, J. A., (1999). Having new eyes: Viewing child sexual abuse as a public health problem. *Sexual Abuse: A Journal of Research and Treatment, 11*, 317-322.

Miranda, A. O., & Corcoran, C. L. (2000). Comparison of perpetration characteristics between male juvenile and adult sexual offenders: Preliminary results. *Sexual Abuse: A Journal of Research and Treatment, 12*, 179-188.

Moffitt, T. E. (1993). Adolescence-limited and life-course-persistent antisocial behavior: A developmental taxonomy. *Psychology Review, 100*, 674-701.

Monroe, R. R. (1978). The medical model in psychopathy and dyscontrol syndromes. In W. R. Reid (Ed.), *The psychopath: A comprehensive study of antisocial disorder and behaviors* (pp. 190-208). New York: Brunner/Mazel.

Patrick, C. J., Bradley, M. M., & Lang, P. J. (1993). Emotion in the criminal psychopath: Startle reflex modulation. *Journal of Abnormal Psychology, 102*, 82-92.

Patrick, C. J., & Zempolich, K. A. (1998). Emotion and aggression in the psychopathic personality. *Aggression and Violent Behavior, 3*, 303-338.

Prentky, R. A. (1996). Community notification and constructive risk reduction. *Journal of Interpersonal Violence, 11*, 295-298.

Prentky, R. A., Harris, B., Frizzel, K., & Righthand, S. (2000). An actuarial procedure for assessing risk with juvenile sex offenders. *Sexual Abuse: A Journal of Research and Treatment, 12*, 71-93.

Prentky, R. A., Knight, R. A., Lee, A. F. S., & Cerce, D. D. (1995). Predictive validity of lifestyle impulsivity for rapists. *Criminal Justice and Behavior, 22*, 106-128.

Quinsey, V. L., Harris, G. T., Rice, M. E., & Cormier, C.A. (1998). *Violent offenders: Appraising and managing risk.* Washington, DC: American Psychological Association.

Raine, A. (1993). *The psychopathology of crime: Criminal behavior as a clinical disorder.* San Diego, CA: Academic Press, Inc.

Rasmussen, L.A. (2004). Differentiating youth who sexually abuse: Applying a multidimensional framework when assessing and treating subtypes. *Journal of Child Sexual Abuse, 13*(3/4), pp. 57-82.

Richardson, G., Kelly, T.P., Bhate, S.R., & Graham, F. (1997). Group differences in abuser and abuse characteristics in a British sample of sexually abusive adolescents. *Sexual Abuse: A Journal of Research and Treatment, 9*, 239-257.

Righthand, S., & Welch, C. (2001). *Juveniles who have sexually offended: A review of the professional literature.* Washington, DC: Office of Juvenile Justice and Delinquency Prevention.

Righthand, S., & Welch, C. (2004). Characteristics of youth who sexually offend. *Journal of Child Sexual Abuse, 13*(3/4), pp. 15-32.

Roberts, C. F., Doren, D. M., & Thorton, D. (2002). Dimensions associated with assessments of sex offender recidivism risk. *Criminal Justice and Behavior, 29*, 569-589.

Robins, L. N., & Radcliff, K. S. (1978-1979). Risk factors in the continuation of childhood antisocial behavior into adulthood. *International Journal of Mental Health, 7*, 96-116.

Rogers, C. M., & Terry, T. (1984). Clinical interventions with boy victims of sexual abuse. In I. Stuart, & J. Geer (Eds.), *Victims of sexual aggression* (pp. 91-104). New York: Van Nostrand Reinhold.

Ryan, G., Lane, S., Davis, J., & Isaac, C. (1987). Juvenile sex offenders: Development and correction. *Child Abuse & Neglect, 11*, 385-395.

Sandberg, D. A., & Lynn, S. J. (1992). Dissociative experiences, psychopathology and adjustment, and childhood and adolescent maltreatment in female college students. *Journal of Abnormal Psychology, 101*, 391-398.

Saunders, E., Awad, G. A., & White, G. (1986). Male adolescent sexual offenders: The offender and the offense. *Canadian Journal of Psychology, 31*, 542-548.

Schram, D. D., Malloy, C. D., & Rowe, W. E. (1992, July). Juvenile sex offenders: A follow-up study of reoffense behavior. *Interchange*, 1-3.

Seghorn, T. K., Prentky, R. A., & Boucher, R. J. (1987). Childhood sexual abuse in the lives of sexually aggressive offenders. *Journal of American Academy of Child and Adolescent Psychiatry, 26*, 262-267.

Weinrott, M. R. (1996). *Juvenile sexual aggression: A critical review.* Boulder, CO: University of Colorado, Institute for Behavioral Sciences, Center for the Study and Prevention of Violence.

Widom, C. S. (1996). Childhood sexual abuse and its criminal consequences. *Society, 33*, 47-53.

Williams, L. M. (1995). *Juvenile and adult offending behavior and other outcomes in a cohort of sexually abused boys: Twenty years later.* Philadelphia: Joseph J. Peters Institute.

Worling, J. R., & Curwen, T. (2000). Adolescent sexual offender recidivism: Success of Specialized treatment and implications for risk prediction. *Child Abuse and Neglect, 24*, 965-982.

Wurtele, S. K., (1999). Comprehensiveness and collaboration: Key ingredients of an effective public health approach to preventing child sexual abuse. *Sexual Abuse: A Journal of Research and Treatment, 11*, 323-325.

ASSESSING SEXUALLY
ABUSIVE YOUTH

Differentiating Youth Who Sexually Abuse: Applying a Multidimensional Framework When Assessing and Treating Subtypes

Lucinda A. Rasmussen

SUMMARY. Recent empirical research has shown that children with sexual behavior problems and adolescents who offend sexually are diverse populations consisting of several subtypes (Hall, Mathews, & Pearce, 2002; Pithers, Gray, Busconi, & Houchens, 1998; Worling, 2001). This article reviews the descriptive and empirical research related

Address correspondence to: Lucinda A. Rasmussen, PhD, Associate Professor, San Diego State University School of Social Work, 5500 Campanile Drive, San Diego, CA 92182-4119 (E-mail: rasmuss2@mail.sdsu.edu).

The author acknowledges Jan Ellen Burton, PhD, and Barbara J. Christopherson, LCSW, for their work in creating the Trauma Outcome Process model and Arthur H. Brown III, PhD, Julie Bradshaw, LCSW, and Steven C. Huke, MS, for contributing to later modifications of the model.

[Haworth co-indexing entry note]: "Differentiating Youth Who Sexually Abuse: Applying a Multidimensional Framework When Assessing and Treating Subtypes." Rasmussen, Lucinda A. Co-published simultaneously in *Journal of Child Sexual Abuse* (The Haworth Maltreatment and Trauma Press, an imprint of The Haworth Press, Inc.) Vol. 13, No. 3/4, 2004, pp. 57-82; and: *Identifying and Treating Youth Who Sexually Offend: Current Approaches, Techniques, and Research* (ed: Robert Geffner et al.) The Haworth Maltreatment and Trauma Press, an imprint of The Haworth Press, Inc., 2004, pp. 57-82. Single or multiple copies of this article are available for a fee from The Haworth Document Delivery Service [1-800-HAWORTH, 9:00 a.m. - 5:00 p.m. (EST). E-mail address: docdelivery@haworthpress.com].

to identifying subtypes of children with sexual behavior problems and adolescents who offend sexually. Examples of clinically and empirically derived typologies are presented. The author discusses how data from the empirically derived typologies can be incorporated within a multidimensional assessment framework based on the Trauma Outcome Process model (Burton, Rasmussen, Bradshaw, Christopherson, & Huke, 1998; Rasmussen, Burton, & Christopherson, 1992; Rasmussen, 1999, 2001, 2002). The application of this framework in assessing and treating children with sexual behavior problems and adolescents who offend sexually is described. *[Article copies available for a fee from The Haworth Document Delivery Service: 1-800-HAWORTH. E-mail address: <docdelivery@haworthpress.com> Website: <http://www.HaworthPress.com> © 2004 by The Haworth Press, Inc. All rights reserved.]*

KEYWORDS. Trauma Outcome Process, sexualized children, children who molest, abuse-reactive children, children with sexual behavior problems, adolescent sexual offender, juvenile sexual offender, typology

Adolescents and children are responsible for nearly half (43%) of the sexual offenses against children ages 6 and younger in the United States (National Center for Juvenile Justice, 1999). It is estimated that juveniles under the age of 18 sexually abuse 70,000 boys and 110,000 girls each year (Ryan & Lane, 1997). Given that sexual offenses perpetrated by adolescents and children are often unreported, the number of victims of these youth may actually be much higher. Of particular concern are reports that children under 12 are increasingly being identified as abusing other children sexually. Juvenile court data has indicated that the arrest rate for sexual offenses committed by children ages 12 and younger increased by 125% between 1980 and 1995 (Butts & Snyder, 1997). Although it is unknown whether these data generalize across all states, it is evident that many children and adolescents abuse other children sexually.

Clinicians, child protective services workers, and juvenile justice professionals need to identify and assess children and adolescents who engage in sexually abusive behavior and provide interventions tailored to their needs. One of the roadblocks to the accurate assessment and appropriate treatment of these youth is that evidence-based treatment models are not readily available. Historically, interventions with children and adolescents who offend sexually were justified as necessary to prevent them from later becoming adult sexual offenders. This assumption was based on retrospective data of samples of adult sexual offenders indicating that about 50% began sexually offending prior to adolescence (Abel, Mittelman, & Becker, 1985; Groth, Longo, & McFadin, 1982). The possibility that children and adolescents who displayed sexually abusive behavior would continue offending into adulthood motivated many practitioners to adapt treatment models used with adult sexual offenders.

A lack of empirically proven models reflects the current state of research literature on youth who offend sexually. Research on adolescents suffers from several methodological limitations (e.g., a lack of treatment outcome studies, few empirically developed typologies, and no actuarial risk assessment) (Becker, 1998; Chaffin & Bonner, 1998; Chaffin, Letourneau, & Silovsky, 2002). Research on children under 12 is even more limited, with only two outcome studies (Bonner, Walker, & Berliner, 1999; Pithers et al., 1998). Without clear, empirically based knowledge about youth who offend sexually, "the field is still using treatment models and assumptions borrowed and adapted from programs developed for incarcerated pedophiles" (Chaffin & Bonner, 1998, p. 314).

These adult-based treatment models may be too confrontational for many youth and can result in unintended and punitive consequences (e.g., excessively restrictive placements, inappropriate application of adult sexual offender registration laws to children and adolescents) (Chaffin & Bonner, 1998; Johnson, 2000). Furthermore, when clinicians rely on treatment models originally established for adult sexual offenders, they may miss attending to the crucial developmental differences between youth who molest children and adult sex offenders. This may exacerbate the problems of these youth, putting them at risk for long-term negative outcomes (Chaffin et al., 2002).

Over the past 25 years, since the first treatment programs were established for children and adolescents who offend sexually, child abuse investigators, clinicians, and researchers have gradually come to recognize a number of important truths. First, adolescents and children do engage in problematic and abusive sexual behaviors. Next, these behaviors exist on a continuum from developmentally expected to sexually abusive (Hall, Mathews, & Pearce, 1998, 2002; Johnson, 1993; Johnson & Feldmeth, 1993). Third, developmentally sensitive interventions are needed. Lastly, sexually abusive youth are a heterogeneous group, and using a one-size-fits-all approach to treatment is therefore inappropriate (Becker, 1998; Chaffin et al., 2002; Veneziano & Veneziano, 2002).

Practitioners need to conduct comprehensive, accurate, and individualized assessments that take into account the developmental distinction between youths and adults, as well as the variations among sexually abusive youth (e.g., child versus adolescent) (Bonner, Marx, Thompson, & Michaelson,

1998; Johnson, 2000; Veneziano & Veneziano, 2002). Differentiating these youth according to their various subtypes can help clinicians to: (a) identify the internal and external risk factors of children and adolescents who engage in sexually abusive behavior, (b) formulate individualized treatment goals, (c) select developmentally appropriate interventions to meet the specific treatment needs of each sexually abusive youth, (d) support the parents of these youth in providing appropriate caregiving and adequate supervision, and (e) implement techniques to teach these youth appropriate social and coping skills and help restore them to a course of normative development (Chaffin et al., 2002; Friedrich, 2002).

The purpose of this article is to review the descriptive literature and recent empirical studies related to defining subtypes of youth who sexually offend. Criteria for defining and describing sexually abusive behavior by children and adolescents are presented. Examples of clinically and empirically derived classification systems (typologies) are reviewed. The Trauma Outcome Process model (Burton et al., 1998; Rasmussen, 1999, 2001; Rasmussen et al., 1992) is then presented. This model provides a multidimensional assessment framework for differentiating subtypes of youth who offend sexually and tailoring interventions to address the needs of different subtypes. It combines practice knowledge of important individual, family, and environmental risk factors with variables shown by recent empirical research to be important in differentiating subtypes, and thus provides a theoretical framework to help guide future research.

DEFINITIONS AND TERMINOLOGY

According to Hall and associates (2002), a definition of children's sexual behavior problems "should not be based on the sexual behavior alone, but should include its context" (p. 293). The definition to be used in this article was based on contextual factors described by Hall, Mathews, Pearce, Sarlo-McGarvey, and Gavin (1996). Problematic or abusive sexual behavior in children under age 12: (a) occurs at a greater frequency or at a much earlier age than would be developmentally expected, (b) interferes with their development, (c) can involve coercion, intimidation, or force, (d) is associated with emotional distress for the children involved, and (e) reoccurs secretly even after caregiver intervention (Silovsky & Niec, 2002).

Clinicians, juvenile justice practitioners, and researchers must consider the potential negative impact of the labels they assign to children and youth who offend sexually. Becker (1998) pointed out, "Labeling young children as child rapists or pedophiles has the potential to stigmatize youth and to isolate them further from peers, adults, and potential to stigmatize youth and to isolate them from potential sources of social and psychological support" (p. 317). Johnson (2000) concurred that mislabeling children as "offenders" can result in drastic consequences (e.g., removal from their homes, not being allowed to be alone with siblings, playmates, or classmates, placement in therapy as an "offender"). Neutral terms used in the literature to describe problematic sexualized behavior include: abuse-reactive, sexually reactive, sexually aggressive, sexually abusive, sexualized children, and children who molest. The term with the widest usage currently is "children with sexual behavior problems" (CSBPs) (Araji, 1997; Bonner et al., 1999; Chaffin & Bonner, 1998; Friedrich, 2002; Hall et al., 2002; Pithers et al., 1998). This term describes children's sexual behavior while avoiding negative labels associated with the legal system (e.g., "perpetrator" or "offender").

CSBP is not an ideal term, however, as it does not distinguish different subtypes of children who display sexualized behaviors. For example, the researchers in two recent outcome studies of children who engaged in sexualized behaviors described *all* the children in their samples as CSBPs (Bonner et al., 1999; Pithers et al., 1998). This was confusing, as each sample was comprised of a heterogeneous group of children, and some children's sexual behaviors were clearly more intrusive or coercive than others (e.g., engaging in oral or anal sex as compared to brief fondling or masturbation, using threats, or force). No attempt was made in either study to discriminate children with multiple victims or incidents of sexualized behavior from children who had one victim or only a few reported incidents. Johnson (2000) cautioned that using the term "children with sexual behavior problems" in this manner might contribute to misdiagnosis and "lead people to see all children with problematic sexual behaviors as offenders" (p. 37).

The term CSBPs can be appropriately used as an umbrella term describing the population of children who engage in sexualized behaviors (Burton et al., 1998). When there is a need to differentiate subtypes, other descriptive terms should be used. "Children who molest" or "sexually abusive children" are appropriate terms when children's sexualized behaviors present harm to others (e.g., threats), are intrusive (e.g., oral, anal, or vaginal penetration), or involve multiple incidents or victims. "Sexualized children" or "children with problematic sexual behaviors" refers to children whose behaviors present harm to self, not others.

Definitions of adolescent sexually abusive behavior typically rely on legal definitions since "child abuse by a teenager is usually defined as a crime by law" (Chaffin et al., 2002, p. 213). These youth have traditionally been referred to in the literature as "adolescent sexual offenders" or "juvenile sexual offenders." On the other hand, some researchers have been concerned about negative labeling and have cautioned against using the term "offender" when referring to adolescents as well as children (Bonner, 1997, as cited in Righthand & Welch, 2001). The author concurs and will use similar terminology in this article to describe adolescents and children. Descriptive terms (e.g., "adolescents who offend sexually" or "adolescents who sexually abuse") will be used in lieu of the terms adolescent or juvenile sexual offender.

According to Ryan (1997), sexually abusive behavior by adolescents is defined according to the degree of equality, consent, and coercion existing in the relationship between the adolescent and others involved in the sexual interaction. Ryan's concept of equality refers to "differentials of physical, cognitive, and emotional development, passivity and assertiveness, power and control, and authority" (p. 3). Consent refers to: (a) the understanding that each participant has of the proposed sexual behavior, (b) knowledge of the societal standards related to the behavior, (c) awareness of potential consequences, (d) mutual respect for agreements or disagreements related to the behavior, (e) voluntary participation in the behavior, and (f) being mentally competent (pp. 4-5). Coercion refers to "the pressures that deny the victim free choice" including power and size differential, bribery, threats, and overt violence (p. 5). Ryan's definitional criteria can assist clinicians in assessing the degree of culpability that an adolescent has for a given sexual interaction and helping youth to accept responsibility for their behavior.

TYPOLOGIES OF CHILDREN
WITH SEXUAL BEHAVIOR PROBLEMS

Typologies are classification systems that attempt to differentiate subtypes of a specified population, based on definitional criteria. Several practitioners have developed typologies describing subtypes of children and adolescents who engage in sexualized and sexually abusive behaviors. Many of these typologies were formulated intuitively through clinical practice experience; others are empirically derived. This article will first review clinical and empirical typologies developed for CSBPs, and will then look at similar efforts to develop typologies of adolescents who offend sexually.

Clinically Derived Typologies of CSBPs

Perhaps the best known of the clinically derived typologies developed for CSBPs is the "Continuum of Sexual Behaviors in Children" formulated by Johnson (Johnson, 1993, 1999, 2000; Johnson & Feldmeth, 1993). This typology is based on clinical observations obtained from "extensive evaluations of children and their families who were referred as a result of the child's sexual behaviors" (Johnson & Feldmeth, 1993, p. 41). It focuses on defining treatment needs, identifying systems interventions, and making certain that "children with less serious sexual behaviors are not misidentified as children who molest" (Johnson, 2000, p. 36). The Continuum consists of four categories that differentiate children along several dimensions based on contextual factors: (a) type of sexual behaviors, (b) intensity of sexual behaviors, (c) sexual arousal, (d) motivation, (e) affect regarding sexuality, (f) response to discovery, (g) planning, (h) coercion, (i) relationship to others involved in sexual behaviors, (j) age difference, (k) interpersonal relationship characteristics, (l) family and environment, (m) possible etiological risk factors, and (n) type of treatment needed.

The first category in Johnson's Continuum, "children who engage in natural and healthy sexual behaviors," consists of children who are motivated by curiosity to engage in sexual behavior as they attempt to explore their own bodies or gather information about gender differences. The children are of "*similar age, size, and developmental level* and participate on a *voluntary* basis" (Johnson, 1999, p. 6). The sexual content of children's play usually depends upon their prior exposure to sexuality (Gil, 1993). Children who have not had excessive sexual exposure are likely to limit any sexualized behavior in their play to developmentally expected activities of undressing, looking, and touching. Children in this category should not be referred to as CSBPs because their behaviors are by definition appropriate for their age and development.

Sexually reactive children, the second category in Johnson's Continuum of Sexual Behaviors in Children, consists of children who do not deliberately intend to hurt others, but engage in sexualized behavior "in response to environmental cues that are overly stimulating or reminiscent of previous abuse or to feelings that reawaken other traumatic or painful memories" (Johnson, 2000, p. 36). Confusing feelings related to their exposure to explicit sexuality often overwhelm these children. Their sexualized behaviors may be either self-focused or interpersonally focused, and may be a way of attempting to reduce their anxiety and cope with their confusion. Some may limit their behavior to self-stimulation (e.g., masturbation, inserting objects in their vagina or rectum). When they do involve other children in their sexually oriented activities, they tend to seek out children whose age is fairly close to their own, and they do not threaten or coerce them into participating in sexualized behavior (Johnson, 1993).

In contrast, the third category in Johnson's Continuum consists of children who "engage in extensive, mutual sexual behaviors." These children lack close, supportive relationships with adults and "use their sexual behaviors to connect with other children" (Johnson, 2000, p. 36). Like sexually reactive children, they may engage in sexual behaviors as a way to cope with confusing feelings, but their feelings also include "abandonment, hurt, sadness, anxiety, and often despair" (p. 36). Most of these children have not resolved their feelings about being sexually and emotionally abused (for an in-depth discussion on the connection between abuse and sexually acting out, see Knight & Sims-Knight, this issue; Righthand & Welch, this issue). Johnson hypothesized that these children were previously "sexually reactive children" who tried to cope with their anxiety/confusion about sexuality by seeking an emotional connection with other similarly lonely children.

The most severe category in Johnson's Continuum, "children who molest," refers to children who have "coercive sexual behaviors far beyond developmentally appropriate childhood exploration" (Johnson & Feldmeth, 1993, p. 51). The sexual behaviors of these children are pervasive, increase over time, and span the full spectrum of sexual behaviors including "oral copulation, vaginal intercourse, anal intercourse, or forcibly penetrating the vagina or anus of another child with fingers, sticks, or other objects" (Johnson, 1993, p. 438). Children who molest may use bribery, trickery, manipulation, or other kinds of emotional and physical coercion to get other children to participate in sexual behaviors. Johnson (2000) emphasized, "sexuality and aggression are closely linked in the thoughts and actions of these children" (p. 36).

Empirically Derived Typologies of CSBPs

Recent randomized clinical trials sponsored by the National Center on Child Abuse and Neglect (NCCAN) (Bonner et al., 1999; Pithers et al., 1998), and a retrospective study (Hall et al., 2002) represent the first attempts to construct typologies of CSBPs based on empirical data. These three studies are reviewed below.

Bonner et al. (1999). These researchers studied 201 children ages 6-12 (126 males and 75 females) referred from mental health agencies, child protective services/foster care, schools, and other sources. The children showed a full spectrum of sexualized behaviors from masturbation to fondling to prolonged sexual contact (e.g., oral sex or vaginal/anal penetration). Bonner et al., conducted a cluster analysis, using data from the Child Sexual Behavior Inventory (CSBI)-Version 2 (Friedrich, Beilke, & Purcell, 1989), which they had used to assess the children's sexualized behaviors. However, since the CSBI-2 did not contain items related to aggressive sexual behavior, the researchers were not able to define any subgroups with clinical validity. Bonner et al. then used a logical analysis of the children's referral sexualized behavior to develop a clinically derived typology of three subgroups: (a) sexually inappropriate, (b) sexually intrusive, and (c) sexually aggressive. Chi-square analysis showed that those in the sexually aggressive subgroup were significantly more likely to be older, male, and aggressive.

Bonner et al. (1999) evaluated treatment outcomes by randomly assigning 110 of the original 201 children in the sample to one of two therapy approaches: (a) cognitive-behavioral (i.e., teaching "sexual behavior rules") or (b) dynamic play therapy (employing toys, puppets, art materials, sand tray, stories, and metaphors). There was no attempt to compare these children according to the researchers' clinically derived typology. Results of the 69 children who completed at least 9 out of 12 weeks of treatment were equivalent. Children in both treatment conditions showed significant reductions in problematic behaviors (as assessed by the CSBI: Version 2 [Friedrich et al., 1989] and the Child Behavior Checklist [Achenbach, 1991]. Structured interviews at 1 and 2 years post treatment showed that children in both treatments had a significant reduction of reported sexual behavior problems (Bonner et al., 1999).

Pithers et al. (1998). In contrast to the difficulty experienced by Bonner et al. (1999) in developing a typology, the researchers in the other NCCAN sponsored study were successful in constructing an empirically derived typology based on a comprehensive set of demographic, family, social, and abuse history characteristics. The Pithers et al. sample consisted of 127 6- to 12-year-old children (83 boys and 44 girls) referred from the child protective services and mental health systems. Their hierarchical cluster analysis included demographic variables and data compiled from a comprehensive battery of assessment measures completed by the children and their parents at intake (e.g., Child Behavior Checklist [parent, teacher, and youth self-report versions; Achenbach, 1991]; Child Sexual Behavior Inventory-Third Edition [Friedrich, 1995; Friedrich et al., 1992]; Eyberg Child Behavior Inventory [Eyberg & Ross, 1978]; Children's Action Tendency Scale [Deluty, 1979]; State-Trait Anxiety Inventory for Children [Spielberger, 1973]; Parenting Stress Index [Abidin, 1990]). The cluster analysis was successful in identifying five subtypes of children, fitting three hypothesized profiles: (a) conduct disordered, (b) highly maltreated and traumatized, and (c) non-disordered.

There was considerable overlap across the subtypes in the Pithers et al. (1998) typology, verifying that it is difficult to clearly differentiate subtypes among the diverse population of children who act out sexually (Chaffin et al., 2002). The first profile, conduct disordered children, consisted of two subtypes: (a) sexually aggressive and (b) rule breakers. These subtypes were comprised of older children (mean age = 9.9 [sexually aggressive] and 9.2 [rule breaker]), who demonstrated significant sexually aggressive behaviors. The sexually aggressive subtype was comprised almost entirely of males (94%), while females made up 42% of the rule breaker subtype. Psychiatric diagnoses for both the sexually aggressive and rule breaker subtypes included Conduct Disorder and Attention Deficit Disorder (ADD). The rule breaker subtype showed severe pathology, with higher levels of general behavior problems, emotional problems, parental stress, and many diagnoses of Oppositional Defiant Disorder (ODD).

The second profile consisted of children who had an extensive history of maltreatment and included two subtypes: (a) highly traumatized and (b) abuse reactive. These subtypes were young children (mean age = 7.8 [highly traumatized] and 8.4 [abuse reactive]), who had extensive histories of maltreatment (Pithers et al., 1998). Two-thirds of the highly traumatized children were male, compared to 96% of the abuse reactive children. Almost all of the highly traumatized children (91%) were diagnosed with Post-Traumatic Stress Disorder (PTSD), compared to only 5% of the abuse-reactive children. On the other hand, 96% of the abuse reactive children were diagnosed with ODD, compared to 18% of the highly traumatized.

The third profile, the non-symptomatic subtype, consisted of children who scored in the non-clinical range on most intake measures. They were young (mean age = 8.6), with more females than males. These children did not have an extensive history of child maltreatment and rarely used coercion in their sexualized behaviors. They scored in the normal range on most measures and were the least likely of all the types to have a history of child maltreatment. Nonetheless, these children appeared to have been exposed to a sexualized environment, with more individuals in their extended families that had perpetrated sexually abusive behaviors than in the families of children in other subtypes (Pithers et al., 1998).

Pithers et al. (1998) completed additional statistical analyses comparing the treatment outcomes of the five subtypes of children to two randomly assigned treatment approaches: (a) a cognitive-behavioral relapse prevention model (adapted from an approach used with adult and adolescent sexual abusers) or (b) expressive play therapy (similar to the dynamic play therapy used by Bonner et al. [1999]). The 127 children in the sample were reassessed on all intake measures (see list above) after 16 weeks of a 32-week course of treatment. Results showed that a greater percentage of the non-symptomatic, highly traumatized, and abuse reactive children attained "clinically significant reductions in their problematic sexual behaviors" (Pithers et al., p. 399) after receiving the relapse prevention therapy. However, only the highly traumatized subtype showed statistically significant results ($p < .005$). Half of the sexually aggressive subtype had significant reductions in sexualized behavior after receiving expressive therapy, while the remaining half who received expressive therapy showed increased sexual behavior problems. The rule breaker subtype did equally well with either treatment approach.

Hall et al. (1998, 2002). The third study to focus on empirically developing subtypes of CSBPs was a retrospective study of the case records of 100 sexually abused children ages 4 to 7. Using contextual factors advocated by Johnson (1993) to identify children's sexual behavior problems, Hall and colleagues (1998) developed a clinically derived typology consisting of three categories: (a) developmentally expected, (b) sexualized self-focused (without any interpersonal contact), and (c) interpersonally focused (engaging in problematic sexual contact/touch).

In a follow-up study, Hall and colleagues (2002) employed cluster analysis to develop an ecologically based typology, using the three clinically derived subgroups from their previous study. The interpersonally focused subgroup was identified as the "research" group, while the other two subgroups comprised the comparison group. A hierarchical cluster analysis was conducted on the research group. To address the limitations of the Pithers et al. (1998) empirical typology, Hall et al. included variables in their cluster analysis relating to child development, family functioning, and care-giving environments, which they drew from their retrospective review of the children's case records (i.e., child maltreatment history, child sexual abuse experience, child behavior, parenting/parent-child relationship, family functioning, family sexual environment, and quality and stability of housing/household). Three stable clusters of CSBPs emerged from the cluster analysis: (a) interpersonal, unplanned, (b) interpersonal, planned (non-coercive), and (c) interpersonal, planned (coercive).

Hall et al. (2002) completed subsequent statistical analyses comparing all five sexual behavior profiles (i.e., the developmentally expected and developmentally problematic subgroups and the three interpersonal sexual behavior clusters). The five sexual behavior profiles were best differentiated by: (a) elements of the child's sexual abuse experience, (b) opportunities to learn/practice problematic sexual behavior, and (c) family variables (i.e., sexual attitudes and interaction styles, violence and criminality, multiple maltreatment histories, and maintenance of appropriate parent-child roles).

Children in the most severe category–interpersonal, planned (coercive)–differed from the other four categories by their degree of planning, coercion and extensive adult-type sexual behavior. These children showed more sexual preoccupation and tended to persist in their sexualized behaviors despite limit setting. They were more likely to have experienced pain and sexual arousal during their own sexual abuse, and to have been abused "within a multi-perpetrator, multi-victim context" in which they were coerced by a perpetrator to commit sexually abusive acts on another child (p. 308). Their own sexual abuse was characterized by the use of sadistic threats by the perpetrator. These children were also more likely to come from families where (a) parental supervision was poor, (b) roles between parents and children were frequently reversed, (c) attitudes in the home supported pairing sex with violence, and

(d) parents resisted counseling due to minimization and denial (for additional discussion of family characteristics of sexually abusive youth, see Righthand & Welch, this issue).

TYPOLOGIES OF ADOLESCENTS WHO OFFEND SEXUALLY

Several researchers have made efforts to develop typologies of adolescents who offend sexually. The following section will review an example of a clinically derived typology for adolescents and will present several of the preliminary efforts to establish empirically derived typologies.

Clinically Derived Typology of Adolescents Who Offend Sexually

Based on their clinical work with adolescents who were referred to the Program for Healthy Sexual Expression (PHASE program) in Minnesota, O'Brien and Bera (1986) developed the first clinically derived typology of adolescents who offend sexually. This personality based typology included several dimensions: (a) motivation for sexually abusive behavior, (b) personality characteristics, (c) family functioning, (d) victim age, (e) delinquency, and (f) sexual history. It consisted of seven types of youth who offend sexually: (a) "Naïve Experimenter," (b) "Undersocialized Child Exploiter," (c) "PseudoSocialized Child Exploiter," (d) "Sexual Aggressive," (e) "Sexual Compulsive," (f) "Disturbed Impulsive," and (g) "Group Influenced." The O'Brien and Bera typology gives useful descriptions of different profiles of adolescents who offend and their families and appears to have face validity (Veneziano & Veneziano, 2002; Weinrott, 1996). However, since it was never empirically validated, the reliability and validity of its categories has not been established.

Empirically Derived Typologies of Adolescents Who Offend Sexually

The typologies developed to date of adolescents who offend sexually "have largely been intuitively derived and have not been adequately empirically validated" (Veneziano & Veneziano, 2002, p. 252). Some typologies focus on offense factors, others on personality.

Sibling incest typology. O'Brien (1991) hypothesized that his sample of 170 adolescents who abused their siblings would show significant differences from (a) adolescents who offended against children other than siblings, (b) adolescents who sexually abused peers or adults, and (c) those whose victims included a mix of siblings, extra-familial children, and/or peers and adults. O'Brien's results confirmed his hypotheses; the adolescents who abused siblings (a) committed the greatest number of abusive acts, (b) had the longest duration of offending, (c) were more likely to vaginally or anally penetrate their victims, and (d) were more likely to have multiple victims. O'Brien's study suggested that victim availability is an important factor in influencing the severity of the sexual offense history of an adolescent who is sexually abusive.

Typologies based on type of offense and victim age. Three studies examined type of offense and victim age as criteria for differentiating adolescents who offend sexually. Graves, Openshaw, Ascione, and Erickson (1996) conducted a meta-analysis of 140 samples involving 16,000 adolescents who offended sexually. Their results identified three types of youth based on type of offense and victim age: (a) pedophilic, (b) sexual assault, and (c) undifferentiated. Pedophilic youth lacked social skills and molested primarily females at least 3 years younger than themselves. Sexual assault youth sexually abused peers or older females. Undifferentiated youth had a variety of offenses and showed no clear pattern in choice of victim.

Prentky, Harris, Frizzell, and Righthand (2000) developed a rationally derived typology that they are using to help develop and validate an actuarial risk assessment for juveniles who offend sexually (Juvenile Sex Offender Assessment Protocol [JSOAP]; for further details concerning the JSOAP, see Prescott, this issue). Their typology consisted of six categories based on type of offense. "Child Molesters" (69% of their sample of 96 youth) molested children ages 11 and younger and at least 5 years younger than themselves. "Rapists" (12.5%) sexually abused victims that were 12 years old or older and less than 5 years younger than themselves. "Sexually Reactive Children" (6.25%) were 11 years old or younger and abused victims that were also younger than 11 years old. "Fondlers" (3%) abused the same age range as Rapists, but their sexual acts were limited to fondling or frottage. "Paraphiliac Offender" (3%) had no physical contact with their victims. The "Unclassifiable" category included 6.25% of the sample. More than half of the sample sexually abused family members, 41% abused acquaintances, and 4% abused strangers.

Hunter, Figueredo, Malamuth, and Becker (2003) made initial efforts toward developing an empirically based typology by comparing 157 adolescent males with a hands-on offense against a male or female child under 12 with 25 adolescent males with a hands-on offense against a male or female 12 years of age or older. They found that adolescents who offended against prepubescent children had "greater deficits in psychosocial functioning, used less aggression in their sexual offending, and were more likely to offend against relatives" (p. 27). Adolescents who offended against children were also found to have a higher incidence of depression. Depressed youth were found to have a higher incidence of experiencing physical abuse and exposure to domestic violence (see Righthand & Welch, this issue). The researchers indicated that they plan to develop an empirically based typology in a subsequent study that will further compare the differences seen in adolescents who sexually offend, as related to age of victim.

Typology based on prior offense history. Butler and Seto (2002) compared 32 adolescents who had committed sex offenses with 48 adolescents who had committed aggressive and non-aggressive criminal offenses, and 34 offenders who had committed non-aggressive criminal offenses. They divided the adolescents who had committed sex offenses into two groups: (a) 22 who had committed sex offenses only, and (b) 10 who had committed other delinquent offenses in addition to the sex offenses. They found that the youth who committed sex offenses had less risk for future delinquency than the two groups of youth who committed other delinquent offenses. They also found that the youth who committed only sex offenses had significantly fewer behavioral problems in childhood, better social adjustment, more prosocial attitudes, and lower risk for delinquency than the youth in the other two groups (i.e., youth who committed other delinquent offenses and youth who committed sex offenses plus other delinquent offenses). The researchers suggested that prior offense history is an important variable to consider when developing an empirical typology of adolescents who offend sexually and assigning them to appropriate interventions (Butler & Seto, 2002).

Personality-based typology. Using cluster analysis of factor-derived scores from the California Personality Inventory, Worling (2001) identified four personality-based subgroups in his sample of 112 adolescent males who offended sexually and specified the treatment needs of each group. There were two "healthier" subgroups (Overcontrolled/Reserved and Confident/Aggressive) and two groups that were more "unhealthy" (Antisocial/Impulsive and Unusual/Isolated). The "unhealthy" subgroups were significantly more likely to have parents who were separated or divorced and were significantly more likely to be charged with a subsequent violent (sexual or nonsexual) or nonviolent offense. The Antisocial/Impulsive and Confident/Aggressive were significantly more likely to be living in a residential setting than the other two subgroups. The Antisocial/Impulsive were the most likely of the subgroups to have been physically abused. This typology holds promise in helping clinicians to identify different etiological factors that influence adolescents who sexually offend and to select and implement individualized interventions that address these factors (for further discussion on personality traits and etiology, see Knight & Sims-Knight, this issue).

COMPARING TYPOLOGIES

The above review affirms that typologies are helpful in identifying the characteristics of CSBPs and adolescents who offend sexually, understanding the risk factors that motivate their behaviors, and guiding the selection of treatment goals and appropriate interventions. The clinically and empirically derived typologies reviewed provide evidence that CSBPs and adolescents who offend sexually are heterogeneous groups who differ in (a) their motivation for engaging in sexualized or sexually abusive behavior, (b) the severity of their sexualized or sexually abusive behavior, (c) their offense patterns and selection of victims, (d) their psychological and personality characteristics, (e) the dynamics of their families and (f) the degree of environmental support that they and their families receive.

Typologies that offer a comprehensive assessment of offense behaviors, contextual factors in the relationship between the children or adolescent involved in a referred sexualized or sexually abusive behavior, and etiological risk factors are the most useful to practitioners. These typologies include two clinically derived typologies: (a) Johnson's clinically derived Continuum of Sexual Behaviors in Children (Johnson, 1993, 1999, 2000; Johnson & Feldmeth, 1993) and (b) O'Brien and Bera's (1986) personality-based typology of adolescents, and two empirically derived typologies: (a) Hall et al.'s (2002) typology of CSBPs and (b) Worling's (2001) personality based typology of adolescents. The empirically derived typology developed by Pithers et al. (1998), while comprehensive in identifying offense characteristics, as well as many of the psychological and family history risk factors, did not consider many of the contextual factors included in Johnson's Continuum of Sexual Behaviors in Children or Hall et al.'s empirical typology (e.g., dynamics in the relationship among children involved in sexually oriented activities, the use of planning and coercion, response to adult limit setting, disturbances in boundaries and other aspects of family functioning, and etiological risk factors in addition to prior trauma). Typologies that consider only one or a few dimensions are less useful to practitioners than those that provide a comprehensive array of characteristics and risk factors.

The development of typologies of adolescents who offend sexually is important, not only as a tool for assessment and treatment planning, but also as a tool for risk assessment and prediction of recidivism (for an in-depth discussion of risk assessment, see Prescott, this issue). Two of the adolescent typologies reviewed (Prentky et al., 2000; Worling, 2001) include risk assessment prediction as one of the purposes for their development. Researchers in the field of adolescents who offend sexually who are interested in developing typologies would do well to look at the two empirically derived typologies for

CSBPs (Hall et al., 2002; Pithers et al., 1998) as models for a comprehensive typology that address a wide array of important variables that impact the functioning of sexually abusive youth and their families. Such comprehensive, multi-dimensional typologies are needed to guide assessment, treatment planning, and selection of interventions.

Unfortunately, no one typology provides a comprehensive framework in itself for assessing CSBPs or adolescents who offend sexually. Johnson's Continuum of Sexual Behaviors in Children comes close, but it is limited by the fact that it is clinically derived and lacks empirical validation. The Hall et al. (2002) typology is a good start toward providing an empirically derived framework that considers most of Johnson's contextual factors. Nonetheless, it was based on a limited sample of preschool sexually abused children, and may not apply to older samples of CSBPs, or to CSBPs who have not been sexually abused. The typologies of adolescents who offend sexually that are currently being developed (Hunter et al., 2003; Prentky et al., 2000; Worling, 2001) hold promise for clinicians, but need to be more comprehensive that what is currently presented in the reports of published research.

THE NEED FOR A MULTIDIMENSIONAL FRAMEWORK

When taken together, clinically derived and empirical typologies emphasize that several dimensions need to be considered when assessing CSBPs and adolescents who offend sexually. First, clinicians who treat CSBPs need to carefully assess the children's sexualized and other problematic behaviors. Similarly, clinicians who treat adolescents who offend sexually need to assess any other problematic behaviors that an adolescent may have, in addition to the referral of sexually abusive behavior.

Second, clinicians need to evaluate the internal and external dynamics and etiological risk factors motivating the sexualized and sexually abusive behaviors of CSBPs and adolescents who offend sexually. They will then be in a better position to effectively plan and implement intervention strategies tailored to address the specific treatment needs of each child or adolescent. Further research is needed to empirically develop typologies that will provide a complete and multidimensional identification of relevant characteristics of CSBPs and adolescents who offend sexually. In the meantime, clinicians will need to rely on existing clinically or empirically derived typologies, or try to find other models that provide a multidimensional assessment framework.

Several practitioners have stressed that a thorough assessment, which includes a comprehensive psychosocial history and standardized measures assessing both the youth and parent(s), is essential when evaluating CSBPs and adolescents who offend sexually (Araji, 1997; Bonner et al., 1998; Burton et al., 1998; Chaffin et al., 2002; Friedrich, 2002; Gil & Johnson, 1993; Rasmussen, 2001, 2002; Righthand & Welch, 2001). The assessment must not be limited to assessing the child or adolescent's sexually abusive behavior, but needs to include a careful evaluation of the youth's emotional and behavioral functioning and identify any salient symptoms of psychological disorders (e.g., Major Depression, Posttraumatic Stress Disorder, Attention-Deficit Hyperactivity Disorder, Conduct Disorder) (Bonner et al., 1998; Friedrich, 2002, Rasmussen, 2001, 2002).

The Trauma Outcome Process (TOP) Model

One treatment model that provides the conceptual framework needed for completing a comprehensive assessment of CSBPs and adolescents who offend sexually, as well as intervention strategies for addressing the special treatment needs of different subtypes of youth is the Trauma Outcome Process (TOP) model (Burton et al., 1998; Rasmussen, 1999, 2001, 2002; Rasmussen et al., 1992). The TOP model is a conceptual framework clinically derived from practice experience. It includes premises and concepts that provide an explanation of the development of sexually abusive behavior (Rasmussen, 1999). Its limitation, like that of Johnson's Continuum of Sexual Behavior in Children (Johnson, 1993, 1999, 2000; Johnson & Feldmeth, 1993), is that it has not been empirically validated. Nevertheless, it is a useful practice model that includes a four-step multidimensional assessment process and intervention strategies for guiding the intake interview and treatment (see Rasmussen, 1999, 2001, 2002 for a full description of the TOP model, its use in assessment, including questions to use in the assessment, and its application in integrating various treatment approaches when treating different subtypes of CSBPs or adolescents who sexually offend).

The TOP model provides a multidimensional framework for identifying areas of concern in CSBPs and adolescents who offend sexually (Rasmussen, 1999, 2001). This framework includes assessing dimensions that were included in establishing subtypes of CSBPs in the Pithers et al. (1998) typology. These include offense characteristics (e.g., type of sexual behavior, number of victims); individual risk factors (e.g., history of sexual abuse, physical abuse, and other types of trauma); and psychological functioning (e.g., applying DSM-IV diagnostic criteria for disorders such as Posttraumatic Stress Disorder, Depression, Attention-Deficit-Hyperactivity Disorder, Oppositional Defiant Disorder, Conduct Disorder). The TOP framework also involves assessing dimensions related to contextual and family factors considered in Johnson's Continuum of Sexual Behaviors in Children (Johnson, 1993, 1999, 2000; Johnson & Feldmeth,

1993) and the Hall et al. (2002) typology. These include the abusive dynamics involved in the child's relationship with other children involved in the referred sexualized or sexually abusive behavior, the child's attachment/separation history, characteristics of the child's sexual abuse experience and secondary wounding following disclosure, disturbances in family boundaries, quality of the family's sexual environment, and environmental support (e.g., household stability).

The TOP model of assessment specifies that intake interviews with CSBPs or adolescents who offend sexually and their families should include "clinical observations of children's verbal statements, nonverbal behaviors, and interaction with their parents" (Rasmussen, 2001, pp. 13-14), as well as biographical data and standardized measures evaluating several areas of child/adolescent and parent functioning. This comprehensive intake assessment is consistent with the process that the Pithers et al. (1998) used in basing their empirical typology on data from several standardized measures.

There are four steps of assessment in the TOP model. First, the clinician identifies the individual, family, and environmental risk and resiliency factors that make children or adolescents vulnerable or resilient to having an excessively negative or maladaptive response to traumatic experiences (for factors associated with resiliency, see Efta-Breitbach & Freeman, this issue). Next, the clinician identifies the emotional, cognitive, and behavioral outcomes that children/adolescents and their families are displaying in response to traumatic experiences. Third, the clinician assesses the youths' self-awareness of their thoughts, feelings, body sensations, motivations, and actions. Finally, the clinician identifies the youths' primary behavioral response to their traumatic experiences (i.e., self-destructive, abusive, or adaptive behavior).

Clinicians who assess CSBPs may use these steps in conjunction with Johnson's Continuum of Sexual Behaviors in Children (Johnson, 1993, 1999, 2000; Johnson & Feldmeth, 1993), as well as with data from the Pithers et al. (1998) and Hall et al. (2002) empirical typologies. Clinicians who assess adolescents who offend sexually may use these steps in conjunction with the O'Brien and Bera (1986) personality-based clinically derived typology and Worling's (2001) personality-based, empirically derived typology.

Assessment of risk factors. The first step of the four-step assessment process in the TOP model is to identify the individual, family, and environmental risk and resiliency factors that make children or adolescents vulnerable or resilient to having excessively negative or maladaptive responses to traumatic experiences (Rasmussen, 1999, 2001). This step is consistent with the ecological perspective taken by Hall and colleagues (2002) when they identified salient individual, family, and community contextual factors influencing CSBPs and used these factors when developing their typology. Rasmussen (2001) identified three individual factors (advocated by Friedrich, 2002) that should be included in the TOP model assessment of children and adolescents: (a) attachment, (b) emotional dysregultion, and (c) self-perceptions.

The empirical typologies developed by Hall et al. (2002) and Pithers et al. (1998) provide objective data validating the need to consider these particular factors when assessing CSBPs and adolescents who offend sexually. For example, in both studies, disrupted attachment was highlighted as a risk factor for the development of sexual behavior problems (for further information on attachment problems, see Longo, this issue). One important finding of the Pithers et al. study was that parents were significantly less attached to the children that the Pithers typology identified as highly traumatized, when compared to the parents of the children in the other four subtypes.

Similarly, Hall and colleagues found that the children in the most severe subtype in their typology (i.e., interpersonal, planned [coercive]) had significantly more cumulative negative events associated with disrupted attachment (e.g., childhood maltreatment, placement in foster care, and permanent loss of a parent). The parents of these children had significantly more problems in functioning and other risk factors (e.g., depression, drug use while pregnant, history of childhood physical and emotional abuse, separation from parents during childhood, parental rejection) than the parents of children in the other subtypes (Hall et al.). These impairments in parental functioning have been shown in other research to be associated with disrupted attachment, particularly disorganized attachment (Davies, 1999). Attachment is assessed in the TOP model assessment by exploring youths' feelings about their parents or other caregivers (e.g., "How do you get along with your Mom (Dad) (Grandmother)?" "Who in your family do you feel closest to?" "Who frightens you?" "Who in your family makes you mad?" "What do they do that you don't like?").

Disruptions in attachment may relate to other family risk factors (e.g., poor boundaries, having a sexualized family environment) that Rasmussen (1999, 2002) indicated were important to evaluate as part of the TOP model's multi-dimensional assessment of risk factors. The Hall et al. (2002) typology provided empirical evidence of the importance of considering boundary and sexuality issues when assessing CSBPs and adolescents who offend sexually. Hall and colleagues found that violations of generational boundaries (i.e., role reversal between parent and child) were most pronounced for children in the interpersonal, planned (coercive) subtype. Problematic sexual attitudes (e.g., pairing of sexuality with violence) were found most frequently in the two most severe subtypes of children (i.e., interpersonal, planned (noncoercive) and interpersonal planned (coercive), but were also frequently found in the subtype of children that showed sexualized self-focused behaviors, with no interpersonal contact. Maternal boundary problems were found in all of the children in the interpersonal, planned (coercive) subtype.

Family boundaries are assessed in the TOP model assessment by observing interactions between family members and asking specific questions related to (a) potential violations of privacy in sleeping arrangements, bathroom use, and dressing; (b) roles in the family, particularly parent and child roles; (c) communication among family members, including use of respectful or disrespectful language and management of conflict and anger; and (d) structural aspects of the house that might violate privacy (e.g., missing doors, holes in walls). The "Boundary Blueprint" exercise provides a format of specific questions for clinicians to use when assessing boundary issues (Burton et al., 1998, pp. 214-223). In addition, the "Safety Checklist" is useful when assessing boundaries or the family's sexual environment (Friedrich, 2002, pp. 289-292).

Rasmussen (2002) stressed the importance of including ecological factors (e.g., poverty, homelessness, parental unemployment) in a comprehensive assessment of CSBPs and adolescents who offend sexually. In the Hall et al. (2002) study, there were no significant differences found between children with developmentally expected sexual behaviors, children with exclusively self-focused sexual behaviors, and children with interpersonal sexual behaviors on most socioeconomic variables. Nonetheless, Hall et al. found that children with interpersonal sexual behavior problems, when compared with children with developmentally expected sexual behaviors and children with exclusively self-focused sexual behavior, had significantly more ($p < .02$) changes in housing. Although this variable was not included in their cluster analysis of the five subtypes of children, Hall et al.'s results suggest that some ecological factors (e.g., stability of housing) may impact whether children's sexual behavior problems are self-focused or interpersonally focused.

In the TOP model assessment, the clinician pays particular attention to assessing the degree of environmental support that children/adolescents and their families have available to them (e.g., extended family, community resources such as school or church, cultural systems). Clinicians should take care to assess whether these resources provide emotional support to children/adolescents and their families, or are non-supportive and provoke addition trauma that interferes with the recovery of youth and their families from traumatic experiences (e.g., the child or adolescent's own victimization, the discovery of the youth's sexually abusive behavior). It is also important to incorporate the family's support system as part of the "prevention team" in helping the child or adolescent to prevent further sexual behavior problems or sexually abusive behavior (Gray & Pithers, 1993). A question to ask family members in the TOP assessment to identify environmental support is, "To whom can you and your family turn during this time (of crisis)?"

Assessment of emotional, cognitive, and behavioral outcomes. The second step of the TOP model assessment is to identify the emotional, cognitive, and behavioral outcomes of youths' traumatic experiences (Rasmussen, 1999, 2001). This involves identifying "signs and symptoms that may represent effects of traumatic experiences" and assessing for "impairment in children's cognitive, emotional, and social functioning" (2001, p. 19). Symptoms of PTSD or other emotional dysregulation are particularly important to assess (Friedrich, 2002; Rasmussen, 2001). The findings of both the Hall et al. (2002) and Pithers et al. (1998) studies documented that symptoms of PTSD are associated with more severe sexual behavior problems. Hall et al. found that the two most severe subtypes (i.e., interpersonal, planned (noncoercive) and interpersonal, planned (coercive) had the greatest percentage of children exhibiting symptoms of PTSD (62% and 91%, respectively). In the Pithers et al. study, children in the highly traumatized subtype were significantly ($p < .0001$) more likely to have a DSM-IV diagnosis of PTSD. As noted previously, the highly traumatized subtype had significantly more perpetrators who sexually abused them ($p < .03$) and more perpetrators who physically abused them ($p < .02$), making them more likely to experience symptoms of PTSD. Two of the typologies reviewed for adolescents who offend sexually (Hunter et al., 2003; Worling, 2001) highlighted depression as an issue that should be routinely assessed, which is consistent with this step of the TOP model assessment.

Assessment of the youth's level of self-awareness. Friedrich (2002) stressed that self-perception is a critical area to assess when evaluating the individual characteristics of CSBPs and adolescents who offend sexually. The third step of the TOP model assessment involves assessing youths' level of self-awareness of thoughts, feelings, body sensations, motivations, and actions (Rasmussen, 1999, 2001). This step is consistent with child characteristics that were assessed in the Hall et al. (2002) study. Although results were not significant, Hall et al. found that the most severe subtype in their typology, children with interpersonal, planned (coercive) sexual behavior, had the highest percentage of children who showed (a) a limited range of affect (91%), (b) hopelessness (80%), (c) a tendency to blame others for misdeeds (61%), and (d) poor internalization of right and wrong (63%). Furthermore, Hall et al. (1998) found that the children's self-perception of who was to blame for their sexual abuse was a significant variable ($p = .00001$) in differentiating children with self-focused sexual behavior problems from children with interpersonally focused sexual behavior problems. Children with developmentally expected sexual behaviors blamed their perpetrator for their abuse, while children with self-focused and interpersonally focused sexual behaviors were ambivalent about whom to blame. Children in the self-focused group often blamed themselves.

The above child characteristics studied by Hall and colleagues (1998, 2002) might be attributed to lack of self-awareness on the part of the child, as hypothesized in the TOP model assessment. In contrast to the Hall et al. studies (1998, 2002), Pithers et al. (1998) did not include in their typology any variables that related to children's self-awareness/self-perceptions. Self-perceptions are addressed in the TOP model assessment by identifying children's/adolescents' thinking errors and teaching them to correct them (Burton et al., 1998; Rasmussen, 2001, 2002–see Burton et al., p. 133, for a list of common thinking errors used by CSBPs and ways to correct them). Similarly, Worling (2001) stressed the need to evaluate social skills and prosocial attitudes of the adolescents who offend sexually and provide interventions to address these areas.

Identifying the youth's primary behavioral response. The final step of the TOP model assessment is to determine whether the youth's behavioral response to traumatic experiences (or to triggers reminding them of traumatic experiences) is self-destructive/internalizing, abusive/externalizing, or adaptive in expressing feelings related to trauma and taking responsibility for one's own recovery (Rasmussen, 1999, 2001). This step is consistent with efforts made by Pithers et al. (1998) to evaluate whether the CSBPs were showing internalizing or externalizing behavior problems. In analyzing assessment results from the Child Behavior Checklist (Achenbach, 1991), Pithers et al. found that children in the rule breaker subtype were significantly ($p < .0001$) more likely to have high internalizing behavior scores than children in the highly traumatized, asymptomatic, and sexually aggressive subtypes. (Children in the abuse reactive subtype did not differ significantly in their internalizing scores from any other subtype.) Similarly, the rule breaker subtype had significantly ($p < .0010$) higher externalizing behavior scores than children in the asymptomatic, sexually aggressive, and abuse reactive subtypes. (Children in the highly traumatized subtype did not differ significantly in their externalizing scores from any other subtype.) These findings are consistent with the premise of the TOP model that it is important to assess whether the behaviors of youths are self-destructive (internalizing), abusive (externalizing), or adaptive (in allowing children to cope effectively with traumatic experiences) (Rasmussen, 1999, 2001).

Interventions. As noted previously, the two NCCAN outcome studies (Bonner et al., 1999; Pithers et al., 1998) found that both cognitive-behavioral and expressive therapies, when applied in short-term intervention (< 32 sessions in the Pithers et al. study; 12 sessions in the Bonner et al. study), were effective in reducing children's sexual behavior problems. The Pithers et al. study found that some interventions were more effective with certain subtypes of children (i.e., the cognitive-behavioral intervention was significantly more effective for the highly traumatized subtype). These results point to a need for integrative models that combine strategies from different therapies and are able to address the treatment needs of different subtypes of CSBPs and adolescents who offend sexually (for discussion of an integrated treatment approach, see Longo, this issue).

CONCLUSION

Children with sexual behavior problems and adolescents who offend sexually are diverse groups. Although clinical typologies describing these children and adolescents are useful schemas to aid assessment, recent empirical typologies provide objective data to help clinicians identify and assess the sexual behaviors, child characteristics, psychological functioning, and family dynamics of different subtypes of children. These data can be incorporated within the context of a multidimensional framework (i.e., Trauma Outcome Process model) to assess children with sexual behavior problems and adolescents who offend sexually, plan treatment, and implement interventions that are tailored to the specific needs of each subtype of children or adolescents.

Treating children with sexual behavior problems and adolescents who offend sexually with integrative practice models such as the Trauma Outcome Process model can best meet their individual needs and prevent recurrence of sexualized and sexually abusive behaviors. Research is needed to further establish empirical typologies for identifying and assessing subtypes of CSBPs and adolescents who offend sexually and to validate the clinically derived conceptual framework presented in this article, the Trauma Outcome Process (TOP) model.

REFERENCES

Abel, G. G., Mittelman, M., & Becker, J. V. (1985). Sex offenders: Results of assessment and recommendations for treatment. In H. H. Ben-Aron, S. I. Hucker, & C. D. Webster (Eds.), *Clinical criminology: Current concepts* (pp. 191-205). Toronto: M & M Graphics.

Abidin, R. R. (1990). *Parenting stress index* (3rd ed.). Charlottesville, VA: Pediatric Psychology.

Achenbach, T. (1991). *Child behavior checklist for ages 4-18.* Burlington, VT: University of Vermont.

Araji, S. K. (1997). *Sexually aggressive children: Coming to understand them.* Thousand Oaks, CA: Sage.

Becker, J. V. (1998). What we know about the characteristics and treatment of adolescents who have committed sexual offenses. *Child Maltreatment, 3*(4), 317-329.

Bonner, B. L., Marx, B. P., Thompson, J. M., & Michaelson, P. (1998). Assessment of adolescent sexual offenders. *Child Maltreatment, 3*(4), 374-383.

Bonner, B. L., Walker, C. E., & Berliner, L. (1999). *Children with sexual behavior problems: Assessment and treatment.* (Final report, Grant No. 90-CA-1469). Washington, DC: Administration for Children, Youth, and Families, Department of Human Services.

Burton, J., Rasmussen, L. A., Bradshaw, J., Christopherson, B. J., & Huke, S. C. (1998). *Treating children with sexually abusive behavior problems: Guidelines for child and parent intervention.* New York: The Haworth Press, Inc.

Butler, S. M., & Seto, M. C. (2002). Distinguishing two types of adolescent offenders. *Journal of the Academy of Child and Adolescent Psychiatry, 41*(1), 83-90.

Butts, J. A., & Snyder, H. N. (1997). The youngest delinquents: Offenders under age 15. *Juvenile Justice Bulletin,* 1-11.

Chaffin, M., & Bonner, B. (1998). "Don't shoot, we're children": Have we gone too far in our response to adolescent sexual abusers and children with sexual behavior problems? *Child Maltreatment, 3,* 314-316.

Chaffin, M., Letourneau, E., & Silovsky, J. (2002). Adults, adolescents, and children who sexually abuse children. In J. E. B. Meyers, L. Berliner, J. Briere, C. T. Hendrix, C. Jenny, & T. A. Reid (Eds.), *The APSAC handbook on child maltreatment* (2nd ed.) (pp. 205- 232). Thousand Oaks, CA: Sage.

Davies, D. (1999). *Child development: A practitioner's guide.* New York: The Guilford Press.

Deluty, R. H. (1979). Children's action tendency scale: A self-report measure of aggressiveness, assertiveness, and submissiveness in children. *Journal of Consulting and Clinical Psychology, 47,* 1061-1071.

Efta-Breitbach, J., & Freeman, K.A. (2004). Recidivism and resilience in juvenile sexual offenders: An analysis of the literature. *Journal of Child Sexual Abuse, 13*(3/4), pp. 257-280.

Eyberg, S. M., & Ross, A. W. (1978). Assessment of child behavior problems. *Journal of Clinical Child Psychology, 7,* 113-116.

Friedrich, W. N. (1995). The clinical use of the child sexual behavior inventory: Frequently asked questions. *The APSAC Advisor, 8,* 1-2, 18-20.

Friedrich, W. N. (2002). *Psychological assessment of sexually abused children and their families.* Thousand Oaks, CA: Sage.

Friedrich, W. N., Beilke, R. L., & Purcell, J. (1989). *The child sexual behavior inventory: Version 2.* Rochester, MN: Psychology Department, Mayo Clinic.

Friedrich, W. N., Grambsch, P., Damon, L., Hewitt, S., Koverola, C., Lang, R., Wolfe, V., & Broughton, D. (1992). The child sexual behavior inventory: Normative and clinical contrasts. *Psychological Assessment, 4,* 303-311.

Gil, E. (1993). Age-appropriate sex play versus problematic sexual behaviors. In E. Gil, & T. C. Johnson (Eds.), *Sexualized children: Assessment and treatment of sexualized children who molest* (pp. 21-40). Walnut Creek, CA: Launch Press.

Gil, E., & Johnson, T. C. (1993). *Sexualized children: Assessment and treatment of sexualized children who molest.* Rockville, MD: Launch Press.

Graves, R. B., Openshaw, D. K., Ascione, F. R., & Ericksen, S. L. (1996). Demographic and parental characteristics of youthful sexual offenders. *International Journal of Offender Therapy and Comparative Criminology, 40,* 300-317.

Gray, A. S., & Pithers, W. D. (1993). Relapse prevention with sexually aggressive adolescents and children: Expanding treatment and supervision. In H. Barbaree, W. Marshall, & S. Hudson (Eds.), *The juvenile sexual offender* (pp. 289-319). New York: Guilford Press.

Gray, A., Pithers, W. D., Busconi, A., & Houchens, P. (1999). Developmental and etiological characteristics of children with sexual behavior problems: Treatment implications. *Child Abuse & Neglect, 23*(6), 601-621.

Groth, A. N., Longo, R. E., & McFadin, J. B. (1982). Undetected recidivism among rapists and child molesters. *Crime and Delinquency, 128*, 450-458.

Hall, D. K., Mathews, F., & Pearce, J. (1998). Factors associated with sexual behavior problems in young sexually abused children. *Child Abuse & Neglect, 22*(10), 1045-1063.

Hall, D. K., Mathews, F., & Pearce, J. (2002). Sexual behavior problems in sexually abused children: A preliminary typology. *Child Abuse and Neglect, 26*, 289-312.

Hall, D. K., Mathews, F., Pearce, J., Sarlo-McGarvey, N., & Gavin, D. (1996). *The development of sexual behavior problems in children and youth.* Ontario, Canada: Central Toronto Youth Services.

Hunter, J. A., Figueredo, A. J., Malamuth, N. M., & Becker, J. V. (2003). Juvenile sex offenders: Toward the development of a typology. *Sexual Abuse: A Journal of Research and Treatment, 15*(1), 27-48.

Johnson, T. C. (1993). Assessment of sexual behavior problems in preschool-aged and latency-aged children. *Child and Adolescent Psychiatric Clinics of North America, 2*, 431-449.

Johnson, T. C. (1999). *Understanding your child's sexual behavior: What's natural and healthy.* Oakland, CA: New Harbinger.

Johnson, T. C. (2000). Sexualized children and children who molest. *Seicus Report, 29*(1), 35-39.

Johnson, T. C., & Feldmeth, J. R. (1993). Sexual behaviors: A continuum. In E. Gil, & T. C. Johnson (Eds.), *Sexualized children: Assessment and treatment of sexualized children who molest* (pp. 41-52). Walnut Creek, CA: Launch Press.

Knight, R.A., & Sims-Knight, J.E. (2004). Testing an etiological model for male juvenile sexual offending against females. *Journal of Child Sexual Abuse, 13*(3/4), pp. 33- 56.

Longo, R.E. (2004). An integrated experiential approach to treating young people who sexually abuse. *Journal of Child Sexual Abuse, 13*(3/4) pp. 193-215.

National Center for Juvenile Justice. (1999). *Juvenile offenders and victims: 1999 national report.* Washington, DC: Office of Juvenile Justice and Delinquency Prevention.

O'Brien, M. (1991). Taking sibling incest seriously. In M. Q. Patton (Ed.), *Family sexual abuse* (pp. 75-92). Newbury Park, CA: Sage.

O'Brien, M., & Bera, W. (1986). Adolescent sexual offenders: A descriptive typology. *Newsletter of the National Family Life Education Network, 1*, 1-5.

Pithers, W. D., Gray, A., Busconi, A., & Houchens, P. (1998). Children with sexual behavior problems: Identification of five distinct child types and related treatment considerations. *Child Maltreatment, 3*(4), 384-406.

Prentky, R., Harris, B., Frizzell, K., & Righthand, S. (2000). An actuarial procedure for assessing risk with juvenile sexual offenders. *Sexual Abuse: A Journal of Research and Treatment, 12*(2), 71-93.

Prescott, D.S. (2004). Emerging strategies for risk assessment of sexually abusive youth: Theory, controversy, and practice. *Journal of Child Sexual Abuse, 13*(3/4) pp. 83-105.

Rasmussen, L. A. (1999). The trauma outcome process: An integrated model for guiding clinical practice with children with sexually abusive behavior problems. *Journal of Child Sexual Abuse, 8*(4), 3-33.

Rasmussen, L. A. (2001). Integrating cognitive-behavioral and expressive therapy interventions: Applying the trauma outcome process in treating children with sexually abusive behavior problems. *Journal of Child Sexual Abuse, 10*(4), 1-29.

Rasmussen, L. A. (2002). An integrated systemic approach to intervention with children with sexually abusive behavior problems. In M. Calder (Ed.), *Young people who sexually abuse: Building the evidence base for your practice.* United Kingdom: RHP Publications.

Rasmussen, L. A., Burton, J., & Christopherson, B. J. (1992). Precursors to offending and the trauma outcome process in sexually reactive children. *Journal of Child Sexual Abuse, 1*(1), 33-48.

Righthand, S., & Welch, C. (2001). *Juveniles who have sexually offended: A review of the professional literature.* Washington, DC: Office of Juvenile Justice and Delinquency Prevention.

Righthand, S., & Welch, C. (2004). Characteristics of youth who sexually offend. *Journal of Child Sexual Abuse, 13*(3/4) pp. 15-32.

Ryan, G. (1997). Sexually abusive youth: Defining the population. In G. Ryan, & S. Lane (Eds.), *Juvenile sexual offending: Causes, consequences, and correction* (Rev. ed.) (pp. 3-9). San Francisco: Jossey-Bass.

Ryan, G., & Lane, S. (1997). *Juvenile sexual offending: Causes, consequences, and correction* (Rev. ed.). San Francisco: Jossey-Bass.

Silovsky, J. F., & Niec, L. (2002). Characteristics of young children with sexual behavior problems: A pilot study. *Child Maltreatment, 7*(3), 187-197.

Spielberger, C. D. (1973). *State-trait anxiety inventory for children: Preliminary manual.* Palo Alto, CA: Consulting Psychologists Press.

Veneziano, C., & Veneziano, L. (2003). Adolescent sexual offenders: A review of the literature. *Trauma, Violence, & Abuse 3*(4), 247-260.

Weinrott, M. (1996). *Juvenile sexual aggression: A critical review.* Boulder: University of Colorado, Institute for Behavioral Sciences, Center for the Study and Prevention of Violence.

Worling, J. R. (2001). Personality-based typology of adolescent male sexual offenders: Differences in recidivism rates, victim-selection characteristics, and personal victimization histories. *Sexual Abuse: A Journal of Research and Treatment, 13*, 149-166.

Emerging Strategies
for Risk Assessment
of Sexually Abusive Youth:
Theory, Controversy, and Practice

David S. Prescott

SUMMARY. Clinicians and other professionals evaluating, managing, and treating sexually abusive youth are frequently called upon to offer judgments regarding risk for sexual reoffense. There are currently no empirically validated methods for accurately classifying risk among this population. Therefore, those faced with this task have an obligation to consider the research on the assessment of risk and recidivism. Five methods of risk assessment are reviewed, and four scales are discussed, with directions on how to obtain them. These include the Juvenile Sex Offender Assessment Protocol (JSOAP), the Protective Factors Scale (PFS), and Estimate of Risk of Adolescent Sex Offender Recidivism (ERASOR). *[Article copies available for a fee from The Haworth Document Delivery Service: 1-800-HAWORTH. E-mail address: <docdelivery@haworthpress.com> Website: <http://www.HaworthPress.com> © 2004 by The Haworth Press, Inc. All rights reserved.]*

Address correspondence to: David Prescott, LICSW, P.O. Box 593, Shaftsbury, VT 05262 (E-mail: vtprescott@earthlink.net).

[Haworth co-indexing entry note]: "Emerging Strategies for Risk Assessment of Sexually Abusive Youth: Theory, Controversy, and Practice." Prescott, David S. Co-published simultaneously in *Journal of Child Sexual Abuse* (The Haworth Maltreatment and Trauma Press, an imprint of The Haworth Press, Inc.) Vol. 13, No. 3/4, 2004, pp. 83-105; and: *Identifying and Treating Youth Who Sexually Offend: Current Approaches, Techniques, and Research* (ed: Robert Geffner et al.) The Haworth Maltreatment and Trauma Press, an imprint of The Haworth Press, Inc., 2004, pp. 83-105. Single or multiple copies of this article are available for a fee from The Haworth Document Delivery Service [1-800-HAWORTH, 9:00 a.m. - 5:00 p.m. (EST). E-mail address: docdelivery@haworthpress.com].

KEYWORDS. Juvenile, sexual, offender, risk, assessment, JSOAP, ERASOR

A remarkable rise in the awareness and development of treatment programs for sexually abusive youth has occurred in the past 30 years (e.g., Safer Society Program, 1993). However, the research into recidivism rates and treatment outcome has not kept pace with this growth of understanding (Worling, 2001; Worling & Curwen, 2000a). Assessment and treatment techniques have been based in large part on strategies developed with adult populations. Examples range from the use of phallometry (Hunter, 1999) to applications of relapse prevention strategies (Gray & Pithers, 1993).

Clinicians, protective service caseworkers, and representatives of the legal system are frequently called upon to provide an opinion, assessment, or prediction regarding the likelihood that a given youth will continue a pattern of sexual aggression. However, at present there remains no empirically validated method for evaluating the likelihood that a youth will recidivate sexually (Prentky, Harris, Frizzell, & Righthand, 2000). The purpose of this article, then, is to provide an overview of recent research and emerging tools that may help the clinician make more informed decisions about how to understand and evaluate risk, as well as to understand the limitations that hinder clinicians' ability to accurately appraise the pro- bability of recidivism (see Hanson, 2000; Monahan, 1981; Quinsey, Harris, Rice, & Cormier, 1998).

WHAT IS RISK?

Different authors have different definitions of risk. Andrews and Bonta (1998) challenge their readers to tailor treatment strategies to the principles of risk, need, and the individual's capacity to respond to interventions. However, the authors of existing risk assessment schemes often include elements that appear to be both markers of risk and areas of treatment need. Examples include the dynamic, or changeable factors such as substance abuse problems, negative mood, and anger/hostility included in Hanson and Harris' (2001) Sex Offender Need Assessment Rating (SONAR) or the distorted attitudes described in Thornton's (2000) Structured Risk Assessment.

Meanwhile, Hart (2001) has challenged many to reconsider what is meant by "risk." He asks whether we are measuring a hazard or a predisposition to a hazard. He offers a definition of risk as "a hazard (potential negative outcome) . . . that is incompletely understood and therefore can be forecast only with uncertainty" (p. 12). He goes on to define risk assessment as "the process of understanding hazards to minimize their negative consequences" (p. 12). This is at variance with risk assessment rating scales such as the Violence Risk Appraisal Guide (VRAG) (Quinsey et al., 1998) that yield only a probability estimate of a violent reoffense. Additionally, this and other scales (see Hanson & Thornton, 1999) often define the hazard measured only in vague terms such as re-arrest or reconviction for "violence" or "sexual offense." Clearly, a definition of risk based on contact with the legal system is under-representative of the incidence of misconduct (Monahan, 1981).

More recently, Webster, Hucker, and Bloom (2002) have recommended criteria for violence risk assessment that include an evidenced-based foundation and an individualized statement of risk. Taken together, these criteria call for an assessor with a solid understanding of the current research into risk assessment as well as a considerable understanding of the individual involved. Evidence suggests that youth can be quite amenable to treatment (Worling & Curwen, 2000b), and so those who assess juveniles ought to understand and assess risk within the context of available treatment services and other factors (e.g., family constellations) that will mitigate their risk in the short and long term.

WHY CONSIDER RISK?

Recent research shows that juveniles commit 20% to 30% of reported rapes and 30% to 60% of child molestation (Hunter, 1999; Weinrott, 1996). There is evidence that different trajectories of sexual aggression may indicate different variations of risk in the short and long term (Hanson, 2002). However, it is important to note that typological studies of adolescents such as those by Knight and Prentky (1993) are still in their infancy.

Retrospective studies of adult pedophiles show that 40% to 50% report a juvenile onset to their offending (Hunter, 1999). Additionally, same-sex pedophilia is associated with an earlier age of onset. There is ample evidence that boy-victim adult pedophiles are at an elevated risk for reoffense (e.g., Hanson & Bussiere, 1998). While there is strong evidence that sexual interest and arousal is fluid and dynamic throughout adolescence (see Hunter, 1999, for a review, as well as Zolondek, Abel, Northey, & Jordan, 2001), it is clear that true sexual disorders can appear in youth.

Studies of juveniles who rape (e.g., Elliott, 1994; Weinrott, 1996) suggest that this form of sexual aggression is less likely to persist into adulthood. However, it is possible that these youth may be at an increased risk for general and violent recidivism (Hanson & Bussiere, 1998; Worling & Curwen, 2000b).

In some instances, sexual aggression may only be part of an emerging pattern of diverse criminality (Forth & Mailloux, 2000; Hare, 1991).

Further evidence exists that behaviors identified by lay adults as indicators of high risk are not always correlated with recidivism. In one study (Prentky et al., 2000), elements related to sexual interest did not differentiate the three re-cidivists from the rest of the sample of 76, while elements related to anti-sociality did. Another study (Daleiden, Kaufman, Hilliker, & O'Neil, 1998) found that juvenile sex offenders had more extensive histories of non-consen-sual sexual experiences and paraphiliac interest when compared to non-of-fending youth, but did not differ in deviant sexual fantasies. In the research on adult sex offenders, elements typically considered as related to recidivism have been found to have little, if any, predictive validity. These include factors such as empathy, denial, and overall psychological maladjustment (Hanson & Bussiere, 1998).

In one study (Curwen, 2000a), self-reported empathy as measured by the Interpersonal Reactivity Index (Salter, 1988) actually had a positive relation-ship with sexual violence. Miner (2000) found that only elements related to impulsivity and attention-seeking (as measured by Multi-Health Systems' Jesness Inventory) were correlated to recidivism. In evaluating California Psychological Inventory (CPI) scores, Worling (2001) found that elevations in the "antisocial/impulsive" and "unusual/isolated" factors were more highly correlated with sexual recidivism than the "confident/aggressive" and "over-controlled/reserved" factors. Although many of these findings may be related to measurement and categorization problems (Lund, 2000), it appears that those seeking to assess risk may best serve youth by remaining wary of factors that would otherwise be relevant to a comprehensive psychosexual evaluation (Ryan & Lane, 1997).

Some other points to consider in assessing risk include results of recent studies showing that confrontational treatment styles can result in poorer out-comes (Marshall, Anderson, & Fernandez, 1999). Additionally, Hanson and Bussiere (1998) found that failure to complete treatment not only predicts reoffense, but can elevate the level of risk in adult offenders (for further dis-cussion on the linkage between failure to complete treatment and recidivism, see Efta-Breitbach & Freeman, this issue). In juvenile populations, a punitive treatment approach can also increase shame, replicate abusive environments, and inhibit healthy sexual development (Prescott, 2001). Although there is ev-idence that many treatment programs are working to reduce shame-based ap-proaches (Curwen, 2000b), an assessment of treatment history may contribute to a more accurate assessment of risk.

Finally, an understanding of base rates is essential to assessing risk (Mona-han, 1981; Serin & Brown, 2000; Webster, Ben-Aron, & Hucker, 1985). However, gaining a sense of the overall base rate of adolescent sexual reoffense can be a frustrating experience. For example, Kenny, Keough, and Seidler (2001) observe that "between 3% and 70% of first-time apprehended juvenile sex offenders reoffend" (p. 131). Table 1 contains information from a number of studies regarding recidivism by adolescents (for an in-depth discussion of factors influencing recidivism, see Efta-Breitbach & Freeman, this issue).

RISK ASSESSMENT METHODS

Although there are many ways to envision the variety of risk assessments (e.g., Hanson, 2000; Monahan, 1981), the following can be useful in addressing the benefits and limitations of single-method approaches.

Anamnestic

Similar to the use of a relapse prevention framework for the prevention of sexual abuse, this method reviews factors related to past misconduct (Gray & Pithers, 1993). It includes a thorough review of the thoughts, feelings, situations, and behaviors that led to past instances of harmful sexual behavior. For example, many youth describe intense anger and/or loneliness as key elements present before their offenses. Others cite peer pressure or areas of their community that compromise their ability to refrain from abusive behavior. It might also include a list of "warning signs" such as interpersonal withdrawal or disruptiveness that might serve to communicate imminence to adults (Quinsey et al., 1998). Such an approach can be of obvious benefit in aiding risk management strategies (Gray & Pithers, 1993), whether initiated by the youth, others, or both. These strategies might include safety plans for home visits and extracurricular activities, or preparations for step-down situations following out-of-home placements.

While relapse prevention has been a hallmark of treatment for many years (Gray & Pithers, 1993), it contains fundamental flaws that can hinder a comprehensive understanding of risk (for additional discussion citing problems with the relapse prevention approach, see Longo, this issue). There are no constraints on weighting and combining factors. There is an implicit assumption that abusive people specialize in one form of abuse (e.g., sexual), and that history will repeat itself in the way that the youth recalls, often well after the fact. There can be an implicit assumption that abusive careers pursue a single trajectory, such as a particular class of behavior or victim, or during certain emotional states and other situations (Pithers, Beal, Armstrong, & Petty, 1989). Finally, while such factors as negative affect, peer pressure, social conflict,

TABLE 1. Selected Base Rates

Citation	Treatment N	Comparison N	Follow-Up Period	Recidivism Measure	Sexual Recidivism	Violent Recidivism	Non-Sexual Recidivism
Alexander (1999)	1025	0	Various, but 453 for more than 5 years	Re-arrest, "whenever possible"	7.1%	N/A	N/A
Becker (1990)	112	0	28 months	Criminal charges	14%	N/A	35%
Borduin, Henggeler, Blaske, & Stein (1990)	8	8	3 years	Criminal charges	12.5% treatment; 75% comparison	N/A	25% treatment; 50% comparison
Brannon & Troyer (1995)	36	0	4 years	Incarcerated as adult	3%	N/A	14%
Bremer (1992)	193	0	several months to 6 years (no M specified)	Self-report	11%	N/A	N/A
Hagan & Cho (1996)	100	0	2-5 years (no M specified)	Convictions	9%	N/A	46%
Kahn & Chambers (1991)	221	0	20 months	Convictions	8%	N/A	45%
Kahn & Lafond (1988)	350	0	several weeks to 5 years (no M specified)	Not specified	9%	N/A	8%
Lab, Shields, & Schondel (1993)	46	109	1-3 years (no M specified)	Convictions	2% treatment; 4% comparison	N/A	22% treatment; 13% comparison
Langstrom & Grann (2000)	46 (age 15-20)	0	72 months (M = 5 years)	Convictions	20%	22%	65%
Mazur & Michael (1992)	10	0	6 months	Parent and self-report	0%	N/A	N/A
Smith & Monastersky (1986)	112	0	28 months	Criminal charges	14%	N/A	35%
Worling (1999)	58	46	2 years- 10 years (M = 6.23)	Criminal charges	5.2% treated; 17.8% non-treated	18.9% treated; 32.2% non-treated	20.7% treated; 50% non-treated

Note. In constructing this table, the author would like to acknowledge the work of James Worling and Tracey Curwen.

David S. Prescott 89

and substance abuse can play a role in one or more offense chains, they also occur alone or in combination, at times when the youth does not go on to sexually aggress. For this reason, an anamnestic approach can be particularly frustrating for the evaluator. For example, Hanson and Bussiere (1998) found no correlation between substance abuse and long-term risk for recidivism. At the same time, Hanson and Harris (2001) have found that substance abuse can be a short-term indicator of reoffense.

Other problems inherent with an anamnestic approach include the absence of any empirical validity, and the fact that they can be very general in nature. There have been no studies to support the use of this method as an accurate assessment of risk across any period of time, much less any establishment of psychometric properties such as inter-rater reliability. It cannot be supported, challenged, or defended.

Finally, anamnestic approaches can be highly subjective and overlook key factors while including interesting but nonessential factors. For example, a history of fire setting may appear to be of significance in assessing risk for sexual recidivism. However, there is evidence in the adult literature that those elements related to risk for fire setting may actually correlate to a reduced risk for violence (Quinsey et al., 1998).

Clinical Judgment

There has been vast debate as to the utility of clinical judgment in assessing risk for violence, sexual aggression, and general criminality. Many authors (e.g., Monahan, 1981; Resnick, 1996) have noted that the prediction of events with low base rates of re-occurrence is problematic, and that the lower the base rate, the more difficult the task of prediction. Quinsey and his colleagues (1998) have observed that those predicting that no one will be violent will be more accurate than those predicting who will be violent.

Hanson (2000) writes:

> Predicting whether sexual offenders are going to recidivate is difficult. There is no shortage of studies in which expert evaluators failed to distinguish between low and high risk offenders. The predictive accuracy of the typical clinical judgment is only slightly above chance levels ($r = .10$). (p. 1)

Quinsey and his colleagues (1998) have stated this less charitably:

> What we are advising is not the addition of actuarial methods to existing practice, but rather the complete replacement of existing practice with actuarial methods. This is a different view than we expressed in Webster, Harris,

Rice, Cormier, and Quinsey (1994), where we advised the practice of adjusting actuarial estimates by up to 10% when there were compelling circumstances to do so . . . Actuarial methods are too good and clinical judgment too poor to risk contaminating the former with the latter. The sorts of compelling circumstances that might tempt one to adjust an actuarial score are better considered separately in deciding on supervisory conditions, interventions designed to reduce risk, and so forth. (p. 171)

In discussing the initial stages of the MacArthur study of mental disorder and violence, Monahan and his colleagues (2001) state, ". . . How best to proceed? More research demonstrating that the outcome of unstructured clinical assessments left a great deal to be desired seemed to be overkill: That horse was already dead" (p. 7).

One might notice that the above commentators are also authors of actuarial scales to which they dedicated years of work and risked their professional reputations. However, one recent meta-analysis (Grove et al., 2001) of clinical versus mechanical forms of prediction in areas ranging from violence to heart disease showed an overall superiority of mechanical methods. Howard Garb (1998), in a review of violence prediction research, concludes: "Though clinicians often make moderately valid short-term and long-term predictions of violence, better results have been obtained with statistical-prediction rules" (pp. 117-118).

Perhaps more insulting to the seasoned clinician, however, is the following observation by Garb (1998):

Predictions of behavior made by clinicians were not more valid than predictions of behavior made by graduate students. For ratings of dangerousness, inter-rater reliability was not better for psychiatrists than for teachers . . . Predictions made by using single items of information have often been more valid than predictions made by clinicians who interviewed patients and reviewed medical records. There is no evidence that predictions based on an evaluation of an individual's personality structure and dynamics are more accurate than predictions based on a limited set of information (e.g., a diagnosis or information about a person's past behavior) . . . Predictions may become more accurate with the improved evaluation of settings. For example, relapse of schizophrenia has been related to characteristics of patients' families. (pp. 117-118)

In summary, then, those entering the world of assessing dangerousness will do best to be humble about their abilities. There is therefore irony in the sometimes-stated view that "those studies of clinical judgment didn't include MY clinical judgment!" Clinical (and even non-clinical) judgment can come in many forms, particularly in providing services to youth. It often appears as an appeal to one's authority or experience (Hanson, 1998). By neglecting the available research, it can be easy to include invalid but seemingly important factors such as overall psychological adjustment or facets of functioning that can serve divergent purposes, such as denial (Bremer, 1998). Like anamnestic risk assessment, it cannot be defended, challenged, or supported, and can be very general in nature.

Actuarial Assessment

In its purest sense, the term "actuarial" refers only to a method of combining data in an explicit, fixed, and objective fashion (Meehl, 1954; 1996). In the area of sex offender recidivism, however, the term can be easily misunderstood as many actuarial scales on a specific sample of offenders. Typically, these samples are of adult males in correctional or forensic psychiatric institutions (e.g., Hanson & Thornton, 2000). The scales typically include mostly "static" factors that are fixed in an offender's history, such as offense history, victim gender, age at release, number of prior sentencing dates, etc. They rely less on "dynamic" or potentially changeable factors such as self-management and substance abuse (Hanson & Harris, 2001). Hanson (2000) draws a distinction between "stable dynamic" variables that tend to remain in place across time (e.g., personality disorders) and "acute dynamic" factors that can change rapidly (e.g., anger).

Sachsenmaier (2001) observes:

> Each item is weighted by statistical analysis. The weights are summed. The total score falls within a risk category, and is tied to a statistical probability that a person will commit a dangerous act, based on a comparison to research sample offenders' actual recidivism at specified follow-up times. (from slide presentation)

A number of points are worth emphasizing. The first is that existing actuarial scales are in essence a comparison of an individual to a sample of offenders. In many cases there is a question of whether the individual is fundamentally different from those in the research sample, and to what extent the individuals in the research sample are different from each other.

For this reason, it is important to remember that a score on a given scale is not an absolute statement of risk. A common analogy is to the actuarial tables used by automobile insurance companies. It is known that young, unmarried males are at elevated risk for accidents, but it is not known *which* of those males will cause accidents. A typical objection to the use of actuarial data is that an individual should be assessed based on his own past misconduct and not that of other individuals. However, it is equally important to remember that many areas of science are based upon the behavior of groups.

Another area of some controversy is whether actuarial scales should be held to the same standards as psychological tests. Grisso (2000) has challenged others to ask themselves whether it is ethical under the standards of the American Psychological Association to use actuarial scales that have not met certain standards such as publication in a peer reviewed journal or included their psychometric properties. At the same time, instruments such as the Rapid Risk Assessment for Sex Offender Recidivism (RRASOR; Hanson, 1997) and Sex Offender Needs Assessment Rating (SONAR; Hanson & Harris, 2001) are, to a large extent, designed for use by probation officers and the like. Wherever one stands on the ethical issues of actuarial methods, it is of vital importance to understand how they are created and what limitations are inherent in their construction.

Presently, two of the leading scales are the Static 99 (Hanson & Thornton, 1999), and the Minnesota Sex Offender Screening Tool-Revised (MnSOST-R; Epperson, 2000). Although cross-validation studies have supported the use of these instruments (Barbaree, Seto, Langton, & Peacock, 2001), their use with juveniles remains contraindicated. They were constructed and validated on adult samples. While one study (Poole, Liedecke, & Marbibi, 2001) of the Static 99 found generally positive results, its authors noted both its small sample size ($N = 49$) and that the items regarding marital status and age at release are biased against the youths who were scored. The authors of the MnSOST-R recommend against its use with incest offenders due to their absence from the construction sample, and Roberts, Doren, and Thornton (2002) have commented on the scale's tendency to weigh antisocial elements more heavily. Ultimately, one can wonder whether the success of these scales is based on their detection of the persistence of sexual deviance and/or antisociality rather than upon its emergence.

In summary, actuarial methods can be a dramatic improvement over clinical judgment. They can be easy to use (Hanson, 1997), and are designed specifically for use in low base-rate situations where clinicians have typically performed at their worst (Monahan, 1981). They are subject to reduced distraction from interesting but non-predictive factors. They are increasingly recognized in diverse settings ranging from community-based treatment to forensic settings.

However, the same scales include inherent disadvantages. The inclusion of seemingly arbitrary items can raise concerns regarding their validity. The nature of relatively rare items, such as sexual sadism, can mask the frequency and severity (and therefore the overall dangerousness) of the risk involved.

Empirically Grounded Structured Assessment

Scales such as the SVR-20 (Boer, Hart, Kropp, & Webster, 1997) and HCR-20 (Webster, Douglas, Eaves, & Hart, 1997) have attracted considerable attention in adult sex offender risk assessment. Generally, they include a specific process for gathering information, but not for weighting it. They focus on both static and dynamic variables. The requirements for decision-making are less formalized than in actuarial scales, and they provide room for new information as it becomes available either through new collateral information, interview data, or observations in a given setting. This method can be particularly useful in larger settings where clinicians wish to use a common language for communicating impressions, formulations, and risk reduction strategies.

There is less research into the predictive validity of these instruments. The available research (e.g., Douglas, Ogloff, Nicholls, & Grant, 1999) suggests that it is the "static" historical factors that have the greatest predictive validity. Given the more subjective nature of the dynamic items (e.g., "lack of insight" in the HCR-20) the reliability and validity of these instruments may vary more across evaluators than the less idiographic actuarial scales.

Clinically Informed Actuarial

Sachsenmaier (2001) has described this as the following:

> Actuarial data are derived from a limited, however large, group of people. An individual may have characteristics relevant to his potential for reoffense not accounted for by the group data. It makes sense to use clinical judgment to augment actuarial determination in reaching a final opinion . . . Clinical judgment CANNOT CHANGE ACTUARIAL SCORES, only the final opinion. (from slide presentation)

In this fashion, an offender who scores lower on an actuarial scale but possesses a rare and particularly harmful condition such as necrophilia or sexual sadism is assessed with different recommendations than a less dangerous offender.

RISK ASSESSMENT OF YOUTH: AGGRAVATING FACTORS

While the previously described methods of assessing risk in adults may appear clear, they become further complicated by the developmental aspects of youth. These range from management of evolving sexuality (Hanson, 2002) to the persistence of antisociality across time (Peters, McMahon, & Quinsey,

1992). Further, youth as a whole are more dependent on their environment than adults, including the influences of family, school, and community. There is evidence that peer groupings may play a more significant role in sexual recidivism (Prentky et al., 2000). As noted earlier, there is evidence that sexual arousal patterns are more fluid and dynamic among adolescents (Hunter, 1999).

Additionally, Kernberg, Weiner, and Bardenstein (2000) have discussed the role of "heterotypic continuity" in youthful development. They observe that the expression of personality pathology can change across the lifespan. For example, an early proneness to boredom can develop into a propensity towards thrill-seeking behavior later on. Finally, Marshall and his colleagues' (1999) findings that confrontational treatment produces less favorable outcomes than warmth and empathy raise questions regarding the effect of the same approaches on youth. Those assessing risk for sexual reoffense among youth may wish to consider to what extent the individual's personality, sense of identity, attitudes, and beliefs are fully formed. More difficult still is the evolving understanding of brain development and plasticity (Siegel, 1999).

On the other hand, given the research described above, youth and community may best be served by risk assessment based largely on historical behaviors (e.g., persisting in a course of sexually abusive behavior despite detection, sanction, and intervention) and reserving more clinically based items for assessing the nature, frequency, and severity of such abuse and the interventions that will best reduce that risk. In any event, further research into this population is needed.

EMERGING STRATEGIES FOR ASSESSING RISK

The following scales are of interest to a broad range of individuals working with sexually abusive youth. Some, such as the ERASOR and Protective Factors Scale, are best used by clinicians having knowledge of adolescent development and sexual aggression, while the JSOAP and Langstrom and Grann's "tentative four-factor risk index" are more easily scored by professionals in other disciplines.

Langstrom and Grann's "Tentative Four-Factor Risk Index" (2000)

This scale's utility and application to North American populations is questionable given the original Swedish demographics. It has not yet been cross-validated, was developed on a small sample ($N = 46$), and has received little attention since its publication in the *Journal of Interpersonal Violence*. However, it is interesting in its simplicity.

The authors used four factors in assessing risk for sexual recidivism: (a) any previous sex offending behavior (including convictions), (b) poor social skills, (c) any male victim, and (d) two or more victims in the index offense ("index" meaning the offense that resulted in the subject becoming a part of the study).

Translated into a 4-point scale, the average recidivist had 2 points (*SD* = .87, range 1-3) while non-recidivists had an average score of .76 (*SD* = .83, range 0-3). The Receiver Operating Characteristic/Area Under the Curve (ROC/AUC) was .84 with a confidence level interval of 95%. The ROC coefficient basically equates to the probability that a randomly chosen recidivist will have a higher score than a randomly chosen non-recidivist. It examines the relationship between true and false positives and negatives with respect to instrument scoring, and is not vulnerable to the effects of low base rates.

Juvenile Sex Offender Assessment Protocol (JSOAP)

This widely-acclaimed instrument was first published as a 26-item scale (Prentky et al., 2000), but has recently been reduced to 23 items (Prentky, 2000). It is currently available from the website of the Center for Sex Offender Management at *www.csom.org*. Although it is regarded by many as an actuarial scale in that it contains fixed and explicit rules for scoring and weighting items, it has not yet been cross-validated and was developed on a small sample of 76 youth including three recidivists at a 1-year follow-up (see Table 2).

As noted above, of the four factors in the scale, it is factor two, the "impulsive, antisocial behavior" constellation that correlated the most highly with recidivism in the small research sample. This is interesting for a number of reasons.

First, the "impulsive, antisocial behavior" factor was, by design, modeled on the Child and Adolescent Taxon Scale (Quinsey et al., 1998). Also known by its acronym, the CATS was developed as a substitute for the Psychopathy Checklist-Revised, (PCL-R; Hare, 1991) or scores in the Violence Risk Appraisal Guide (VRAG; Quinsey et al., 1998). In this case, the CATS proved to be effective as easy to score from file review and/or self-report, and for many applications can be more cost-effective than the PCL-R. More recently, the CATS was used to provide evidence of an underlying antisociality taxon among children (Skilling, Quinsey, & Craig, 2001).

Second, the "sexual drive/preoccupation" factor was less correlated with recidivism in the research sample. Reasons for this are not known. It may be speculated that the nature of the youths' sexual crimes, fantasies, and drives result in many of the more dangerous youths not being released from institutions and therefore unavailable for follow-up. It may also be that the brief

TABLE 2. Items in the Juvenile Sex Offender Assessment Protocol (JSOAP)

Factor 1: Sexual Drive/Preoccupation
• Prior charged sex offenses
• Duration of sex offense history
• Evidence of sex preoccupation
• Planning in sexual development
• Sexualization of victim (e.g., atypical acts, sadism, protracted confinement, use of victim in pornography)

Factor 2: Impulsive, Antisocial Behavior
• Caregiver instability
• History of expressed anger
• School behavior problems (K-8)
• School suspensions or expulsions (K-8)
• History of Conduct Disorder (< age 10)
• Juvenile antisocial behavior (age 10-17)
• Charged or arrested before age 16
• Multiple types of offenses
• Impulsivity
• History of substance abuse
• History of parental substance abuse

Factor 3: Clinical/Treatment
• Accepts responsibility for offenses
• Internal motivation for change
• Understands sexual assault cycle and relapse prevention
• Evidence of empathy, remorse, guilt
• Absence of cognitive distortions

Factor 4: Community Stability/Adjustment (past 6 months)
• Evidence of poorly managed anger in the community
• Stability of current living situation
• Stability of school
• Support systems in community
• Quality of peer relationships

Note. These items cannot properly be scored without the instructions that are available from the original articles.

length of the follow-up played a role. Hanson and Bussiere (1998) found that, on average, rapists recidivated more rapidly than child molesters.

In summary, the JSOAP can be an effective aid to those assessing risk among youth. Clinical items such as empathy, remorse, guilt, and cognitive distortions are included but not weighted heavily when compared to historical items. Unfortunately, the specific role of these clinical items is not discussed fully. Many evaluators have met youth who freely admit their offenses out of pride and the arousal associated with recalling them. Other evaluators are familiar with the fact that strongly expressed remorse in a clinical interview does not mean that the same remorse will prevent future offenses (see the item description for remorse in Hare, 1991). Similarly, an internal motivation for change can change with time.

The JSOAP is relatively easy to score and contains many items associated with juvenile recidivism in the literature. It does not contain seemingly arbitrary items. It is already considered essential to understanding sexually abusive youth in many quarters. Like the SVR-20 and HCR-20 it can contribute to a common expression of findings and methods of treatment planning among groups of clinicians and other service providers.

The Protective Factors Scale (PFS)

This scale (see Table 3) is available from its author, Janis Bremer, PhD, of Project Pathfinder, Inc. in St. Paul, Minnesota. It measures key areas of functioning that serve to protect youth from further sexual misconduct. Although the instrument remains in development, it is a departure from more traditional approaches to risk assessment. By emphasizing those factors that mitigate risk, the PFS lends itself to a broad range of treatment approaches and strength-based risk management strategies.

In a draft version, Bremer (2001) states:

> The Protective Factors Scale was initially designed as a way to evaluate the adequacy of initial placement orders for treatment. The results of the pilot study indicate that the PFS did predict at what level of placement a youth would successfully complete treatment. It is a placement tool that fits a unique niche. Community safety involves more than simply sexual recidivism. A means of where to place a youth on a continuum of care (Bengis, 1997) is quite useful. The continuum of care places a youth on a range of service from short-term psycho-educational community-based through intensive outpatient treatment, placement in the community, placement out of the community and correctional secure placement. (p. 1)

With the PFS, Bremer emphasizes that thinking exclusively in terms of "risk" is not sufficient to reduce that risk. Many users resonate with the focus on those factors that prevent youth from reoffense. Others find this in line with Andrews and Bonta's (1998) recommendation that the principles of need and responsivity be considered alongside risk.

In summary, The Protective Factors Scale is easy to use and focuses on elements that can help prevent sexual recidivism by building on the strengths of the youth, their family, and community. In this way, it can contribute meaningfully to risk reduction strategies and methods. Initial results show that it can be effective in decisions regarding level of care. It contains items shown to be related both to increased risk and the healthy development of youth. Beyond its use as a scale, it can serve as a useful group of elements for clinicians to consider in developing treatment plans and interventions. It should not be used in isolation from other risk assessment methods.

TABLE 3. Items Currently in the Protective Factors Scale (PFS)

Factor 1: Sexuality • Identified concern characteristics • Personal boundaries • Sexual preference
Factor 2: Personal Development • General behavior • School attendance • Social adjustment • Emotional adjustment
Factor 3: Environmental Support • Caregiver stability • Family style • Cooperation

Note. These items cannot properly be scored without the instructions that are available form the original articles. At this writing, the scale is still in development and available from its author. These items are included only to encourage readers to consider protective factors in assessments of risk.

Estimate of Risk of Adolescent Sex Offender Recidivism (ERASOR)

This scale is available from its principle author, James Worling, at The Safe-T Program, Thistletown Regional Centre, 51 Panorama Court, Toronto, Ontario, Canada, M9V 4L8.

Modeled on the HCR-20 and SVR-20, where items are scored as present, absent, and partially/possibly present, the ERASOR (Worling & Curwen, 2000a) is an example of an empirically grounded structured risk assessment method. Although its items (see Table 4) may appear easy to score, many require a great deal of consideration. At this writing, there is no available information on inter-rater reliability, predictive validity, or other psychometric properties.

Advantages of the ERASOR include the ability to consider a wide range of information in forming impressions and recommendations. It can be used as a tool for evaluation, treatment planning, and delivery. Like other structured assessment methods, it enables the use of a common language among groups of clinicians. Many of the items have the potential to be used for evaluating treatment outcomes.

Perhaps the greatest advantage of the ERASOR is its manual and the item descriptions themselves, which provide an extensive overview of the literature as well as the difficulties inherent in adolescent sexual abuser risk assessment. In its present form, it represents the current state of the art.

The items in the ERASOR reflect several possible pathways to reoffense. In keeping with current research, these can include pathways reflective of an emerging sexual disorder, antisociality, or chronic detachment (Roberts, Doren, & Thornton, 2002). The ERASOR includes both static and dynamic factors, in-

TABLE 4. Items from Estimate of Risk of Adolescent Sex Offender Recidivism (ERASOR)

- Deviant sexual interest (younger children, violence, or both)
- "Obsessive" sexual interests/Preoccupation with sexual thoughts
- Attitudes supportive of sexual offending
- Unwillingness to alter deviant sexual interests/attitudes
- Ever assaulted 2 or more victims
- Ever assaulted same victim 2 or more times
- Prior adult sanctions for sexual assault(s)
- Threats of, or use of, violence/weapons during sexual offense
- Ever sexually assaulted a child
- Ever sexually assaulted a stranger
- Indiscriminate choice of victims
- Ever sexually assaulted a male victim (male offenders only)
- Diverse sexual-assault behaviors
- Antisocial interpersonal orientation
- Lack of intimate peer relationships/social isolation
- Negative peer associations and influences
- Interpersonal aggression
- Recent escalation in anger or negative affect
- Poor self-regulation of affect and behavior (Impulsivity)
- High-stress family environment
- Problematic parent-offender relationships/parental rejection
- Parent(s) not supporting sexual-offense-specific assessment/treatment
- Environment supporting opportunity to offend
- No development or practice of realistic prevention plans/strategies
- Incomplete offense-specific treatment

Note. Reading the item descriptions is of primary importance. The items above are included only to give the reader a rough idea of areas to be assessed in the ERASOR.

cluding those that are relatively stable over time (e.g., incomplete offense-specific treatment) and those that can change acutely and rapidly (e.g., recent escalation in anger or negative affect). The manual provides a comprehensive yet succinct set of descriptions of the individual items.

Each of these scales is informed by the research into this population, and each is fairly easy to use. None have been subjected to a significant level of scrutiny such as cross-validation, but ongoing study into them continues. Scales such as the PFS and ERASOR require some level of clinical skill, while the JSOAP and Langstrom and Grann's tentative four-factor scale can be used as brief screening tools for non-clinical purposes. However, their limitations should be fully understood by those who employ them and communicate their findings.

CONCLUSIONS

Those working with sexually abusive youth, whether at the front lines of community, residential, or secure treatment, are frequently asked to render judgment regarding risk. Although there remains no empirically validated means of classifying long-term risk among adolescent sexual abusers, those assessing risk will serve both the individual and their communities best by being familiar with the emerging research and strategies regarding this most difficult population.

This article highlights a number of emerging tools that are grounded in recent research. Approaching the problem of risk assessment from three different directions, (a) actuarial/semi-actuarial (JSOAP, tentative four-factor scale), (b) empirically grounded structured assessment (ERASOR), and (c) protective factors (PFS), these scales are the current state of the art in adolescent risk assessment.

As much of an "improvement over chance" as these scales may represent, they are not yet at an acceptable level of competence in assessing risk among adolescents. Many potential markers of sexual recidivism remain un-addressed, including the lack of knowledge regarding the role of intelligence, neurological insult, and personality development. Under these conditions, the best efforts of risk assessors should be directed toward communicating risk in such a way that our youth and their communities do not suffer any unnecessary harm.

REFERENCES

Alexander, M. (1999). Sexual offender treatment efficacy revisited. *Sexual Abuse: A Journal of Research and Treatment, 11*, 101-116.

Andrews, D.A., & Bonta, J.L. (1998). *The psychology of criminal conduct* (2nd ed.). Cincinnati: Anderson Publishing.

Barbaree, H.E., Seto, M.C., Langton, C., & Peacock, E. (2001). Evaluating the predictive accuracy of six risk assessment instruments for adult sex offenders. *Criminal Justice and Behavior, 28*, 490-521.

Becker, J.V. (1990). Treating adolescent sexual offenders. *Professional Psychology: Research and Practice, 21*, 362-365.

Bengis, S. (1997). Comprehensive service delivery within a continuum of care. In G. Ryan, & S. Lane (Eds.), *Juvenile sexual offending: Causes, consequences, and correction* (pp. 211-218). San Francisco: Jossey-Bass.

Boer, D.P., Hart, S.D., Kropp, P.R., & Webster, C.D. (1997). *Sexual violence risk-20: Professional guidelines for assessing risk of sexual violence.* Burnaby, British Columbia, Canada: The Mental Health, Law, and Policy Institute of Simon Fraser University.

Borduin, C.M., Henggeler, S.W., Blaske, D.M., & Stein, R.J. (1990). Multisystemic treatment of adolescent sexual offenders. *International Journal of Offender Therapy and Comparative Criminology, 39*, 317-326.

Bremer, J.F. (1992). Serious juvenile sex offenders: Treatment and long-term follow-up. *Psychiatric Annals, 22,* 326-32.

Bremer, J.F. (1998). Challenges in the assessment and treatment of sexually abusive adolescents. *Irish Journal of Psychology, 19,* 82-92.

Bremer, J.F. (2001, May). The protective factors scale: Assessing youth with sexual concerns. Plenary address presented at the 16th annual conference of the National Adolescent Perpetration Network, Kansas City, MO.

Curwen, T. (2000a, May). Utility of the interpersonal reactivity index (IRI) as a measure of empathy in male adolescent sex offenders. Paper presented at the 6th International Conference on the Treatment of Sexual Offenders, Toronto, Ontario.

Curwen, T. (2000b). *A survey of residential programs for sexually offending adolescents.* Mississauga, Ontario: Peel Collaborative Child and Adolescent Treatment Program.

Daleiden, E.L., Kaufman, K.L., Hilliker, D.R., & O'Neil, J.N. (1998). The sexual histories and fantasies of youthful males: A comparison of sexual offending, nonsexual offending, and non-offending groups. *Sexual Abuse: A Journal of Research and Treatment, 10,* 195-209.

Douglas, K. S., Ogloff, J. R. P., Nicholls, T. L., & Grant, I. (1999). Assessing risk for violence among psychiatric patients: The HCR-20 risk assessment scheme and the Psychopathy Checklist: Screening Version. *Journal of Consulting and Clinical Psychology, 67,* 917-930.

Efta-Breitbach, J., & Freeman, K.A. (2004). Recidivism and resilience in juvenile sexual offenders: An analysis of the literature. *Journal of Child Sexual Abuse, 13*(3/4), pp. 125-138 .

Elliott, D.S. (1994, November). *The developmental course of sexual and non-sexual violence: Results from a national longitudinal study.* Paper presented at the meeting of the Association for the Treatment of Sexual Abusers' 13th Annual Research and Treatment Conference, San Francisco, CA.

Epperson, D. (2000, March). *The Minnesota sex offender screening tool-revised.* Paper presented at Sinclair Seminars' Sex Offender Reoffense Risk Prediction Symposium, Madison, WI.

Forth, A.E., & Mailloux, D.L. (2000). Psychopathy in youth: What do we know? In C.B. Gacono (Ed.), *The clinical and forensic assessment of psychopathy* (pp. 25-54). Mahwah, NJ: Lawrence Erlbaum Associates.

Garb, H. (1998). *Studying the clinician: Judgment research and psychological assessment.* Washington, DC: American Psychological Association.

Gray, A.S., & Pithers, W.D. (1993). Relapse prevention with sexually aggressive adolescents and children: Expanding treatment and supervision. In H.E. Barbaree, W.L. Marshall, & S. Hudson (Eds.), *The juvenile sex offender* (pp. 289-320). New York: Guilford Press.

Grisso, T. (2000). Ethical issues in sex offender reoffense risk prediction, in *Sex offender reoffense risk assessment* [videotape presentation]. (Available from www.sinclairseminars.com).

Grove, W.M., Zald, D.H., Boyd, S., Lebow, S., Snitz, B.E., & Nelson, C. (2001). Clinical versus mechanical prediction. *Psychological Assessment, 12*(1), 19-30.

Hagan, M.P., & Cho, M.E. (1996). A comparison of treatment outcomes between adolescent rapists and child sexual offenders. *International Journal of Offender Therapy and Comparative Criminology, 40,* 113-122.

Hanson, R.K. (1997). *The development of a brief actuarial risk scale for sexual offender recidivism* (User Report 1997-04). Ottawa: Department of the Solicitor General of Canada.

Hanson, R.K. (1998). *Predicting sex offender recidivism* [videotape presentation]. Madison, WI: Wisconsin Sex Offender Treatment Network.

Hanson, R.K. (2000). *Risk assessment.* Beaverton, OR: Association for the Treatment of Sexual Abusers.

Hanson, R.K. (2002). Recidivism and age: Follow-up data from 4,673 sex offenders. *Journal of Interpersonal Violence, 17,* 1046-1062.

Hanson, R.K., & Bussiere, M.T. (1998). Predicting relapse: A meta-analysis of sexual offender recidivism studies. *Journal of Consulting and Clinical Psychology, 66* (2), 348-362.

Hanson, R.K., & Harris, A.J.R. (2001). A structured approach to evaluating change among sexual offenders. *Sexual Abuse: A Journal of Research and Treatment, 13,* 105-122.

Hanson, R.K., & Thornton, D. (1999). *Static 99: Improving actuarial risk assessments for sex offenders* (User Report 1999-02). Ottawa: Department of the Solicitor General of Canada.

Hanson, R.K., & Thornton, D. (2000). Improving actuarial risk assessments for sex offenders, *Law and Human Behavior, 24,* 119-136.

Hare, R.D. (1991). *The Hare psychopathy checklist-revised.* Toronto: Multi-Health Systems, Inc.

Hart, S.D. (2001, June). *Complexity, uncertainty, and the reconceptualization of violence risk assessment.* Paper presented at the meeting of the European Association of Psychology and Law, Lisbon, Portugal.

Hunter, J. (1999). *Understanding juvenile sexual offending behavior: Emerging research, treatment approaches, and management practices.* Washington, DC: Center for Sex Offender Management.

Kahn, T.J., & Chambers, H.J. (1991). Assessing reoffense risk with juvenile sex offenders. *Child Welfare, 70,* 333-345.

Kahn, T.J., & Lafond, M.A. (1988). Treatment of the adolescent sexual offender. *Child and Adolescent Social Work, 5,* 135-148.

Kenny, D.T., Keough, T., & Seidler, K. (2001). Predictors of recidivism in Australian juvenile sex offenders: Implications for treatment. *Sexual Abuse: A Journal of Research and Treatment, 13,* 131-148.

Kernberg, P.F., Weiner, A.S., & Bardenstein, K.K. (2000). *Personality disorders in children and adolescents.* New York: Basic Books.

Knight, R.A., & Prentky, R.A. (1993). Exploring characteristics for classifying juvenile sex offenders. In H.E. Barbaree, W.L. Marshall, & S. Hudson (Eds.), *The juvenile sex offender* (pp. 45-83). New York: Guilford Press.

Lab, S.P., Shields, G., & Schondel, C. (1993). Research note: An evaluation of juvenile sexual offender treatment. *Crime and Delinquency, 39,* 543-553.

Langstrom, N., & Grann, M. (2000). Risk for criminal recidivism among young sex offenders. *Journal of Interpersonal Violence, 15,* 855-871.

Longo, R.E. (2004). An integrated experiential approach to treating young people who sexually abuse. *Journal of Child Sexual Abuse, 13*(3/4), pp. 193-215.

Lund, C. A. (2000). Predictors of sexual recidivism: Did meta-analysis clarify the role and relevance of denial? *Sexual Abuse: A Journal of Research and Treatment, 12,* 275-288.

Marshall, W.L., Anderson, D., & Fernandez, Y. (1999). *Cognitive behavioral treatment of sexual offenders.* Chichester, UK: Wiley.

Mazur, T., & Michael, P.M. (1992). Outpatient treatment for adolescents with sexually inappropriate behavior: Program description and six-month follow-up. *Journal of Offender Rehabilitation, 18,* 191-203.

Meehl, P. (1954/1996). *Clinical versus statistical prediction.* Northvale, NJ: Jason Aronson.

Miner, M.H. (2000, May). *Can we find the active ingredients in sex offender treatment?: A preliminary analysis.* Paper presented at the 6th International Conference on the Treatment of Sexual Offenders, Toronto, Ontario.

Monahan, J. (1981). *The clinical prediction of violent behavior.* Northvale, NJ: Jason Aronson Inc.

Monahan, J., Steadman, H.J., Silver, E., Applebaum, P.S., Robbins, P.C., Mulvey, E.P., Roth, L.H., Grisso, T., & Banks, S. (2001). *Rethinking risk assessment: The Macarthur study of violence and mental disorder.* New York: Oxford University Press.

Peters, R.D., McMahon, R.J., & Quinsey, V.L. (1992). *Aggression and violence throughout the life span.* Newbury Park, CA: Sage Publications.

Pithers, W.D., Beal, L.S., Armstrong, J., & Petty, J. (1989). Identification of risk factors through records analysis and clinical interview. In D.R. Laws (Ed.), *Relapse prevention with sex offenders* (pp. 77-87). New York: Guilford Press.

Poole, D., Liedecke, D., & Marbibi, M. (2001). *Risk assessment and recidivism in juvenile sex offenders: A validation study of the static 99.* Austin, TX: Texas Youth Commission.

Prentky, R. (2000, March). *Juvenile sex offender assessment protocol (JSOAP).* Paper presented at the Sinclair Seminars' Sex Offender Reoffense Risk Prediction Symposium, Madison, WI.

Prentky, R., Harris, B., Frizzell, K., & Righthand, S. (2000). An actuarial procedure for assessing risk with juvenile sex offenders. *Sexual Abuse: A Journal of Research and Treatment, 12,* 71-94.

Prescott, D.S. (2001). Collaborative treatment for sexual behavior problems in an adolescent residential treatment center. *Journal of Psychology and Human Sexuality, 13,* 43-58.

Quinsey, V.L., Harris, G.T., Rice, M.E., & Cormier, C.A. (1998). *Violent offenders: Managing and appraising risk.* Washington DC: American Psychological Association.

Resnick, P. (1996). *The clinical prediction of violence* [audiotaped lecture]. (Available from Specialized Training Services, www.specializedtraining.com).

Roberts, C.F., Doren, D.M., & Thornton, D. (2002). Dimensions associated with sex offender recidivism risk. *Criminal Justice and Behavior, 29,* 569-589.

Ryan, G., & Lane, S. (1997). *Juvenile sexual offending: Causes, consequences, and correction.* San Francisco. Jossey-Bass.

Sachsenmaier, S.J. (2001, November). *Expert witness testimony and sex offender risk assessment.* Paper presented at the 20th Annual Research and Treatment Conference of the Association for the Treatment of Sexual Abusers, San Antonio, TX.

Safer Society Program. (1993). *Juvenile and adult female sex offender treatment programs identified by safer society program* (Information sheet). Brandon, VT: Author.

Salter, A.C. (1988). *Treating child sex offenders and victims.* Newbury Park, CA: Sage Publications.

Serin, R.C., & Brown, S.L. (2000). The clinical use of the Hare psychopathy checklist-revised in contemporary risk assessment. In C.G. Gacono (Ed.), *The clinical and forensic assessment of psychopathy* (pp. 251-268). Mahwah, NJ: Lawrence Erlbaum Associates.

Siegel, D.J. (1999). *The developing mind: Toward a neurobiology of interpersonal experience.* New York: Guilford Press.

Skilling, T.A., Quinsey, V.L., & Craig, W.M. (2001). Evidence of a taxon underlying serious antisocial behavior in boys. *Criminal Justice and Behavior, 28,* 450-470.

Smith, W.R., & Monastersky, C. (1986). Assessing juvenile sexual offenders' risk for reoffending. *Criminal Justice and Behavior, 13,* 115-140.

Thornton, D. (2000, March). *Structured risk assessment.* Paper presented at Sinclair Seminars' Sex Offender Reoffense Risk Prediction Symposium, Madison, WI.

Webster, C.D., Ben-Aron, M.H., & Hucker, S.J. (1985). *Dangerousness: Probability and prediction, psychiatry, and public policy.* Cambridge, MA: Cambridge University Press.

Webster, C.D., Douglas, K.S., Eaves, D., & Hart, S.D. (1997). *HCR-20: Assessing risk for violence.* Burnaby, British Columbia, Canada: The Mental Health, Law, and Policy Institute of Simon Fraser University.

Webster, C.D., Harris, G.T., Rice, M.E., Cormier, C.A., & Quinsey, V.L. (1994). *The violence prediction scheme: Assessing dangerousness in high risk men.* Toronto: Centre of Criminology, University of Toronto.

Webster, C.D., Hucker, S.J., & Bloom, H. (2002). Transcending the actuarial versus clinical polemic in assessing risk for violence. *Criminal Justice and Behavior, 29,* 659-665.

Weinrott, M.R. (1996). *Juvenile sexual aggression: A critical review.* Boulder CO: Center for the Study and Prevention of Violence.

Worling, J.R. (1999, November). *Beyond the looking glass: Predicting adolescent sex offender recidivism from the results of a 10-year treatment study.* Paper presented at the 18th Annual Research and Treatment Conference of the Association for the Treatment of Sexual Abusers, Lake Buena Vista, FL.

Worling, J.R. (2001). Personality-based typology of adolescent male sexual offenders: Differences in recidivism rates, victim-selection characteristics, and personal victimization histories. *Sexual Abuse: A Journal of Research and Treatment, 13,* 149-166.

Worling, J.R., & Curwen, T. (2000a). *Estimate of risk of adolescent sexual offense recidivism (ERASOR)*. Toronto, Canada: Thistletown Regional Centre for Children and Adolescents, Ontario Ministry of Community and Social Services.

Worling, J.R., & Curwen, T. (2000b). Adolescent sexual offender recidivism: Success of specialized treatment and implications for risk prediction. *Child Abuse and Neglect, 24*, 965-982.

Zolondek, S.C., Abel, G.G., Northey, W.F., & Jordan, A.D. (2001). The self-reported behaviors of juvenile sex offenders. *Journal of Interpersonal Violence, 16*, 73-85.

Interviewing Strategies
with Sexually Abusive Youth

Ian Lambie
John McCarthy

SUMMARY. Adolescents who have sexually abused may pose a serious problem for both the community and the treatment provider concerning the management of risk and the application of effective intervention strategies. Fundamental to providing good clinical treatment is an assessment that results in an individualized treatment plan specifically tailored to the young person's needs. An integral but often overlooked part of this involves interviewing clients in a way that elicits accurate information and facilitates the development of a therapeutic relationship upon which effective therapy can be undertaken. This article will describe interviewing strategies and highlight the importance of the

---

Address corespondence to: Ian Lambie, PhD, Psychology Department, University of Auckland, Private Bag 92019, Auckland, New Zealand (E-mail: i.lambie@auckland.ac.nz).

Submitted for publication 7/30/03; revised 1/8/04; accepted 1/20/04.

[Haworth co-indexing entry note]: "Interviewing Strategies with Sexually Abusive Youth." Lambie, Ian, and John McCarthy. Co-published simultaneously in *Journal of Child Sexual Abuse* (The Haworth Maltreatment and Trauma Press, an imprint of The Haworth Press, Inc.) Vol. 13, No. 3/4, 2004, pp. 107-123 and: *Identifying and Treating Youth Who Sexually Offend: Current Approaches, Techniques, and Research* (ed: Robert Geffner et al.) The Haworth Maltreatment and Trauma Press, an imprint of The Haworth Press, Inc., 2004, pp. 107-123. Single or multiple copies of this article are available for a fee from The Haworth Document Delivery Service [1-800-HAWORTH, 9:00 a.m. - 5:00 p.m. (EST). E-mail address: docdelivery@haworthpress.com].

client-therapist relationship in providing effective therapeutic interventions. *[Article copies available for a fee from The Haworth Document Delivery Service: 1-800-HAWORTH. E-mail address: <docdelivery@haworthpress. com> Website: <http://www.HaworthPress.com> © 2004 by The Haworth Press, Inc. All rights reserved.]*

KEYWORDS. Interviewing, therapist-client relationship, motivation, motivational interviewing, family therapy, interviewing strategies

One of the most distinguishing factors in counseling adolescents who have sexually abused is their relatively insistent desire to deny and minimize their offending behavior. Such processes serve to protect them from facing the full extent of what they have done from both a legal and personal perspective. This is inherently a natural response that all humans may at least contemplate when faced with an adverse situation. Namely, it minimizes the perceived or actual harm they may face.

For this reason, many clinicians choose not to work with this population or do not remain in this type of work for long periods. Numerous studies have consistently suggested that client characteristics are important in determining the outcome of psychotherapy (e.g., Anderson & Lambert, 1995). These factors include the type, severity, and complexity of the presenting problem, the client's motivation, past trauma and current coping styles, and the client's level of responsibility for the change process.

In the treatment of sexually abusive youth, therapists must be aware of the risk factors and particular client variables that are likely to affect the adolescent and their family's responsivity to treatment and subsequent treatment outcome (e.g., motivation, family support, stability, and type of living placement). This article will outline the key issues that clinicians face when working with this population and provide practical strategies to assist clinicians in working effectively with adolescents in denial.

THE PROCESS OF CHANGE

Despite the fact that treatment of adolescent sexual offenders dates back to the early 1980s, there is surprisingly little literature available on treatment modalities that have been found effective with this group. It is widely accepted that adolescent sex offender treatment has been informed by adult sex offender treatment, which in turn has shaped programs for younger children. Yet the question remains, are models and methods used by adults appropriate for younger populations?

What is apparent in working with any client group is the role that psychotherapeutic factors play in assisting change within the client. A significant body of research indicates that the effectiveness of therapy may in fact have more to do with process issues (e.g., client-therapist relationship), as opposed to therapeutic techniques (Hubble, Duncan, & Miller, 1999). In 1936, Saul Rosenzweig provided what was thought to be the first systematic argument suggesting that the effectiveness of therapy may have more to do with the therapeutic process as opposed to different theoretical orientations (Luborsky, Singer, & Luborsky, 1975). From scientific studies on psychotherapy outcome research, Lambert (1992) proposed that therapy composed of four therapeutic factors. He called these: (a) extra-therapeutic factors, (b) therapeutic techniques, (c) relationship factors, and (d) expectancy or placebo factors.

Extra-Therapeutic Factors

Lambert (1992) argued that extra-therapeutic factors, or client factors, are the most important of the factors that exist amongst psychotherapies. Extra-therapeutic factors are what clients bring with them to therapy as well as environmental influences. They may include the client's strengths, social supports, the sense of personal responsibility, the severity and type of problem, the motivation to change, the strength of social supports, and the presence or absence of co-morbidity.

Commonly, adolescent offenders may present with co-morbid disorders that may include Conduct Disorder, Attention-Deficit Hyperactivity Disorder, substance abuse, and Posttraumatic Stress Disorder (Bourke & Donohue, 1996; Lightfoot & Barbaree, 1993; Morenz & Becker, 1995; Ryan, Miyoshi, Metzner, Krugman, & Fryer, 1996). The presence of these disorders and the aforementioned factors can affect whether there is a positive or negative outcome in psychotherapy. Co-morbid disorders left untreated can lead to significant impairment and distress that likely impact negatively on treatment. High levels of trauma reported by these adolescents are also likely to impact negatively on the outcome of treatment, possibly through subsequent dysregulation of emotional states and a resulting hyper-arousal to stimulus in their environment (Friedrich, 1995).

Research suggests that client factors change at varying rates and may account for as much as 40% of the outcome in psychotherapy (Bergin & Garfield, 1994). For example, motivation may vary quite rapidly as opposed to personality variables that may remain relatively stable over time. What is evident is that clients who show the most improvement believe the results of their gains are primarily due to themselves as opposed to therapist or other external factors (for an in-depth discussion of factors associated with both recidivism and resiliency in adolescents who sexually offend, see Efta- Breitbach & Freeman, this issue).

Therapeutic Techniques

Therapeutic techniques are factors that are specific to the therapy the client is undergoing. It includes the therapy model (e.g., in adolescent sexual offender treatment the predominant models are cognitive-behavioral and family systems). Despite many studies being undertaken comparing one model with another, surprisingly little evidence has been found for one model being superior over another (Lambert, 1992). In the field of adolescent sex offender treatment, the research is still in its infancy, and comparative studies of one therapeutic model over another have yet to be undertaken. Lambert (1992) suggested that the therapeutic technique may account for approximately 15% of the outcome in psychotherapy.

Relationship Factors

Another significant factor that contributes to the process of change in clients is the relationship between therapist and client. These include a positive regard towards the client, genuineness, and congruence with the client. Other factors such as being able to express empathy and affirmation towards the client when appropriate also impact on treatment outcome. Relationship factors are thought to account for up to 30% of the treatment outcome in counseling. Some of these factors include warmth, caring, empathy, acceptance, mutual affirmation, and encouragement. Lambert and Bergin (1994) proposed that these probably account for the most gain in psychotherapy.

Bordin (1976) suggested that there are three important components of the therapeutic alliance that impact the outcome: (a) goals, (b) tasks, and (c) bonds. The goals of therapy are the objectives that both the client and therapist agree on, while the tasks are the nuts and bolts of a therapy session that include both behaviors and processes. For a strong therapeutic alliance to happen, it is important that both therapist and client view these as important. Finally, therapeutic bonds are the positive relationship between a client and therapist that includes trust, confidence, and acceptance (for additional discussion of the therapeutic relationship, see Longo, this issue).

Expectancy/Placebo Factors

The final set of factors is placebo, hope, and expectancy. This involves clients gaining improvement based on their knowledge that they are being treated and their assessment that the therapist is credible. One common factor that influences all medicine and psychotherapeutic outcomes is that treatment in itself offers people hope that change can take place. Lambert (1992) argued that hope and expectancy of change may be as important in producing change as technique. It is thought to account for up to 15% of the variance in client change. Lambert, Weber, and Sykes (1993) reviewed studies looking at the effect sizes of psychotherapy, placebo, and no-treatment controls. They found that the average client placed in placebo treatment has a 66% greater improvement compared with no-treatment controls, while an average client undergoing psychotherapy is better off than 79% of clients who do not receive any treatment.

Conclusions

The fact that client outcome is principally determined by client variables and extra-therapeutic effects as opposed to the therapist or therapy techniques adds further support to the role that risk factors play in the treatment outcome of adolescent sexual offenders. While the therapeutic relationship is important in supporting change in psychotherapy, in our opinion, one of the challenges of sex offender treatment is that few clients in the early stages of treatment possess any real *desire* to change.

MOTIVATIONAL INTERVIEWING

An important development in the rehabilitation of sexual offenders has been the work on motivational interviewing by Prochaska and DiClemente (1984), Garland and Dougher (1991), and Miller and Rollnick (2002). Motivational interviewing is a model of assisting clients who may be experiencing resistance to change. It relies on a variety of techniques by which the clinician can increase the internal motivation of the client towards change and assist them in sustaining new behaviors and avoiding relapse.

Burke, Arkowitz, and Dunn's (2002) review of adapted motivational interviewing (defined by the presence of feedback or other additional features alongside the core components of motivational interviewing) reported widespread empirical support with a range of disorders, including alcohol and substance abuse, the treatment of diabetes, hypertension, dual diagnosis disorders, and bulimia. However, no studies using purely motivational interviewing have been conducted. Burke and colleagues concluded that motivational interviewing is superior to no-treatment control groups and has often been as effective as more standard treatments that are two or three times longer.

Two key assumptions of motivational interviewing are that (a) a client's resistance typically stems from his/her environment and (b) motivation to change behavior (or to overcome their resistance) is elicited from within the client rather than externally. While these issues may pertain to adolescents, there are also maturational processes that may be unique to this client population, such as anti-authoritarian issues. In addition, an adolescent's initial engagement in therapy is often mandated, and motivation may increase over time.

The role of the clinician is not to persuade the client to change or resolve the client's ambivalence. Rather, the clinician's task is to quietly direct the client towards examining that ambivalence and to develop discrepancy and dissonance in the client about his/her situation. Arguments with clients are to be avoided; resistance is not to be directly confronted. Instead, the clinician is encouraged to argue indirectly—to 'roll' with the client's resistance in much the same way as a martial arts fighter might roll with his opponent's momentum and use it to make his opponent's position less secure. At the same time, clinicians must operate from a position of empathy with their client. They must create for the client a sense that change is both desirable and achievable, and that efforts towards change will be based on a collaborative effort rather than imposed and directed by the clinician.

STAGES OF CHANGE

Six stages of change have been identified through which clients may progress during the process of change (Miller & Rollnick, 1991). These stages are often referred to as the "wheel of change."

Pre-Contemplation

At this first stage in the cycle of change, a client has not yet realized the need for change, although someone else may be aware that they have a problem. If pointed out by someone else, the client may be surprised and bewildered but not defensive. Clients at this stage require information and feedback in order to raise their level of awareness.

Contemplation

Clients in the contemplation stage present with a reasonable understanding of what has brought them to treatment, but they may still feel ambivalent about change. They may be weighing the pros and cons of the status quo as compared to making the required changes. Clients at this stage need gentle challenging so that any comparisons arrived at are realistic. They also need encouragement to see that change is possible.

Preparation

After some time, clients may come to feel as though the reasons for changing their behavior outweigh the reasons for keeping it the same. They become increasingly interested in and ready to change. They may begin to experiment with change, or make plans to change; they may even make some initial changes. At some point during this stage, they have made a decision to change. Clients at this stage require reassurance and support that they have made the right decision.

Action

Clients in the action stage are in the process of making changes and trying out new ways of behaving. Again, considerable support may be necessary for clients, particularly for those who lack the necessary self-esteem or for whom the changes may result in major lifestyle consequences (e.g., leaving a long-term relationship).

Maintenance

The maintenance stage involves clients attempting to sustain their changes and beginning to implement strategies that will prevent their relapsing into old behaviors. This may lead to permanent change. However, there may also be occasional 'lapses' back into the old ways. Lapses are temporary slippages, and while they may be frustrating and demoralizing, they are not unexpected or unusual. Usually with a lapse, the client's desire to change remains.

Relapses

'Relapses' are different from the occasional 'lapses' described above. In addition to the old behaviors returning for a longer period of time, a relapse is usually accompanied by a return to earlier change stages such as pre-contemplation, during which clients question their motivation and rationale for change.

Following a relapse, the client will need to re-visit all the stages of the wheel of change rather than simply begin again at the action stage. This is necessary in order to ensure that their readiness and motivation to change is as strong as possible.

INTERVIEWING STRATEGIES

A number of techniques from the Motivational Interviewing model may be used effectively with sexually abusive youth and are outlined in the following strategies.

Read the Background Notes

Prior to the interview, read all documentation available on the adolescent, his/her family, and the victim's disclosure.

Establish Rapport

Putting the client first will increase the likelihood of honesty and compliance in counseling.

Show Respect

The clinician should create a context for respectful behavior in the interview and model this for the adolescent. For example, only respectful language should be allowed (no sexually aggressive terms for body parts, etc.). If challenging the adolescent's cognitive distortions, clinicians should tell the adolescent that they have concerns for them and respect them as a person, but have no respect for their offending behavior (e.g., "I respect you and believe you deserve a better life than that of continuing your sexually abusive behavior, so I want to be really honest with you about your offending"). By doing this, the clinician models both respect and honesty.

Take Care in Expressing Emotion

The clinician should take care not to distance the adolescent by showing strong emotional reaction to their disclosures.

Create a Context for Honesty

The clinician should preface the interview by talking about the importance of honesty and the consequences for the offender of not being honest. It can be helpful if the clinician is able to use some form of leverage with the offender if they are not honest. Bearing in mind that the adolescent may be fearful of the consequences if the offending is admitted, it is crucial to have obtained from the family strong statements of their support for the adolescent being honest. It might be useful to inform the adolescent that they may change their account later to a more honest one. The clinician should support and reinforce even the smallest admission of offending by the adolescent with praise for being honest. This increases the likelihood that the adolescent will be more honest in the future.

Clinicians should also be aware of the importance not only of under-disclosing but of over-disclosing, as the young person may want to please the professional and say what he/she thinks the clinician wants to hear. Remember, more does not necessarily equal a more honest disclosure.

Establish Credibility and Control of the Interview

Clinicians should state from the beginning of the interview that they have experience with other adolescents who have sexually abused. Clinicians can seem especially credible if they can predict what the adolescent might be thinking and the extent of the adolescent's offending.

Open-Ended Questions

Asking open-ended questions is especially important in allowing the adolescent to talk about their offending in as much detail as possible and to allow them sufficient time to do this.

Be Sexually Explicit

The clinician needs to be prepared to be sexually explicit in the interview. Similarly, adolescents may need some warning that they will be expected to discuss their sexual behavior in detail and that this may be embarrassing for them.

Anticipate Embarrassment

Adolescent sex offenders may have their own stereotype that sexually abusive adolescents are totally deviant and worthless. The clinician can help facilitate disclosure by downplaying that stereotype. The clinician can also compare the adolescent's discomfort experienced now with the probable increased discomfort that would be experienced if the adolescent's offending were to continue. It is also a well-known phenomenon that many offenders feel a sense of relief when they finally disclose their offending.

Offer Hope Through Therapy

It can be comforting for the adolescent and his/her family if therapy is discussed as a positive experience. The clinician must outline the positive aspects of therapy, as well as the consequences for refusing it. They could also use examples of other adolescents for whom therapy has been successful. It might be useful to say things such as, "You're really lucky to have this opportunity to change. Many adult offenders did not have this chance and have led really unhappy lives. You have many positive things going for you and you deserve better than this. Your life can be different."

Predict Cognitive Distortions

The adolescent may come to the interview with his/her story better prepared than the clinician's. The adolescent's stance can be undermined if the clinician is able to predict the kind of excuses the offender will use. The clinician could then say for example, "If you say to me that you didn't know it was wrong or it was the younger child's fault, then you will be saying the same things that other kids that offend say. What do you think your family would say to that? What do you think I'll think?"

Challenge Cognitive Distortions

Working through cognitive distortions is essential in ensuring that offenders change their behavior. However, as was described earlier, the challenging should not be forceful or hostile in order to effect change. Creating dissonance by repeating, reframing, rephrasing, interrupting, and giving information are all useful ways to challenge the young person's thoughts and offending behavior. Ways of challenging while maintaining rapport include: (a) acting more warmly at the time, (b) using plenty of humor and making joining comments, and (c) using simple, non-jargon language.

Working with Denial

The clinician should be careful when directly challenging an offender's account of an offending incident. Often a direct challenge such as "you're lying" only serves to place the young person further in denial. It is often more successful to resort to a face-saving maneuver or to simply note the discrepancy in the statement and return to it later.

Adolescents Tell "Their Story"

Even if the clinician already has a good account of the offending incidents, the adolescent should be encouraged to describe the offending. This assists the offender both in being honest and in accepting responsibility for his/her actions. Talking about the incidents for the first time allows them to think about them in a different way, and offenses they may not have previously thought about may be recalled.

Reframing

Examples of helpful reframing statements that the clinician can use are that therapy is not an imposition but an opportunity to make a different life, and therapy does not indicate failure, but a success on which the adolescent can be congratulated for being brave enough to attend. Reframing can also include ways of working with cognitive distortions. For example, adolescents who may deny planning their offending (e.g., saying, "it just happened") might be challenged by suggesting that if they have no control over their sexual behavior, they may need institutional care; or the question could be asked, "Why didn't you offend on a busy street?"

Assume the Adolescent Has a History of Offending

The clinician should take a cautious position and assume that the adolescent has a history of sexually abusive behavior. It is possible that they have been sexually offending for some time prior to getting caught. Rather than asking questions such as, "Did you do. . .?," the clinician could ask, "When did you first offend?" and "How many months or years have you been doing this for?"

Check Suicidal Ideation and Depression

While the clinician should request a mental health assessment if there are genuine concerns for the offender's mental health, it is always useful to at least assess for depression and suicidality. This would include current and past mood level and mental state, detailing any current suicide plans, past attempts, whether there is positive family history and whether they have known someone who has committed suicide. Suicidal ideation and/or intent should not be downplayed or ignored and clinicians should always seek further specialist assessment.

There is a need to be aware that on very rare occasions, adolescents *may* use the threat of suicide in an attempt to manipulate the clinician's sympathies and as a way of taking the pressure off themselves. An important part of any risk assessment for depression and suicide is case consultation and supervision, and this should be routinely undertaken.

Face-Saving Maneuvers

It is rare that an adolescent is able to be totally honest in the initial interview due to the shame, embarrassment and/or denial they may have. Face-saving maneuvers that the clinician may offer include suggesting a second interview at which time the adolescent will have "remembered" more of their offending, because this normally occurs. The clinician may also suggest to the offender some of the excuses he/she may have used at the time of the offending and allow the offender to make those excuses in the interview (e.g., "You may not have realized that what you did was really abusive . . . but it sounds like you did something to the child"). The clinician "sidelines" the cognitive distortions in order to get an admission. However, the distortions should be noted for follow-up later in therapy.

Provide Information

It is useful for clinicians to offer adolescents and their family a prediction, based on the clinical research and the clinician's experience with other adolescents, of their likely future and consequent need for therapy. The clinician should always provide information on what help is available to the offender. Even if they are still denying any abusive behavior at the end of the initial interview, the clinician should take the opportunity to educate about the effects of sexually abusive behavior on both victims and perpetrators.

Express Concern for the Young Person Without Therapy

By keeping abreast with current and relevant research and proven clinical expertise, the clinician is better able to discuss potential outcomes for adolescent sexual offenders who do not wish to engage in treatment.

Addiction as a Metaphor

For adolescents who deny the need for help on the basis that they will never reoffend, it can be useful to compare sexual offending with alcohol addiction (i.e., it may be difficult to stop without professional assistance; one must learn how to deal with temptation in high risk situations; one needs to change lifestyle problems that may have contributed to the problem). However, the addiction metaphor needs always to be used with care in case the adolescent or family is left with the impression that the offending was beyond the adolescent's control or responsibility, or that he has an 'illness' that is incurable.

INTERVIEWING THE FAMILIES OF SEXUALLY ABUSIVE ADOLESCENTS

The families of sexually abusive youth can be a powerful force to support and confront the offender in admitting the abusive behavior (Stevenson, Castillo, & Seforbi, 1989). As a consequence, it is essential that the family be involved in the early stages of interviewing the adolescent. As a rule, it is advisable to meet first with the adolescent and family together, then have a period alone with the adolescent, and finally bring them all back together (for more extensive discussion of the initial contact phase with families, see Kolko, Noel, Thomas, & Torres, this issue).

Frequently, the family will be having great difficulty in accepting the reality of the adolescent's behavior. If the family and adolescent both strongly deny the offending despite conclusive evidence to the contrary, it is useful to interview them separately early in the interview process.

Throughout the interview with the family there are a number of strategies that can help prepare the adolescent to disclose offending.

Prepare the Family for the Shock of Disclosure

It is essential that the family be prepared in the event that an adolescent is likely to disclose his/her offending.

Create a Context for Honesty

This can be facilitated by joining with the family in the first instance, and then acknowledging the anger, disbelief, shame, and embarrassment of learning that their child has sexually abused. The clinician should offer hope, dispel myths, give information, be educational, and particularly be supportive and show compassion. The clinician should constantly be trying to encourage the family to make supportive comments about the adolescent being honest. The type of questions the clinician might ask include, "Would you rather your son was honest or dishonest about his behavior?" and "Would you respect your son if he was more honest?"

Explain to the family that their reaction will greatly affect the adolescent's ability to be honest. Support the family in their being able to tell the adolescent that they will be able to handle the disclosure. Present to the family the consequences of not getting the necessary help. The clinician might say, "Would you want your son to have a future where he grows up to be an adult sex offender and ends up in jail?" In some situations, the use of some form of leverage may be needed to convince the family of the seriousness of the issue.

Prepare the Family for Talking Explicitly About Sex

For many adolescents who sexually offend, their families may be ambivalent about discussing sexuality. By preparing the family for detailed discussions on sexual matters, the clinician is also giving permission for the adolescent to speak explicitly and possibly break the family norms (for additional details on discussing sexuality, see Zankman & Bonomo, this issue).

Be Sensitive to Other Victims in the Family

Often, victims of abuse within the family will be present and understandably may find these sessions extremely difficult. Sometimes their experiences can be helpful in confronting the offender. Their personal stories can begin to create a climate for further honest disclosures from the adolescent. Respect for the feelings of victims must be shown at all times. It would be inappropriate to have both the offender's siblings and victims of abuse at a family interview.

Inform the Family of Potential Relapse

Always discuss with the family the risk of the adolescent re-offending. If the victim is within the same household, discuss the need for the adolescent to spend some time outside the home. This is especially relevant in the initial stages of counseling and if younger children are living at home. The family must have safety rules in place around the adolescent, and these rules need to be discussed with the clinician. It is also important that the family understand that maintaining safety is ultimately the offender's rather than the family's responsibility and that their role is to support him/her in carrying this out.

Discuss Ongoing Support

Once therapy begins, the main focus will be on the adolescent. Some family members can become resentful of him/her receiving all of the attention. It is important that the family is also offered support (for specific strategies, see Nahum & Brewer, this issue). This enables them to continue to see treatment as valuable, to motivate the adolescent towards change, and to more effectively monitor the adolescent's behavior in the family.

CONCLUSION

The purpose of this article is not to offer a one-size-fits-all approach when interviewing sexually abusive youth, but rather to offer a range of effective techniques and practical strategies clinicians can adopt in their work.

When compared with adult sexual offenders, the majority of adolescent sex offenders have been offending for a fraction of the time. A difference is that adult offenders have often developed elaborate cognitive distortions to deny and minimize their behavior. This serves as a way to reduce internal and external inhibitors and rationalize their behavior. In contrast, adolescents often have relatively simple cognitive distortions and are consequently more responsive to making changes in counseling. This message should be given to adolescent offenders and their families to increase their hope and motivation for change.

An adolescent's developmental stage is one where he/she is making dramatic changes. What may complicate therapy is a rebellious nature that some adolescents have as they make the transition from dependence to independence. In the process of assessment and therapy, creative ways need to be employed that not only engage the adolescent but also allow for the important issues in sex offender treatment to be addressed.

Development and maintenance of the therapeutic relationship with the adolescent is key in ensuring the success of future interventions. The use of motivational interviewing techniques is part of a 'tool kit' that allows clinicians to systematically work with adolescents towards increasing their motivation for engaging in therapy and thereby increasing the likelihood of sustained change. Furthermore, by involving the adolescent's family and providing ongoing support, the clinician further sets the scene in assisting the adolescent towards change and reducing future risk.

REFERENCES

Anderson, E.M., & Lambert, M.J. (1995). Short-term dynamically oriented psychotherapy: A review and meta-analysis. *Clinical Psychology Review, 9*, 503-514.
Bergin, A.E., & Garfield, S.L. (Eds.). (1994). *Handbook of psychotherapy and behavior change* (4th ed.). Washington, DC: American Psychological Association.

Bordin, E.S. (1976). The generalizability of the psychoanalytic concept of the working alliance. *Psychotherapy: Theory, Research, and Practice, 16*, 252-260.

Bourke, M.L., & Donohue, B. (1996). Assessment and treatment of juvenile sex offenders: An empirical review. *Journal of Child Sexual Abuse, 5*, 47-70.

Burke, B., Arkowitz, H., & Dunn, C. (2002). The efficacy of motivational interviewing. In W.R. Miller, & S. Rollnick (Eds.), *Motivational interviewing: Preparing people to change addictive behavior* (2nd ed.) (pp. 217-250). New York: Guilford Press.

Efta-Breitbach, J., & Freeman, K.A. (2004). Recidivism and resilience in juvenile sex offenders: An analysis of the literature. *Journal of Child Sexual Abuse, 13*(3/4), pp. 125-138.

Friedrich, W.N. (1995). *Psychotherapy with sexually abused boys: An integrated approach.* Thousand Oaks, CA: Sage.

Garland, R.J., & Dougher, M.J. (1991). Motivational interviewing in the treatment of sex offenders. In W.R. Miller, & S. Rollnick (Eds.), *Motivational interviewing: Preparing people to change addictive behavior* (pp. 303-313). New York: Guilford Press.

Hubble, M.A., Duncan, B.L., & Miller, S.D. (1999). Introduction. In M.A. Hubble, B.L. Duncan, & S.D. Miller (Eds.), *The heart and soul of change: What works in therapy* (pp. 1-32). Washington, DC: American Psychological Association.

Kolko, D.J., Noel, C., Thomas, G., & Torres, E. (2004). Cognitive-behavioral treatment for adolescents who sexually offend and their families: Individual and family applications in a collaborative outpatient program. *Journal of Child Sexual Abuse, 13*(3/4), pp. 157-192.

Lambert, M.J. (1992). Implications of outcome research for psychotherapy integration. In J.C. Norcross, & M.R. Goldstein (Eds.), *Handbook of psychotherapy integration* (pp. 94-129). New York: Basic Books.

Lambert, M.J., & Bergin, A.E. (1994). The effectiveness of psychotherapy. In A.E. Bergin, & S.L. Garfield (Eds.), *Handbook of psychotherapy and behavior change* (4th ed.) (pp. 143-189). New York: Wiley.

Lambert, M.J., Weber, F.D., & Sykes, J.D. (1993, April). *Psychotherapy versus placebo.* Poster presented at the annual meeting of the Western Psychological Association, Phoenix, Arizona.

Lightfoot, L.O., & Barbaree, H.E. (1993). The relationship between substance use and abuse and sexual offending in adolescents. In H.E. Barbaree, W.L. Marshall, & S.M. Hudson (Eds.), *The juvenile sex offender* (pp. 203-224). New York: Guilford.

Longo, R.E. (2004). An integrated experiential approach to treating young people who sexually abuse. *Journal of Child Sexual Abuse, 13*(3/4), pp. 193-215.

Luborsky, L., Singer, B., & Luborsky, L. (1975). Comparative studies in psychotherapy. *Archives of General Psychiatry, 32*, 995-1008.

Miller, W.R., & Rollnick, S. (1991). *Motivational interviewing: Preparing people to change addictive behavior.* New York: Guilford Press.

Miller, W.R., & Rollnick, S. (2002). *Motivational interviewing: Preparing people to change addictive behavior* (2nd ed.). New York: Guilford Press.

Morenz, B., & Becker, J. (1995). The treatment of youthful sexual offenders. *Applied and Preventive Psychology, 4*, 247-256.

Nahum, D., & Brewer, M.M. (2004). Multi-family group therapy for sexually abusive youth. *Journal of Child Sexual Abuse, 13*(3/4), pp. 215-243.

Prochaska, J.O., & DiClemente, C.C. (1984). *The transtheoretical approach: Crossing the traditional boundaries of therapy.* Malabar, FL: Krieger.

Ryan, G., Miyoshi, T.J., Metzner, J.L., Krugman, R.D., & Fryer, G.E. (1996). Trends in a national sample of sexually abusive youths. *Journal of the American Academy of Child and Adolescent Psychiatry, 35*(1), 17-25.

Stevenson, H., Castillo, E., & Seforbi, R. (1989). Treatment of denial in adolescent sex offenders and their families. *Journal of Offender Counseling, Services, and Rehabilitation, 14*(1), 37-50.

Zankman, S., & Bonomo, J. (2004). Working with parents to reduce juvenile sex offender recidivism. *Journal of Child Sexual Abuse, 13*(3/4), pp. 139-156.

TREATING YOUTH WHO SEXUALLY OFFEND

Treatment of Juveniles Who Sexually Offend: An Overview

Jill Efta-Breitbach

Kurt A. Freeman

SUMMARY. Juvenile sexual offending is increasingly being recognized as a serious crime among youth. The prevalence of sexual offending and sexual reoffending suggests that many juvenile sex offenders (JSOs) may repeat their offending behaviors if not treated. However, clinical trials evaluating specific interventions are virtually nonexistent. Instead, the literature on the treatment of JSOs is marked by discussions of strategies that are hypothesized to be beneficial, as well as descriptions of treatment programs that exist across the country. Fur-

Address correspondence to: Jill Efta-Breitbach, PsyD, Womack Army Medical Center, Fort Bragg, NC 28310 (E-mail: Jill.Breitbach@na.amedd.army.mil).

[Haworth co-indexing entry note]: "Treatment of Juveniles Who Sexually Offend: An Overview." Efta-Breitbach, Jill, and Kurt A. Freeman. Co-published simultaneously in *Journal of Child Sexual Abuse* (The Haworth Maltreatment and Trauma Press, an imprint of The Haworth Press, Inc.) Vol. 13, No. 3/4, 2004, pp. 125-138; and: *Identifying and Treating Youth Who Sexually Offend: Current Approaches, Techniques, and Research* (ed: Robert Geffner et al.) The Haworth Maltreatment and Trauma Press, an imprint of The Haworth Press, Inc., 2004, pp. 125-138. Single or multiple copies of this article are available for a fee from The Haworth Document Delivery Service [1-800-HAWORTH, 9:00 a.m. - 5:00 p.m. (EST). E-mail address: docdelivery@haworthpress.com].

Digital Object Identifier: 10.1300/J070v13n03_07

ther, while existing literature suggests that treatment for JSOs may deter future sexual offending behaviors, it is unclear which, if any, aspects of these treatments promote the development of positive behaviors. A discussion of existing treatment approaches, effectiveness, and treatment considerations follows. *[Article copies available for a fee from The Haworth Document Delivery Service: 1-800-HAWORTH. E-mail address: <docdelivery@ haworthpress.com> Website: <http://www.HaworthPress.com> © 2004 by The Haworth Press, Inc. All rights reserved.]*

KEYWORDS. Juvenile, youth, sexual, offender, recidivism, treatment

Treatment of juvenile sex offenders (JSOs) involves multiple and complex components. The goals of treatments may vary as a function of the referral source, the facility in which intervention is provided, the pre-intervention assessment conducted, and the intervention modality used. Attempting to formulate treatments for JSOs while considering necessary biopsychosocial aspects is an elaborate task. Treatment involves more than just the JSO, and can be administered in several different contexts (e.g., inpatient, outpatient). Further, assessing what the JSO's treatment should include is a difficult task as a variety of interventions and modalities are available. In this article, an introduction of JSO treatment literature is provided. It is important to note that there are very few empirical studies that examine the treatments described. When specific empirical support was found in the literature, it is noted.

GOALS OF JSO TREATMENT

The primary goal of sexual offender therapy is for offenders to safely reintegrate into society as productive individuals (Dewhurst & Nielsen, 1999; DiGiorgio-Miller, 1994; Lee & Olender, 1992; Ryan, 1999; Sapp & Vaughn, 1990; Swenson, Henggeler, & Schoenwald, 1998). According to the National Adolescent Perpetrator Network (1988, as cited in Becker, 1990), 19 issues should be addressed in the treatment of JSOs: (a) accepting responsibility without externalizing blame; (b) identification of the cycle of offense behavior; (c) development of the ability to interrupt the cycle before an offense occurs; (d) the JSO's own victimization; (e) victim awareness or empathy; (f) power and control issues; (g) the role and reduction of deviant arousal; (h) a positive sexual identity for the JSO; (i) understanding the consequences of an offense to the JSO, the JSO's family, the victim, and the victim's family;

(j) family dysfunction that supports or triggers offending; (k) cognitive distortions; (l) identification and expression of feelings; (m) appropriate social relationships with peers; (n) levels of trust in relating to adults; (o) addictive/compulsive qualities contributing to deviancy; (p) skill deficits that interfere with successful functioning; (q) relapse prevention; and (r) options for restitution to victims and community. An ideal treatment program would address all of these issues and combine various modalities with emphasis on the specific needs of each JSO. However, each treatment location, intervention, and modality includes specific treatment goals, along with the overarching goal of reintegrating JSOs into society as productive individuals.

OTHER PARTIES INVOLVED IN TREATMENT

Although a JSO him- or herself may be the identified client in need of therapeutic services, the reality is that many others are also typically involved in some way in the treatment. In the research literature, there are no indications that JSOs in treatment were self-referred. Therefore, involvement of referral sources and other parties complicates developing a positive working alliance with JSOs. One of the primary pathways for JSOs to access treatment is via the court system (Bremer, 1998). Although this could potentially interfere with the development of a strong therapeutic relationship, many will argue that a referral by the court system actually increases the likelihood of treatment success. One of the benefits of having adjudicated referrals for treatment is that post-treatment monitoring is commonplace through interactions with probation officers (Gerdes, Gourley, & Cash, 1995).

In addition to those parties involved in the process of referring an offending youth to treatment, one must also consider that often times a JSO's family members may be involved in ongoing therapeutic services. Having family members involved in the treatment of JSOs is beneficial because of aftercare monitoring and supervision, although special considerations are warranted if the victim of the abuse is in the JSO's immediate family (DiGiorgio-Miller, 1994).

Finally, the therapist(s) or treatment team requires consideration. Because establishing a relationship is presumed to be an important variable impacting treatment success (Becker, 1990), it is helpful to consider the JSO preferences for therapeutic interactions. For example, Kaplan, Becker, and Tenke (1991) found that JSOs victimized by males and family members showed the greatest preference for female therapists. While limited data are available to guide such decisions, attending to all parties involved in the treatment of JSOs ensures that treatment not only addresses relevant needs of those involved, but also provides an opportunity to develop a social support network beyond existing structures.

DETERMINING PROPER TREATMENT PROGRAMS

Treatment programs cannot be effective unless the clients referred to them have treatment needs that match the program's aims and the level of restriction associated with the program (Bremer, 1998). It should be noted that there is a limited amount of research that examines outcomes based on treatment settings. For example, in their review of the literature, Ertl and McNamara (1997) found no methodologically sound empirical studies examining differences in outcome based on treatment setting. However, Kahn and Chambers (1991) did note that JSOs treated in institutional programs were somewhat more likely to reoffend non-sexually than those treated in community programs. Those researchers, however, did not control for demographic differences that may have existed between the two types of programs (Ertl & McNamara, 1997).

Further, Bremer (1992) found that all youths spending more than 15 months in their inpatient program had no reported reoffenses. However, Rasmussen (1999) found that first time JSOs had lower rates of recidivism when treated in a community-based program, as opposed to restrictive settings, although the author suggests that obtained findings may reflect the fact that more serious offenders are placed in restrictive settings. In summary, research has not adequately supported the ability of one treatment location to prevent recidivism over another.

TYPES OF INTERVENTIONS

Existing research literature suggests a comprehensive treatment program consisting of a variety of therapeutic interventions used simultaneously (Bourke & Donohue, 1996). For example, Sapp and Vaughn (1990) conducted a nation-wide survey of correctional facilities treating JSOs. They found that treatment modalities reflected extensive use of psychological therapy and behavior modification, with a total of 338 different therapies and techniques included. Furthermore, program directors indicated that they would like to add 190 additional treatment elements, for a total of 528. This suggests that of the JSO treatment programs included in Sapp and Vaughn's sample, each program would like to implement an average of 17.6 different therapies. From this research one can extrapolate that JSO treatment is variable and includes a variety of therapeutic techniques.

Existing research has identified that the primary interventions practiced across treatment settings consist of a combination of various cognitive-behavioral techniques as well as psychoeducational and pharmacological/biological interventions (Bourke & Donohue, 1996; Ertl & McNamara, 1997; Hunter & Santos, 1990). The modalities where intervention techniques are applied include individual, family, and group therapy settings, as well as inpatient (i.e., residential or correctional) settings (Camp & Thyer, 1993). Of note, one of the most recent meta-analyses on effectiveness of JSO treatments suggests that cognitive-behavioral treatments and systemic interventions are associated with reduction in both sexual and nonsexual recidivism (Hansen et al., 2002; for further support, see Walker, McGovern, Poey, & Otis, this issue).

Cognitive-Behavioral Techniques

Relapse prevention. Cognitive-behavioral interventions are common in the treatment of JSOs (e.g., Bourke & Donohue, 1996; Davis & Leitenberg, 1987; Ertl & McNamara, 1997). Perhaps most salient is the relapse prevention technique, which has been suggested as the most common cognitive-behavioral approach used in JSO treatment (Dewhurst & Nielsen, 1999). Relapse prevention as applied to treatment with JSOs was adapted from the addiction field and teaches offenders to deconstruct their sexual offenses into component parts (i.e., thoughts, feelings, behaviors, and triggers). It requires JSOs to identify all of the internal and external factors involved in the original offending process and then determine strategies to reduce the salience of triggering cues. The goal is to enable offending youth to manage future situations (Dewhurst & Nielsen, 1999). Further, the relapse prevention model helps the JSO acquire new skills and teaches him/her to challenge inappropriate beliefs and attitudes (for specific relapse prevention strategies, see Kolko, Noel, Thomas, & Torres, this issue).

Modifying cognitive distortions. According to Ertl and McNamara (1997), treatments with a focus on modifying an offender's maladaptive beliefs and cognitive distortions are highly advocated for when working with this population. Thus, cognitive restructuring is a popular intervention among treatment programs (Davis & Leitenberg, 1987; for specific strategies, see Kolko et al., this issue; Longo, this issue; Nahum & Brewer, this issue).

Clinical theory suggests that JSOs should become aware of thoughts before, during, and after their offense in order to begin to recognize how their thinking contributed to the offense (DiGiorgio-Miller, 1994). JSOs often recognize their behavior as either entirely congruent or painfully dissonant with their sense of the world, yet very few have a sense of responsibility for the harm they cause (Ryan, 1999). Thus, having the juvenile accept responsibility for behavior is often the first step in cognitive-behavioral treatments (Becker &

Hunter, 1997). Accepting responsibility is encouraged through addressing shame, embarrassment, and fear of consequences.

Therapeutic work challenging self-statements that grant permission or provide excuses for sexual abuse may also be helpful when attempting to have a youth accept responsibility for his or her offense. Role-playing is an example of one method used to confront cognitive distortions and maladaptive beliefs (Becker, 1990). Further, values clarification, which involves asking the JSO what he or she identifies as important, increases the youth's awareness of how his or her actions are non-congruent with beliefs (Kahn & LaFond, 1988). In summary, modifying cognitive distortions addresses the goals of accepting responsibility, increasing awareness, and correcting cognitive distortions that support or trigger offending.

Building empathy. Research has shown significant differences in reported empathy of JSOs versus non-offending peers (Burke, 2001). Given this, building empathy for victims and potential victims is incorporated into many cognitive-behavioral treatments. Along with recognizing and addressing faulty thinking patterns that contribute to offending behavior, JSOs are thought to benefit from exploring what their victims may have been thinking during a sexual offense. As part of the process of strengthening empathy, the JSO will often write letters to the victims expressing regret, empathy, and sorrow for committing the offense (DiGiorgio-Miller, 1994). The focus on helping JSOs experience empathetic responses is theoretically beneficial because it can help the offending youth become more sensitive to the negative outcomes that he/she and his/her family could experience should he/she reoffend, as well as what the potential victims and their families will endure (for specific empathy-building strategies, see Longo, this issue).

Impulse control. Many cognitive-behavioral methodologies aim to ameliorate impulse control problems and deviant sexual arousal. These techniques have demonstrated efficacy in reduction of overall arousal to deviant cues (Becker, Kaplan, & Kavoussi, 1988; Hunter & Santos, 1990). One type of cognitive technique designed to reduce arousal and impulsivity is satiation training. Satiation training generally involves instructing a JSO to masturbate to ejaculation while thinking about or watching a scene of a non-deviant sexual content and continuing to masturbate post-ejaculation while thinking about or watching a scene involving deviant sexual content (Ertl & McNamara, 1997). This process continues until the JSO's arousal to deviant stimuli becomes impossible, or de-conditioned (Bourke & Donohue, 1996). While research demonstrates some success of this intervention with adult sex offenders, using it with JSO populations presents more ethical concerns for the treating therapist or team (Becker & Kaplan, 1993; Hunter & Santos, 1990). For example, some individuals feel that exposing juveniles to deviant sexual content is unethical. One modification of satiation training, using verbal satiation versus masturbatory satiation, appears less controversial. Verbal satiation teaches the JSO how to use repetitive verbalizations to satiate arousal to deviant stimuli (Becker, 1990).

Another technique for reducing impulsivity is covert sensitization. In covert sensitization, the JSO uses verbal imagery to reduce arousal and impulsivity. The JSO imagines and verbalizes the feelings and emotions experienced prior to and during a sexual offense. This is followed by imagery of aversive images that reflect negative consequences as a result of the sexual offense (Hunter & Santos, 1990; Kahn & Lafond, 1988). Aversive images can range from harsh treatment in correctional facilities to having peers and family members find out about the offense (Becker, 1990). Visualization of positive rewards for exercising control or escaping the potential offense situation may also be utilized (Hunter & Santos, 1990). It is important to note that there have been no empirical studies with JSOs to determine overall effectiveness of covert sensitization or aspects of this intervention that may deter future offending behavior (Bourke & Donohue, 1996).

A third cognitive-behavioral technique designed to reduce impulsivity and deviant arousal is systematic desensitization. In this procedure, the JSO performs progressive muscle relaxation and then visualizes behavior that has precipitated deviant sexual behavior in the past (Bourke & Donohue, 1996). The JSO then gradually increases the intensity of the imagined behaviors as he/she progresses through the stages of his/her sexual offense, remaining relaxed through the entire visualized sequence of events. Prior to visually committing the offense, the JSO is to modify the scenario so he/she does not feel compelled to finish the act. The purpose of this intervention is to allow the JSO to remain calm and relaxed and modify his/her need to commit the sexual offense. In their review, Ertl and McNamara (1997) note that although preliminary research indicates that systematic desensitization may be more effective than covert sensitization, it is being used less frequently in treatment programs.

Skills training. Finally, it should be noted that some specialized trainings designed for use in cognitive-behavioral modalities are utilized in JSO treatments. Specifically, social skills training is often integrated to teach JSOs about "normal" development and functioning (Bourke & Donohue, 1996). Social skills deficits are targeted through identification of a specific skill, modeling the skill, instructing the JSO to role-play the skill, and providing praise and feedback after the skill is performed. Targeted skills are in categories such as relationship and dating skills, communication skills, empathy skills, conflict resolution, compliment training, assertiveness skills, and personal care skills (Kahn & Lafond, 1988). The effectiveness of social skills training in the treatment of JSOs has yet to be empirically studied (Bourke & Donohue, 1996). However, despite the fact that there is no empirical evidence to support its use, over 86% of treatment programs surveyed by Sapp and Vaughn (1990) reported using social skills training.

Psychoeducation Techniques

Psychoeducational techniques have been integrated with cognitive-behavioral techniques to combat cognitive distortions and maladaptive beliefs (Bourke & Donohue, 1996). The goal of psychoeducation is to provide JSOs and their families with information about factors associated with sexual offending. However, there is no empirical research that suggests these techniques are directly related to reduction in recidivism.

Sex education. Sex education, one popular psychoeducation topic, is designed to teach the JSOs about their own sexual development and sexuality and improve sexual knowledge (Camp & Thyer, 1993). Sex education includes a variety of topics such as common sexual myths, information about pubertal development and sexually transmitted diseases, and a focus on sexual communication (Becker, 1990). Further, because it has been proposed that JSOs are often confused about their own sexuality (DiGiorgio-Miller, 1994), information regarding sexual and gender identity development may be appropriate. The psychoeducation approach (i.e., sharing information) can offer JSOs a safe environment and opportunity to ask treatment providers about appropriate sex behaviors, developmental issues, and sexual reproduction (DiGiorgio-Miller, 1994; for additional discussion, see Kolko et al., this issue).

Anger management. Teaching JSOs how to control their anger is another psychoeducational technique often used in treatment. JSOs frequently use physical aggression as their primary form of problem solving (Becker et al., 1988). Therefore, anger is a feeling many sex offenders commonly recall when discussing their offenses (Lombardo & DiGiorgio-Miller, 1988). One of the primary goals of anger control training is to teach offenders to recognize when they are angry so that they can then practice using more appropriate methods of problem solving (Ertl & McNamara, 1997). JSOs are also encouraged to practice listening, empathy, and attending skills (Becker & Kaplan, 1993). As with other forms of psychoeducation, the effectiveness of anger control training in the treatment of JSOs is unknown (for additional anger control techniques, see Kolko et al., this issue; Longo, this issue).

Pharmacological and Biological Treatments

Biological treatment operates from the underlying assumption that abnormal sexual aggression results from hormonal imbalances (Camp & Thyer, 1993). Biological interventions typically include castration, pharmacological hormone treatments, and sterotaxtic neurosurgery (Camp & Thyer, 1993; Ertl & McNamara, 1997; Sapp & Vaughn, 1990). Use of biological and pharmacological treatments in the United States, specifically with adolescent perpetrators, remains controversial and, thus, is infrequent (Camp & Thyer, 1993; Ertl & McNamara, 1997; Hunter & Lexier, 1998). Concern and controversy likely comes from the realization that many JSOs could experience devastating side effects from use of these interventions. Finally, ethical concerns may arise from the ability of JSOs to understand and consent to these treatments (for more details about aspects of biological treatments, see Sapp and Vaughn, 1990).

TREATMENT MODALITIES

Therapeutic services provided to JSOs may be implemented in several different formats. Discussions found in the literature describe implementation of services through individual therapy, group therapy, family therapy, and therapy involving various systems and care providers (e.g., Bourke & Donohue, 1996; Veneziano & Veneziano, 2002). As with most topics regarding the treatment of JSOs, there exists no empirical literature to guide the selection of the modality of intervention. Thus, decisions regarding this topic are often left to individual providers, are dictated by legal decisions (e.g., incarceration of youth), or are dictated by specific program stipulations. Each of the general modalities of treatment is described below.

Individual Therapy

Some juvenile sex offenders receive treatment through individual psychotherapy. It should be noted that theoretical approaches of individual therapy have received varying degrees of support from research. Cognitive-behavioral approaches have demonstrated effectiveness in JSO treatments (Ertl & McNamara, 1997). However, psychoanalytic and other insight-oriented approaches have not proven effective and are not recommended for use with JSOs (Bourke & Donohue, 1996).

Treatment goals addressed in individual therapy may include dealing with personal victimization, correcting cognitive distortions, and accepting responsibility. However, these goals are often integrated into other modalities, as well.

Group Therapy

For many treatment programs, the primary therapeutic modality is group-based interventions (Bremer, 1992; Davis & Leitenberg, 1987). A major goal of group treatment is identifying and expressing feelings, as well as developing social skills and appropriate relationships with peers. However, the content and goals of the group therapy sessions can be highly variable depending on goals of treatment, setting of the treatment program, and therapeutic orientation of the intervention providers (Bourke & Donohue, 1996).

One benefit of using group therapy with JSOs is that the setting and process of interaction provides many opportunities for vicarious learning and modeling from peers (Vizard, Monck, & Misch, 1995). Peer pressure can be utilized as a means of helping the JSO to abandon his or her denial of culpability in the offending behavior (Camp & Thyer, 1993). Addressing other addictions or negative behaviors may also be useful adjunctive interventions appropriate for group therapy (Ertl & McNamara, 1997). Confrontation techniques put senior group members in positions to point out discrepancies in thinking for younger or unmotivated JSOs (Bourke & Donohue, 1996). Dysfunctional attitudes can then be replaced with accurate information and positive messages, increasing self-esteem in the process (Kahn & LaFond, 1988).

Family Therapy

Family therapy is a major component of many JSO treatment programs (Becker et al., 1988) and often is used in conjunction with individual and/or group therapy (Camp & Thyer, 1993). Including family therapy as a modality for interventions is important because the family forms part of the environment in which the JSO operates and will likely influence post-treatment functioning (Vizard et al., 1995). Further, family therapy provides the JSO and his/her family the opportunity to address family issues that may have contributed to the juvenile's sexual offending (Ertl & McNamara, 1997). Other components of therapy may include victim confrontation when the victim is in the family, value clarification exercises, and psychodrama (Camp & Thyer, 1993). However, there have been no specific investigations to determine the effectiveness of family therapy with this population (Ertl & McNamara, 1997; for further discussion of family interventions, see Kolko et al., this issue; Nahum & Brewer, this issue; Zankman & Bonomo, this issue).

Multisystemic Therapy

There is evidence suggesting that including family, school, and peer systems in JSO treatment is an effective strategy (Bentovim, 1998; Borduin, Henggeler, Blaske, & Stein, 1990). Bentovim suggested that systemic therapy should include individual or group treatment for perpetrators and focus on the perpetrator's denial of responsibility, abuse of power, personal trauma experiences, and personal attachment. It is also suggested that family therapy be used to focus on protection of victims and siblings, role clarification, facilitation of an apology on the part of the JSO, and fostering parental support of JSO. Thus, treatment programs conceptualized within a systemic framework involve individual or group therapy for the perpetrators, victims, siblings, and parents, with concurrent family intervention that may involve dyadic, group, and whole-family sessions.

Multisystemic therapy (MST) addresses the JSO's cognitive deficits such as denial, empathy, family relations such as cohesion and parental supervision, and dysfunctional peer relationships (Borduin et al., 1990). For example, Bourke and Donohue (1996) suggest that a MST therapist might first attempt to identify and correct weaknesses in the JSO's cognitive processing. Next, the family system might be addressed. Also, assisting in the development of communication skills for increased peer relationship success would be addressed. Finally, examining relationships between school officials and the JSO's parents would be targeted.

To date, the only empirical study that compared treatment outcomes for JSOs utilized MST. In a 3-year longitudinal study conducted by Borduin and colleagues (1990), the 16 JSOs assigned to MST groups showed lower recidivism rates than the 16 JSOs who only received individual therapy. While preliminary and in need of systematic replication, these data provide evidence for implementation of intervention that addresses the multiple systems that are involved in a JSO's life. Further, MST has been shown to be effective with other types of adolescent offenders (e.g., Borduin, 1999; Borduin, Mann, Cone, & Henggeler, 1995), adding support to its benefit with JSOs.

CONCLUSIONS

In the current article, we provided an introductory review of existing published information regarding the treatment of JSOs. While there is a growing literature that involves discussion of treatment options, programs, modalities, and strategies, clinical trials systematically evaluating various treatments are virtually nonexistent. Published reports that exist on the treatment of JSOs suggest that cognitive-behavioral therapy, through an integrative systems approach involving the various mesosystems of JSOs, may be the most advantageous method of applying treatment to JSOs. However, this comment is obviously tempered by the dearth of empirical evidence.

Based on this introductory review of the literature on the treatment of JSOs, it is evident that much remains to be done to establish empirical foundations for the treatment of this clinical population. Unfortunately, the literature evaluating treatment outcomes has lagged behind the recognition of this clinical phenomenon and the resulting development and implementation of programs to address JSOs. As a result, while research shows that lack of successful treatment predicts higher rates of recidivism (e.g., Studer & Reddon, 1998), little is known about what "successful treatment" entails. Further, intra- and interpersonal, demographic, and other variables that impact treatment have not been well established. Clearly, more needs to be done to determine how to best treat youth who commit sexual offenses.

Ideally, providers of treatment programs targeting JSOs would have empirical literature to guide decisions and would be afforded the time, financial resources, and opportunity to apply interventions at the individual, family, and systems levels. Realistically, however, treatment providers are left to differentiate which aspects of the treatments previously described are possible, practicable, and as close to a "perfect fit" as possible. Continued research is needed to help strengthen intervention efforts with this clinical population.

REFERENCES

Becker, J.V. (1990). Treating adolescent sexual offenders. *Professional Psychology: Research and Practice, 21,* 362-365.

Becker, J.V., & Hunter, J.A. (1997). Understanding and treating child and adolescent sexual offenders. *Advances in Clinical Child Psychology, 19,* 177-197.

Becker, J.V., & Kaplan, M.S. (1993). Cognitive behavioral treatment of the juvenile sex offender. In H.E. Barbaree, W.L. Marshall, & S.M. Hudson (Eds.), *The juvenile sex offender* (pp. 278-288). New York: The Guilford Press.

Becker, J.V., Kaplan, M.S., & Kavoussi, R. (1988). Measuring the effectiveness of treatment for the aggressive adolescent sexual offender. *Annals of the New York Academy of Science, 528,* 215-222.

Bentovim, A. (1998). Family systemic approach to work with young sex offenders. *The Irish Journal of Psychology, 19,* 119-135.

Borduin, C.M. (1999). Multisystemic treatment of criminality and violence in adolescents. *Journal of the American Academy of Child and Adolescent Psychiatry, 38,* 242-249.

Borduin, C.M., Henggeler, S.W., Blaske, D.M., & Stein, R.J. (1990). Multisystemic treatment of adolescent sexual offenders. *International Journal of Offender Therapy and Comparative Criminology, 34,* 105-113.

Borduin, C.M., Mann, B.J., Cone, L.T., & Henggeler, S.W. (1995). Multisystemic treatment of serious juvenile offenders: Long-term prevention of criminality and violence. *Journal of Consulting & Clinical Psychology, 63,* 569-578.

Bourke, M.L., & Donohue, B. (1996). Assessment and treatment of juvenile sex offenders: An empirical review. *Journal of Child Sexual Abuse, 5,* 47-70.

Bremer, J.F. (1992). Serious juvenile sex offenders: Treatment and long-term follow-up. *Psychiatric Annals, 22,* 326-332.

Bremer, J.F. (1998). Challenges in the assessment and treatment of sexually abusive adolescents. *The Irish Journal of Psychology, 19*, 82-92.

Burke, D.M. (2001). Empathy in sexually offending and nonoffending adolescent males. *Journal of Interpersonal Violence*, 16, 222-233.

Camp, B.H., & Thyer, B.A. (1993). Treatment of adolescent sex offenders: A review of empirical research. *The Journal of Applied Social Sciences, 17*, 191-206.

Davis, G.E., & Leitenberg, J. (1987). Adolescent sex offenders. *Psychological Bulletin, 101*, 417-427.

Dewhurst, A.M., & Nielsen, K.M. (1999). A resiliency-based approach to working with sexual offenders. *Sexual Addiction & Compulsivity: The Journal of Treatment and Prevention, 6*, 271-279.

DiGiorgio-Miller, J. (1994). Clinical techniques in the treatment of juvenile sex offenders. *Journal of Offender Rehabilitation, 21*, 117-126.

Ertl, M.A., & McNamara, J.R. (1997). Treatment of juvenile sex offenders: A review of the literature. *Child and Adolescent Social Work Journal, 14*, 199-221.

Gerdes, K.E., Gourley, M.M., & Cash, M.C. (1995). Assessing juvenile sex offenders to determine adequate levels of supervision. *Child Abuse & Neglect, 19*, 953-961.

Hanson, R. K., Gibson, A., Harris, A., Marques, J., Murphy, W., Quinsey, V., & Seto, M. (2002). First report of the collaborative outcome data project on the effectiveness of psychological treatment for sex offenders. *Sexual Abuse: A Journal of Research and Treatment, 14*, 169-194.

Hunter, J.A., & Lexier, L.J. (1998). Ethical and legal issues in the assessment and treatment of juvenile sex offenders. *Child Maltreatment, 3*, 339-349.

Hunter, J.A., & Santos, D.R. (1990). The use of specialized cognitive-behavioral therapies in the treatment of adolescent sexual offenders. *International Journal of Offender Therapy and Comparative Criminology, 43*, 239-248.

Kahn, T.J., & Chambers, H.J. (1991). Assessing reoffense risk with juvenile sexual offenders. *Child Welfare, 70*, 333-345.

Kahn, T.J., & Lafond, M.A. (1988). Treatment of the adolescent sexual offender. *Child and Adolescent Social Work, 5*, 135-148.

Kaplan, M.S., Becker, J.V., & Tenke, C.E. (1991). Treatment of adolescent sexual offenders. *Journal of Interpersonal Violence, 17*, 3-11.

Kolko, D.J., Noel, C., Thomas, G., & Torres, E. (2004). Cognitive-behavioral treatment for adolescents who sexually offend and their families: Individual and family applications in a collaborative outpatient program. *Journal of Child Sexual Abuse, 13*(3/4), pp. 157-192.

Lee, D.G., & Olender, M.B. (1992). Working with juvenile sex offenders in foster care. *Community Alternatives: International Journal of Family Care, 4*, 63-75.

Lombardo, R., & DiGiorgio-Miller, J. (1988). Concepts and techniques in working with juvenile sex offenders. *Journal of Offender Counseling, Services, & Rehabilitation, 13*, 39-53.

Longo, R.E. (2004). An integrated experiential approach to treating young people who sexually abuse. *Journal of Child Sexual Abuse, 13*(3/4), pp. 193-215.

Nahum, D., & Brewer, M.M. (2004). Multi-family group therapy for sexually abusive youth. *Journal of Child Sexual Abuse, 13*(3/4), pp. 215-243.

Rasmussen, L. A. (1999). Factors related to recidivism among juvenile sexual offenders. *Sexual Abuse: A Journal of Research and Treatment, 11*, 69-86.

Ryan, G. (1999). Treatment of sexually abusive youth: The evolving consensus. *Journal of Interpersonal Violence, 14*, 422-436.

Sapp, A.D., & Vaughn, M.S. (1990). Juvenile sex offender treatment at state-operated correctional institutions. *International Journal of Offender Therapy and Comparative Criminology, 34*, 131-146.

Studer, L.H., & Reddon, J.R. (1998). Treatment may change risk prediction for sexual offenders. *Sexual Abuse: Journal of Research & Treatment, 10*, 175-181.

Swenson, C.C., Henggeler, S.W., & Schoenwald, S.K. (1998). Changing the social ecologies of adolescent sexual offenders: Implications of the success of multisystemic therapy in treating serious antisocial behavior in adolescents. *Child Maltreatment, 3*, 330-339.

Vizard, E., Monck, E., & Misch, P. (1995). Child and adolescent sex abuse perpetrators: A review of the research literature. *Journal of Child Psychology and Psychiatry, 36*(5), 731-756.

Walker, D.F., McGovern, S.K., Poey, E.L., & Otis, K.E. (2004). Treatment effectiveness for male adolescent sexual offenders: A meta-analysis and review. *Journal of Child Sexual Abuse, 13*(3/4), pp. 281-294.

Zankman, S., & Bonomo, J. (2004). Working with parents to reduce juvenile sex offender recidivism. *Journal of Child Sexual Abuse, 13*(3/4), pp. 139-156.

Working with Parents to Reduce Juvenile Sex Offender Recidivism

Scott Zankman
Josephine Bonomo

SUMMARY. Although there is very little research in the area of including parents in juvenile sex offender treatment, one of the factors that might be worth exploring is how the parental relationship may aid in successful relapse prevention. Since the family environment is a potential risk factor for adolescent sex offenders, integration of relapse prevention into daily family life may be a significant part of these youths' success or failure in the community. This article focuses on the concept of including parents in juvenile sex offender treatment. Issues addressed include what treatment providers can do to involve parents in relapse prevention, treatment providers' misconceptions about the inclusion of parents in treatment, a rationale for including parents in treatment, and research regarding different parenting styles. *[Article copies available for a fee from The Haworth Document Delivery Service: 1-800-HAWORTH. E-mail address: <docdelivery@haworthpress.com> Website: <http://www.Haworth Press.com> © 2004 by The Haworth Press, Inc. All rights reserved.]*

Address correspondence to: Scott Zankman, MA, 2722 Colby Avenue, Suite 402, Everett, WA 98201 (E-mail: zankman@att.net).

The authors thank Doug Sprenkle, PhD, for his assistance in manuscript preparation and Jeffrey Badger for his research assistance.

[Haworth co-indexing entry note]: "Working with Parents to Reduce Juvenile Sex Offender Recidivism." Zankmen, Scott, and Josephine Bonomo. Co-published simultaneously in *Journal of Child Sexual Abuse* (The Haworth Maltreatment and Trauma Press, an imprint of The Haworth Press, Inc.) Vol. 13, No. 3/4, 2004, pp. 139-156; and: *Identifying and Treating Youth Who Sexually Offend: Current Approaches, Techniques, and Research* (ed: Robert Geffner et al.) The Haworth Maltreatment and Trauma Press, an imprint of The Haworth Press, Inc., 2004, pp. 139-156. Single or multiple copies of this article are available for a fee from The Haworth Document Delivery Service [1-800-HAWORTH, 9:00 a.m. - 5:00 p.m. (EST). E-mail address: docdelivery@haworthpress.com].

Digital Object Identifier: 10.1300/J070v13n03_08

KEYWORDS. Juvenile sex offender treatment, family treatment, relapse prevention

The predominant model used at this time in working with juvenile sex offenders is a psychoeducational, individually focused, cognitive-behavioral approach. This approach focuses on identifying a sexual abuse cycle, isolating risk factors, challenging thinking errors in the cycle, and developing a relapse prevention plan to avoid high-risk situations and decrease dynamic risk factors. Dynamic risk factors are factors that can be affected through treatment, such as low self-esteem, social isolation, and deviant sexual arousal.

The sexual abuse cycle has been described in the literature as an essential element in understanding juvenile sex offending behavior (Lane, 1997; Ryan, 1999). In general, these youth have cognitive schemas that are based on negative experiences from the past. Their cognitive schemas are often the basis for negative expectations for future experiences, and these expectations result in withdrawal behavior. When this withdrawal strategy for affect management is not effective, resentment mounts, and fantasy and power-based solutions are developed. This eventually leads to abusive behaviors. At this point in the cycle, these youth attempt to manage fears of being caught and then reframe their sexual behavior in an attempt to regain some level of normalcy. This sexual abuse cycle is maintained by thinking errors, which are reinforced by feelings of control or power over previously negative experiences or relationships.

A case example may help clarify the progression through the cycle. Sean is a 15-year-old youth who is socially isolated from his peers in school. He is curious about sexual experiences with peer age females, yet he does not believe that any females his age would be interested in dating him. The tension between sexual interests and social isolation is a difficult and daily struggle for Sean. Sean decides to keep his struggle to himself.

One of Sean's jobs at home is to baby-sit his younger brother while his mother is at work. Once his mother leaves, he sets his brother in front of the television and downloads pornography from the Internet in his bedroom. Sean becomes sexually aroused as he imagines sexual experiences with the women in the photos. Sean's brother knocks on the door to see what his brother is doing. Sean realizes that his brother is younger and will do whatever Sean wants. He quickly imagines his brother doing sexual acts to him similar to the experiences he just fantasized about, and he ends up sexually abusing his brother. After the incident, he tells his brother that they will both get in trouble if he tells anyone. Sean decides to be nice to his brother so he does not draw negative attention to himself when his mother arrives home.

The juvenile sex offender relapse prevention plan has also been described in the literature (Gray & Pithers, 1993). Relapse prevention tends to be described in general terms that include the application of treatment to potential risk factors that might increase the likelihood for relapse. Specific focus is given to identifying high-risk situations for sexual recidivism and developing skills to intervene in these situations.

Therapists' perspectives regarding treatment approach is based on the discussion and implementation of broad and essential concepts such as the sexual abuse cycle and relapse prevention. Thus, therapists must grapple with questions of how best to impact youth during a therapy session in ways that help the youth apply lessons from treatment to daily life. Therapists must implement therapeutic interventions effectively to reduce dynamic risk factors as one aspect of eliminating relapse. Interventions are developed based on the needs and context of each adolescent's current life situation. Specific skills taught to address dynamic risk factors include: (a) thought-stopping techniques to interrupt deviant arousal, (b) psychoeducational techniques that target appropriate social skills and various pro social aspects of life, (c) victim empathy exercises to address self-centered attitudes, and (d) self-disclosure exercises to challenge cognitive distortions and interrupt isolation.

THEORETICAL RATIONALE FOR INCLUDING PARENTS

Adolescents are embedded in a socio-ecological context that is crucial to examine in order to fully understand their development and treatment. This contextual perspective is often assessed and noted when using traditional juvenile sex offender treatment (Butler & Seto, 2002; Ryan, 1999; Valliant & Bergerson, 1997; Worling & Curwen, 2000). Yet, multiple systems such as family, peer, and school relations may not be addressed as directly or immediately as possible without parents' presence in juvenile sex offender treatment. This is not to say that these multiple systems are ignored. However, juvenile sex offender treatment providers might have the strongest influence in interrupting the sexual abuse cycle and designing more effective relapse prevention plans if there is support from the youth's natural environment. Taking this systemic, socio-ecological approach and interweaving cognitive behavioral interventions might be the most comprehensive and effective treatment. In fact, there has been a growing belief within the field that effective treatment of juvenile sex offenders should include some level of parental and family involvement (Barbaree, Marshall, & McCormick, 1998; Butler & Seto, 2002; Rasmussen, 1999; Swenson, Henggeler, Schoenwald, Kaufman, & Randall, 1998; Worling & Curwen, 2000). Unfortunately, except for a study using multisystemic therapy (Bourdin, Henggeler, Blaske, & Stein, 1990), randomized, controlled research on treatment effectiveness is lacking in the juvenile sex offender treatment field.

Furthermore, including parents as part of the juvenile sex offender treatment can aid in effectively addressing dynamic risk factors. First, in most cases parents tend to play an important role in the progression of the sexual abuse cycle due to the nature of youth's development (Ryan, 1997). Youths rarely identify their sexual abuse cycle without including their parental relationship in some stage of the cycle. Therefore, if parents play a significant role in the abuse cycle development, they can also play a role in the interruption of the cycle. The cognitive-behavioral interventions of thought-stopping and social skills training, for example, can be done in a family context where the youth can be supported at the same time that the parents become part of the therapy process.

Second, although a family is not responsible for a youth's decision to assault sexually, they are an important system in the youth's life (Rasmussen, 1999; Worling & Curwin, 2000). Parents have a significant amount of influence over the youth in daily life activities. Developmentally, youth are in a fluid state of learning new ways of interacting and thinking, and parents can have significant impact on their social and cognitive development. When parents are included in therapy, the change process can become more meaningful and relevant to the youth since their parents are central to their everyday environment. In addition, including parents in therapy allows for problems to be redefined relationally, which may increase the motivation to change for all involved (Sexton & Alexander, 2003). The need to include parents in treatment of youth with Conduct Disorder has been shown to be essential in empirically validated family treatments (e.g., Alexander, Pugh, Parsons, & Sexton, 2000; Henggeler, Schoenwald, Borduin, Rowland, & Cunningham, 1998).

Third, Hunter and Figueredo (1999) found that youths' attitudes of openness and accountability in treatment are the best predictors of a positive treatment outcome. They stated that these attitudes tended to be more closely related to external influences such as parental openness to treatment rather than underlying psychopathology. Although external influences such as court and legal contingencies are key factors in increasing accountability to treatment, parents also have a significant amount of influence over the attitudes that a youth brings to treatment. In many cases, when the parents are closed to treatment, the adolescent will adopt a similar attitude. Clinically, it is difficult to motivate a youth towards treatment progress when parents do not support what is happening in sessions.

Last, parents will have continued contact with the youth beyond the limited time frame of treatment. If relapse prevention is to be ongoing, it is important to develop a support system for the youth to deal effectively with risk factors.

Parents are ideal candidates for this support since they will be the ones monitoring and supervising their youth.

COMMON ARGUMENTS AGAINST PARENTAL INCLUSION

There are some strongly held beliefs about juvenile sex offender treatment, the youth who participate in it, and their families. The following is a list of possible issues that may detract from including parents and other family members in juvenile sex offender treatment.

Issues of Responsibility

It is important that juvenile sex offenders take responsibility for their abusive sexual history. Hunter and Figueredo (1999) found that youths' denial states about their sexual offenses were predictive of who successfully complied with treatment, with those not in denial being more likely to comply with treatment. Likewise, by taking responsibility for past assaultive behaviors, youths are better able to understand their past behaviors and use this information to reduce risk for a repetition of these patterns.

At the same time, it is important to distinguish between the need to take responsibility for past behaviors and the need to take responsibility for present relapse prevention concerns. When practitioners put the burden of responsibility on the youth to interrupt the abuse cycle, they run the risk of underutilizing the resources available to the youth, and fail to recognize the complexity of relationships that keep the negative patterns in process. Similarly, practitioners may unknowingly ask the youth to take responsibility for negative family patterns while not including the parents' part in the problem.

Addressing risk factors in the families of juvenile sex offenders is often conducive to changing problematic behaviors. It is difficult to identify an abuse cycle for a youth without including some connection to parents' behaviors. Because of this, it is important to explore how parents' behaviors continue to keep the cycle going in the youth's daily life. In other words, when we make relapse prevention a family issue, the youth is able to focus on the aspects of change that are obtainable, and other family members can also make changes in order to support the success of the youth.

An example might clarify this point. Denise is a 15-year-old who lives with her father; she committed a sex offense when she was 14. In the past, Denise would react to her father's intense worrying by interacting with delinquent peers, which increased the likelihood for criminal behaviors. While worrying, her father would repeatedly ask a version of the same question or drive back and forth past the house where he believed his daughter was spending her time. Denise would see her father driving by and become more agitated, thus increasing her reactivity. She would react to her father's behavior by either impulsively leaving the house and making poor decisions or running away with peers. These decisions eventually led to illegal behaviors such as drug use, theft, and sexual contact with younger females and males.

While it is essential that Denise find ways to manage her impulsivity, it would be remiss not to address the systemic influences in her family context that were part of the sexual abuse cycle. When her father was able to acknowledge his part in the cycle, he made changes by finding ways to worry about his daughter that did not trigger Denise's potentially negative responses. Once Denise understood that her father would never stop worrying about her, she could do certain things to reduce her father's worry. By identifying their joint responsibility in the cycle, Denise was actually able to use her father's support to think before acting, thus reducing her risk for making poor decisions and increasing her probability of avoiding high-risk situations. If a practitioner were only to work with Denise, he/she would fail to recognize the influence that Denise's father has to help her disrupt negative patterns.

Parental Incompetence

There are times when youths' parents are assessed as having their own symptomology such as anxiety or depression. Often, therapists tend not to include the parent in the treatment sessions due to concern that the parent will "get in the way" of what they are trying to do in treatment.

It is important to remember that the youth has a lifetime of experience managing the context of his family relationships. Likewise, when a youth leaves the therapy session, he/she eventually returns home. Although practitioners may support the youth in taking on new skills and belief systems distinct from the parent's beliefs, the youth still must find a way to operate with new skills in the home environment. Not including parents in sessions may set the youth up for isolation from those who are important to him/her. The effect of this type of isolation may not be evident while the youth is in treatment since there is ongoing support from the therapist and members of the treatment group. However, once the youth graduates from treatment, there may not be as strong a connection between the youth and family.

Likewise, when practitioners do not include the "difficult to treat" parents in therapy, they may fail to help the youth develop and practice the skills needed to deal effectively with parents. While practitioners can have conversations with the youth about how to deal with parents, there is a difference between talking about dealing with parents and actually practicing skills with parents in the room.

Family Chaos

Similar to issues of parental incompetence, there are times when there is so much chaos in a family due to drug addiction, parental conflict, parental withdrawal, unemployment, or mental health issues that it seems more reasonable to remove the child from the family due to concerns that the family will continually disrupt treatment progress.

Therapists may try to mold families into their own definitions of what is "normal," which makes change nearly impossible to achieve. Because this does not always seem possible, the recommendation might be to remove the youth from the home. The problem with this outlook is that although the therapist may not agree with the families' methods of managing life, the family is still the youth's home environment. At these times, expectations for change must be realistic. Therapists might want to examine the realistic changes the youth and the youth's parents can make that might interrupt the cyclical patterns that eventually lead to abusive behaviors. Trying to address three generations of drug addiction and neglect in a family in a few treatment sessions is not realistic. However, finding safe ways for the youth's parents to help the youth with treatment homework while the television is continuously turned on might be the first step towards building a support system for the youth. As each small step is met with success and confidence, more suggestions can be made. When the therapist develops plans for all family members to be successful, shame is reduced and trust is developed.

Parental Dominance

Cashwell and Caruso (1997) discussed the possibility that some parents may react to their children in ways that interfere with the treatment process. Many parents have high degrees of denial, guilt, shame, confusion, and anger about their child's assaultive behavior due to feelings of responsibility for their child's behavior or struggles with their own abusive past. There is realistic concern that the parents may dominate the treatment sessions with their own intra-psychic needs. At these times, the therapist may feel protective of the youth's needs and treatment goals and attempt to insulate treatment by excluding the parents from sessions.

There are two important points to consider with this type of situation. First, as stated previously, the youth still needs to address the parental relationship. If therapists do not include parents in sessions, they may lack understanding of how to support and educate the youth in interacting with parents. Second, there are times when a high degree of emotionality between family members points to a high degree of connectedness between them. In these situations, it might better suit the youth to help negotiate his/her own needs versus the needs of the parent. Likewise, when practitioners include parents in treatment, they are in a position to model for the youth how to negotiate and manage his/her parents' needs by showing, for instance, how to communicate differently. Also, giving parents some time for their feelings in sessions may build a stronger alliance with them and increase the likelihood that they will be more motivated to follow treatment goals.

There is Enough to Deal with Already

There are many aspects of treatment for a youth to complete. There are risk factors to address and a significant amount of information to share as part of the psychoeducational aspect of treatment. In addition, this does not even take into account that many of the youth who commit sexual offenses have other issues to address such as their own victimization history, drug and alcohol abuse, or mental health disorders. Furthermore, the therapist must interface with so many important people in the youth's life, including schoolteachers, probation officers, psychiatrists, and other family members that might want to talk with them. To make matters more complex, most therapists are working with large and difficult caseloads that can be potentially traumatic for them (Ennis & Horne, 2003). In light of these factors, the thought of including the parents in therapy might seem overwhelming and unrealistic.

However, Rasmussen (1999) points out that therapeutic changes experienced by the family often parallel changes experienced by the youth. There is a mutual influence one has on the other. In other words, when the family experiences a change in motivation or involvement, the youth will be affected by this shift in the family. Thus, while working with families might appear to be adding more work for therapists, doing so may actually make working with this population more manageable.

Uncomfortable Issues

Many times, therapists struggle to motivate parents to discuss sex offender treatment because parents are uncomfortable talking about issues of sexual arousal, masturbation, or pornography. Likewise, the youth is often embarrassed when it is suggested that parents be included in sessions. Many therapists also hold the belief that they should not "make" the youth talk about sexuality to parents. At these times, there are ways to talk about sensitive issues such as sexual arousal in more general ways that help address sexual issues. In fact, it is at these times that parents may especially need to be included in sessions, since all family members involved may need guidance about how to talk about such issues.

The therapist can be a guide or role model to show ways to talk about these issues. For instance, a therapist may want to discuss one way of interrupting a potentially risky interactional cycle by having parents ask certain questions in ways that are supportive of their youth when they notice a change in the youth's affect. The questions to be asked do not need to be specific, but rather a way of monitoring and supervising the youth's behaviors. For example, a parent may ask, "I'm wondering if what happened at school today has made you tempted to escape into the Internet." The family can then participate in a discussion of how to deal with different possible responses from the youth. If parents are not included in these types of interventions, the youth is only talking with the therapist, and when therapy is completed, there is no generalization of skills to the youth's home environment where change can be supported and sustained.

Issues of Causality

Because family relationships appear not to be the cause of sexual abuse, there is a tendency to minimize their importance. Treatment providers often show more interest in risk factors that are more directly connected to sexual behavior. These risk factors are usually intra-psychic such as deviant sexual arousal and cognitive distortions. While these factors are important, opportunities to interrupt negative interactional patterns can also play a significant role in interrupting abusive behaviors.

Relationship Complexity

Sometimes practitioners hesitate to include parents in treatment because family relationships can be so complex. It can be difficult to even know where to begin. This complexity is even more highlighted when it becomes apparent that there are offense specific issues to address, particularly when the abuse is incestuous. There are no easy answers for parents who are struggling with how to support both their child who is the victim and their child who is the offender. Yet, the complexity of family patterns may be a large contributing risk factor in the youth's life. Therapists provide a great service to the youth and parents when they are able to manage the complexity in the therapy room. At these times, therapists become both role models for how to deal with complexity and inspirations for finding solutions to their problems.

JUVENILE SEX OFFENDER TREATMENT AS A SPECIALTY FIELD

A relevant debate in the juvenile sexual offender field is whether adolescents who commit sexual offenses exhibit unique characteristics different from youth who commit general nonsexual crimes. This question is significant in that the identification of unique factors for juvenile sex offenders highlights possible etiological sources, thus leading to clearer intervention strategies (For an in-depth discussion of the etiological sources of juvenile sex offending, see Knight & Sims-Knight, this issue). A review of the literature on both sides of this debate will be explored briefly as a way to discuss including parents in juvenile sex offender treatment.

Milloy (1998) takes the position that the literature on juvenile sex offenders does not point to strong evidence of a unique profile compared to nonsexual delinquents. The differences are clearer when non-delinquent youth are compared to the delinquent group, whether they are sexual or nonsexual offenders. It is also important to mention that many juveniles who commit sexual offenses also commit nonsexual crimes. In fact, the sexual recidivism rate among juveniles who have committed sexual offenses is only about 14%. However, their recidivism rate for nonsexual offenses is about 54% (Rasmussen, 1999). Thus, it appears that juveniles who commit sexual offenses do not, in most cases, commit further future sexual offenses. Rather, they appear to move on to more nonsexual delinquent crimes. In this way, they resemble general delinquents. This is key in conceptualizing treatment options.

Milloy (1998) continues on this theme when she reports that the literature does not support the premise that juveniles specialize in one type of crime. Rather, the evidence suggests that delinquent behavior is primarily non-patterned and that juveniles are versatile offenders. Pure sex offenders, even among juveniles, are rare.

Jacobs, Kennedy, and Meyer (1997) did not find significant differences between adolescent sex offenders and general delinquent offenders. They concluded that rape committed by a juvenile is one delinquent behavior of a juvenile's general delinquency pattern. Their results did not support the assumption that juvenile sex offenders are a unique subgroup of delinquency offenders. Thus, treatment should focus not only on specific sex offender concerns but also on other aspects of their delinquency patterns.

The other side of the discussion states that there are differences between juvenile sex offenders and general nonsexual delinquents. Research has found adolescent sex offenders to be more assaultive, socially introverted, resentful, and more directly hostile than general offender groups (Valliant & Bergerson, 1997). Higher levels of anxiety and social estrangement have also been found in juvenile sex offenders compared to nonsexual adolescent offenders (Blaske, Borduin, Henggeler, & Mann, 1998). Finally, sexual interest in children was a factor that distinguished between adolescent sex offenders and general offenders (Worling & Curwen, 2000).

In summary, there is a need for further research in this area, as there is not clear agreement whether juvenile sex offenders are a unique subgroup. Likewise, there is not clear agreement among the researchers who support the uniqueness of adolescent sex offenders as to what these distinguishing characteristics are.

In either case, adolescent sex offenders need to be understood within the developmental and systemic contexts in which they exist. In fact, there is a growing trend within the field of adolescent sex offender treatment to intervene from within this more holistic perspective (Blaske et al., 1998; Butler & Seto, 2002; Hunter, Figueredo, Malamuth, & Becker, 2003; Rasmussen, 1999; Ryan, 1999; Swenson et al., 1998). One key system is the adolescent sex offender's family. From either side of this debate, there is a need to include parents or parental figures in treatment. The juvenile sex offender treatment field would greatly benefit from research focused on when and how to incorporate parents and other systems into the treatment process.

SEXUAL AROUSAL CONCERNS

While a comprehensive discussion concerning sexual arousal patterns for juvenile sex offenders is beyond the scope of this article, it is important to identify some emerging ideas on this subject and why the inclusion of parents in treatment may influence a youth's relationship to sexual patterns (for additional discussion of sexual arousal patterns, see Righthand & Welch, this issue). This is not to suggest that including parents in treatment should be used as the sole intervention when addressing arousal concerns. However, not considering sexual arousal issues within a developmental and systemic context might limit the ability to influence and sustain change.

The development of sexual deviance is most likely due to experiences in the person's early family life, most specifically related to the parent-child dynamics (Barbaree et al., 1998). Possibly, the identification of the parent-child dynamics in the child's early experiences and the interruption of these dynamics in the adolescent's current life may provide the opportunity for more effective behavioral interventions. The difference between juvenile arousal and adult arousal is important to this discussion because juvenile sexual interests and arousal are more fluid and varied than adults (Hunter & Becker, 1994; Hunter, Goodwin, & Becker, 1994). This fluidity implies the ability to be influenced by internal (e.g., cognitions) and external (e.g., family) sources. Because these external sources might influence a youth's sexual arousal patterns, integrating these systems into treatment seems like an important aspect of sexual arousal intervention.

TARGETING PARENTING RISK AND PROTECTIVE FACTORS

Family factors such as spousal violence, child abuse, and low warmth and cohesion have been shown to be related to both general juvenile offenders and juvenile sex offenders (Bishof, Stith, & Whitney, 1995; Ryan & Lane, 1997). While these family factors are addressed in family-based interventions for general juvenile offenders, the study of parental inclusion in the treatment of juvenile sex offenders is lacking.

In order to understand how parents can be included in treatment of juvenile sex offenders, it is important to be able to identify ways in which parental risk factors are decreased at the same time that parental protective factors are increased. Therefore, an investigation into the role of parents is important in adolescence. Adolescence is often thought of as a time in which peer influence supersedes parental influence. However, parental influence has been found to be important in relation to delinquency (Baumrind, 1991; Brown, Mounts, Lamborn, & Steinberg, 1993). Since research has indicated a relationship between youths' low self-control and poor parenting (Gottfredson & Hirschi, 1990), addressing the parental role in therapy can aid in utilizing parents as resources for intervention in relapse prevention for the juvenile sex offender. Addressing parental influence could include teaching parenting skills to decrease delinquent youths' low levels of self-control, which is characteristic of these youth.

The parenting styles literature is often based on Baumrind's (1996) model, which suggests that effective parenting includes parents being both demanding and responsive, or what the author calls "the authoritative" parenting style (Baumrind, 1991). The demanding component includes parents' ability to include the youth as part of the family, supervise, discipline, and confront when the youth disobeys (Maccoby & Martin, 1983). The responsive component includes encouraging individuality, paying attention to the youth's unique needs, and being supportive (Baumrind, 1991; Maccoby &

Martin, 1983). In general, findings have shown that authoritative parents are more likely to have youth with higher social competence, including having self-control, compared to parents with authoritarian, permissive, or rejecting-neglecting styles (Baumrind, 1991; Logue, 1996).

Because parenting styles are related to self-control in youth, including parents in family therapy with juvenile sex offenders would seem important. The parents' ability to provide an environment where the youth feels both supported but also held responsible allows for reciprocal influence between the youth and parent. Hostile and neglectful parenting has been related to antisocial behaviors (Weiss, Dodge, Bates, & Petit, 1992). Family therapy with juvenile sex offenders can enhance the parent's ability to support, monitor, and supervise the juvenile sex offender and reduce hostility or blaming.

The knowledge that parents influence self-control in youth can improve work with parents to help juvenile sex offenders break abuse cycles, and change daily interactions within the family context and other social systems. When parents can change the way they view their role in the treatment of their youth, the likelihood that they will become involved will most likely increase. Thus, for instance, teaching parents skills of giving support while also providing supervision (authoritative parenting style) will empower them to be part of interrupting the abuse cycle. Parenting practices will influence the probability that the youth will go to parents and announce that a "temptation" has occurred. Parents can then be coached in the two essential areas discussed by Baumrind (1991). First, parents can be given the skills to respond encouragingly to the youth since he reported such a thought in the progress of breaking the abuse cycle. At the same time, parents can be given skills to respond with appropriate monitoring and supervision to ensure safety and protection for all involved. By teaching parents more authoritative parenting practices, day-to-day behaviors most likely will include more positive interactions and fewer negative interactions. This will help create a more positive, non-hostile family environment that allows for more pro-social behaviors (Weiss et al., 1992).

Last, authoritative parenting practices would logically seem to impact parents' ability to intervene in relapse prevention. Parents can be taught to be able to observe "red flags" or "triggers" of potential relapse and to intervene accordingly. So, in addition to teaching juvenile sex offenders to track and monitor their own thoughts and behaviors in the cycle to prevent relapse, parents also have the opportunity to be included in the relapse prevention plan.

CASE EXAMPLE

Jeff is a 16-year-old youth who spent 6 months in the juvenile institution for raping a neighborhood boy on several occasions. Jeff was 15 at the time, and the victim was 7. Besides Jeff's history of sexual offending behavior, he also has a history of property damage in his home along with some physical altercations with his mother. Jeff openly admits to excessive pornography use and social isolation. Jeff identifies a general abuse cycle. He is triggered by a variety of issues, but a significant concern for him is his insecurity around peer-age females and also his ability to feel connected to a particular social group at school. Jeff's anxiety about these concerns became the foundation of the schema he expects to experience in situations and relationships in school. Jeff attempts to manage his anxiety at school by avoiding contact with others, but he is unsuccessful. He continues feeling frustrated and powerlessness when he arrives home to an environment where he does not feel he can share his worries. In fact, interactions between him and his parents escalate his feelings of powerlessness and helplessness, so Jeff may find comfort in searching the Internet for pornography as a way to manage his affect. Deviant arousal may occur, and Jeff may soon find himself engaging in inappropriate sexual behavior with an underage boy.

Through treatment sessions with his parents, Jeff is able to identify that he does not handle stress very well. He ruminates obsessively, hoping to find a solution to handling his stress. Jeff's mother is similar to Jeff in that she also spends a lot of her time ruminating about her stressors. When she is anxious and feeling powerless, she tends to make demands on Jeff and follows him around to make sure he does things correctly. When Jeff's father comes home, he immediately hears about their fight and often intensifies the conflict by making comments that alienate either his son or wife.

Although Jeff's parents are not the cause of his sexual offense behavior or continuation through the cycle, they play a part in the early phases of it. Jeff's parents can see this and begin to make changes in how they relate to Jeff. These changes are based on feedback from Jeff, the therapist, and their own insights. Jeff's mother decides that it is not helpful to be so intently focused on Jeff when she needs something even though it is important to her. Jeff's father sees that although he is overworked and needing space when he comes home, he needs to prepare himself to give Jeff a short amount of his time. Because Jeff is interested in what his parents are saying, he begins to participate further in the discussion. He begins to see that sometimes he just needs to vent and talk about his day. Because he seems to have already thought through the issue so thoroughly, he does not really need feedback about how to handle a situation. More importantly, when Jeff is able just to talk, his anxiety decreases and he is better able both to listen to what his responsibilities are around the house and to think through more easily his school problems and act on what he believes might work.

Jeff realizes that besides peer relationships, he has other issues that produce anxiety for him. He realizes that although some of the subject matter is uncomfortable, he needs to find a way to talk about these things so he can make healthy decisions more clearly. Jeff's parents realize that the content of what Jeff is actually talking about is irrelevant as far as how to support him. It is more important to them that they avoid giving him too much feedback and mostly just listen to him so he can talk.

In this example, Jeff's abuse cycle is interrupted as each family member involved in the treatment learns new skills. Although the skills learned are not addressing causal issues related to sexual offending, they are effectively using the skills to stop the cycle. Jeff may still struggle with pornography use, but the use begins to take on new meaning since it is no longer connected to the abuse cycle.

CONCLUSION

We suggest that abuse cycle interruption and relapse prevention integration is effectively addressed when they incorporate working with family interaction patterns, particularly the youth's interactions with parents. The skills taught to both the youth and parents constitute the foundation of a relevant and meaningful relapse prevention plan. Once skills have been taught to both the youth and the parents concerning the interruption of a specific interaction pattern, then these same skills can be generalized to address other dynamic risk factors as they are identified. In a sense, treatment can be looked at as the family's continual progression of independence away from needing the support of the treatment provider. As the parents learn ways to support the interruption of the cycle, there is less need for therapeutic involvement in this area. Even though there is a focus on relational patterns between specific family members, there remains the same cognitive/behavioral foundation as the standard treatment approach.

Family interventions in the treatment of juvenile delinquency have been lauded for their effectiveness (Henggeler et al., 1998; Sexton & Alexander, 2003). Because the family context is important in conceptualizing youth at-risk behaviors for both sexual and nonsexual juvenile offenders, it would seem important to note the use of parents in juvenile sex offender intervention. Just as the juvenile sex offender treatment field has borrowed the relapse prevention model from the substance abuse field, it may be appropriate to revisit what the substance abuse field has been doing in intervention for juveniles.

Studies of parental inclusion in juvenile sex offender treatment are lacking. However, one study compared multisystemic therapy (MST), a family based intervention, to individual counseling in treating juvenile sex offenders. The MST group had recidivism rates of 12.5% for sexual offenses and 25% for nonsexual offenses. The individual counseling group had recidivism rates of 75% for sexual offenses and 50% for nonsexual offenses (Bourdin et al., 1990). While this study had a small sample size of 16, further investigation in using family treatment is warranted. It appears that sex offender treatment could be significantly enhanced by the inclusion of interventions used in the generalist delinquency field (Bischof et al., 1995). The juvenile sex offender field may consider reviewing how family interventions have worked effectively with the general delinquent population in order to provide some insight on how to incorporate parental involvement in treatment without abandoning the predominant cognitive-behavioral approach.

REFERENCES

Alexander, J.F., Pugh, C., Parsons, B., & Sexton, T. (2000). *Blueprints for violence prevention: Book three: Functional family therapy.* Boulder, CO: University of Colorado, Institute for Behavioral Sciences, Center for the Study and Prevention of Violence.

Barbaree, H.E., Marshall, W.L., & McCormick, J. (1998). The development of deviant sexual behavior among adolescents and its implications for prevention and treatment. *The Irish Journal of Psychology, 19*(1), 1-31.

Baumrind, D. (1991). The influence of parenting style on adolescent competence and substance use. *Journal of Early Adolescence, 11,* 56-95.

Baumrind, D. (1996). Parenting: The discipline controversy revisited. *Family Relations, 45,* 405-414.

Bischof, G.P., Stith, S.M., & Whitney, M.L. (1995). Family environments of adolescent sex offenders and other juvenile delinquents. *Adolescence, 30*(117), 157-171.

Blaske, D.M., Borduin, C.M., Henggeler, S.W., & Mann, B.J. (1998). Individual, family, and peer characteristics of adolescent sex offenders and assaultive offenders. *Developmental Psychology, 25*(5), 846-855.

Borduin, C.M., Henggeler, S.W., Blaske, D.M., & Stein, R. (1990). Multisystemic treatment of adolescent sexual offenders. *International Journal of Offender Therapy and Comparative Criminology, 35,* 105-114.

Brown, B.B., Mounts, N., Lamborn, S.D., & Steinberg, L. (1993). Parenting practices and peer group affiliation in adolescence. *Child Development, 64,* 467-482.

Butler, S. M., & Seto, M.C. (2002). Distinguishing two types of adolescent sex offenders. *Child & Adolescent Psychiatry, 41*(1), 83-90.

Cashwell, C.S., & Caruso, M.E. (1997). Adolescent sex offenders: Identification and intervention strategies. *Journal of Mental Health Counseling, 19*(4), 336-349.

Ennis, L., & Horne, S. (2003). Predicting psychological stress in sex offender therapists. *Sexual Abuse: A Journal of Research and Treatment, 15*(2), 149-156.

Gottfredson, M., & Hirschi, T. (1990). *A general theory of crime.* Stanford, CA: Stanford University Press.

Gray, A.S., & Pithers, W.D. (1993). Relapse prevention with sexually aggressive adolescents and children: Expanding treatment and supervision. In H.E. Barbaree, W.L. Marshall, & S.M. Hudson (Eds.), *The juvenile sex offender* (pp. 264-277). New York: The Guilford Press.

Henggeler, S.W., Schoenwald, S.K., Borduin, C.M., Rowland, M.D., & Cunningham, P.E. (1998). *Multisystemic treatment of antisocial behavior in children and adolescents.* New York: Guilford Press.

Hunter, J.A., & Becker, J.V. (1994). The role of deviant sexual arousal in juvenile sexual offending: Etiology, evaluation, and treatment. *Criminal Justice and Behavior, 21*(1), 132-149.

Hunter Jr., J.A., & Figueredo, A. J. (1999). Factors associated with treatment compliance in a population of juvenile sexual offenders. *Sexual Abuse: A Journal of Research and Treatment, 11*(1), 49-67.

Hunter Jr., J.A., Figueredo, A.J., Malamuth, N.M., & Becker, J.V. (2003). Juvenile sex offenders: Toward the development of a typology. *Sexual Abuse: A Journal of Research and Treatment, 15*(1), 27-48.

Hunter, J.A., Goodwin, D.W., & Becker, J.V. (1994). The relationship between phallometrically measured deviant sexual arousal and clinical characteristics in juvenile sexual offenders. *Behavior Research and Therapy, 32*, 533-538.

Jacobs, W.L., Kennedy, W.A., & Meyer, J.B. (1997). Juvenile delinquency: A between group comparison study of sexual and nonsexual offenders. *Sexual Abuse: A Journal of Research and Treatment, 3*(3), 201-217.

Knight, R.A., & Sims-Knight, J.E. (2004). Testing an etiological model for male juvenile sexual offending against females. *Journal of Child Sexual Abuse, 13*(3/4), pp. 33-56.

Lane, S. (1997). The sexual abuse cycle. In G. Ryan, & S. Lane (Eds.), *Juvenile sexual offending: Consequences, causes, and correction* (pp. 77-121). San Francisco: Jossey-Bass Publishers.

Logue, A.W. (1996). Self-control: An alternative to self-regulation framework applicable to human and nonhuman behavior. *Psychological Inquiry, 7*, 68-72.

Maccoby, E.E., & Martin, J.A. (1983). Socialization in the context of the family: Parent-child interaction. In E. Hetherington (Ed.), & P. Mussen (Series Ed.), *Handbook of child psychology, vol. 4, socialization, personality, and social development* (pp. 1- 101). Boston: Allyn & Bacon.

Milloy, C.D. (1998). Specialized treatment for juvenile sex offenders. *Journal of Interpersonal Violence, 13*(5), 653-657.

Rasmussen, L.A. (1999). Factors related to recidivism among juvenile sexual offenders. *Sexual Abuse: A Journal of Research and Treatment, 11*, 69-85.

Righthand, S., & Welch, C. (2004). Characteristics of youth who sexually offend. *Journal of Child Sexual Abuse, 13*(3/4), pp. 15-32.

Ryan, G. (1997). The families of sexually abusive youth. In G. Ryan, & S. Lane (Eds.), *Juvenile sexual offending: Consequences, causes, and correction* (pp. 136-154). San Francisco: Jossey-Bass Publishers.

Ryan, G. (1999). Treatment of sexually abusive youth: The evolving consensus. *Journal of Interpersonal Violence, 14*(4), 442-436.

Sexton, T.L., & Alexander, J.F. (2003). Functional family therapy: A mature clinical model for working with at-risk adolescents and their families. In T.L. Sexton, G.R. Weeks, & M.S. Robbins (Eds.), *Handbook of family therapy: The science and practice of working with families and couples* (pp. 323-351). New York: Brunner-Routledge.

Swenson, C.C., Henggeler, S.W., Schoenwald, S.K., Kaufman, K.L., & Randall, J. (1998). Changing the social ecologies of adolescent sexual offenders: Implications of the success of multisystemic therapy in treating serious antisocial behavior in adolescents. *Child Maltreatment, 3*(4), 330-338.

Valliant, P.M., & Bergerson, T. (1997). Personality and criminal profile of adolescent sexual offenders, general offenders in comparison to nonoffenders. *Psychological Reports, 81*, 483-489.

Weiss, B., Dodge, K.A., Bates, J.E., & Petit, G.S. (1992). Some consequences of early harsh discipline: Child aggression and a maladaptive social information processing style. *Child Development, 63*, 1321-1335.

Worling, J. R., & Curwen, T. (2000). Adolescent sexual offender recidivism: Success of specialized treatment and implications for risk prediction. *Child Abuse and Neglect, 24*(7), 965-982.

Cognitive-Behavioral Treatment for Adolescents Who Sexually Offend and Their Families: Individual and Family Applications in a Collaborative Outpatient Program

David J. Kolko
Colleen Noel
Gretchen Thomas
Eunice Torres

SUMMARY. This article describes an outpatient treatment program for adolescent sexual abusers that was established by a mental health

---

Address correspondence to: David J. Kolko, PhD, Director, Services for Adolescent and Family Enrichment (*SAFE*), Western Psychiatric Institute and Clinic, 3811 O'Hara Street, Pittsburgh, PA 15213 (E-mail: kolkodj@upmc.edu).

The authors acknowledge the collaboration and support of their colleagues Dr. Jack Rozel, Dr. Oscar Bukstein, Dan Fernandez, Amy Gradnik, and Matthew Hennessy from the SAFE Program, and MaryLee Tracy, David Mink, Teri Vangenewitt, and Clyde Schneider from the Special Services Unit, Juvenile Court, Allegheny County (Pittsburgh).

This collaborative program is supported, in part, by a grant from the Juvenile Court of Allegheny County (Jim Rieland, Director, Court Services).

[Haworth co-indexing entry note]: "Cognitive-Behavioral Treatment for Adolescents Who Sexually Offend and Their Families: Individual and Family Applications in a Collaborative Outpatient Program." Kolko, David J. et al. Co-published simultaneously in *Journal of Child Sexual Abuse* (The Haworth Maltreatment and Trauma Press, an imprint of The Haworth Press, Inc.) Vol. 13, No. 3/4, 2004, pp. 157-192; and: *Identifying and Treating Youth Who Sexually Offend: Current Approaches, Techniques, and Research* (ed: Robert Geffner et al.) The Haworth Maltreatment and Trauma Press, an imprint of The Haworth Press, Inc., 2004, pp. 157-192. Single or multiple copies of this article are available for a fee from The Haworth Document Delivery Service [1-800-HAWORTH, 9:00 a.m. - 5:00 p.m. (EST). E-mail address: docdelivery@haworthpress.com].

157

agency in collaboration with a specialized probation program in the juvenile court. Individualized treatment is based on a comprehensive clinical assessment with the youth and guardian, for which examples are provided. Given the heterogeneity of this population, we describe several treatment strategies directed to various individual or family clinical targets, including psychiatric disorders, sexual deviance and sexuality, normal adolescent development and adaptive skills, and parent and family relationships. Ongoing collaborative and coordination issues are also reviewed. The integration of mental health and probationary services provides a balanced approach to the community management and treatment of the low-risk, primarily first-time, adolescent sexual offender. *[Article copies available for a fee from The Haworth Document Delivery Service: 1-800-HAWORTH. E-mail address: <docdelivery@ haworthpress.com> Website: <http://www.HaworthPress.com> © 2004 by The Haworth Press, Inc. All rights reserved.]*

KEYWORDS. Adolescent sexual offenders, cognitive-behavioral treatment, outpatient treatment, interventions for adolescent sexual offenders, individual and family treatment

There is increasing recognition of the prevalence, origins, impact, and treatment of adolescent sexual offenders. Empirical studies have highlighted considerable heterogeneity in putative risk factors, offense histories, personalities and clinical functioning, treatment regimens, and outcomes of adolescents with sexually abusive behavior (Center for Sex Offender Management [CSOM], 1999; Veneziano & Veneziano, 2002), among other characteristics (Hunter, Hazelwood, & Slesinger, 2000). Several characteristics are potential targets for intervention, such as details about the offense (Hunter, Figueredo, Malamuth, & Becker, 2003), prior victimization (Ford & Linney, 1995), psychological or personality traits (Worling, 2001), social competence and adaptive skills (Barbaree, Marshall, & McCormick, 1998), and parental and family dysfunction (Ford & Linney, 1995; Kobayashi, Sales, Becker, Figueredo, & Kaplan, 1995).

One implication of the varied clinical backgrounds of this population is the importance of assessing and possibly treating a broad array of child, parent, and family characteristics believed to be associated with sexual offender recidivism and/or appropriate adolescent and family functioning. Given the absence of clear guidelines in this area, various intervention procedures may be considered to increase the level of participation and/or outcome for any given adolescent and his family, especially those who are maintained in the community. Although most of the treatment materials for adolescent offenders are applied in residential programs, we describe an outpatient program that draws upon relevant cognitive-behavioral treatments used with adult sexual offenders (Marshall, Anderson, & Fernandez, 1999) and juvenile offenders (CSOM, 1999).

This article provides an overview of the context, content, and process of treatment provided to adolescents with sexually abusive behavior who receive treatment in the community. The adolescents were participants in a collaborative treatment program that provides integrated probationary and clinical services to adolescent offenders and their families. We describe the organization and structure of this program, relevant assessment measures, and selected child and family treatment methods. Based on preliminary program evaluation data, we offer some general suggestions for outpatient treatment programs.

PROGRAM DESCRIPTION

Overview and Context

The collaborative treatment program described herein (the "SSU/SAFE Program") integrates the efforts of trained probation officers from the Special Services Unit (SSU) of the Northern probation office of the Juvenile Court, Allegheny County (Pittsburgh, Pennsylvania) and clinicians from Services for Adolescent and Family Enrichment (SAFE) at Western Psychiatric Institute and Clinic, University of Pittsburgh School of Medicine. The program serves children and adolescents ages 10-18 who remain in the community following their adjudication of a sexual offense through the Juvenile Court of Allegheny County. The program was developed to integrate probationary (e.g., monitoring, sanctions, sexual offender group) and mental health/clinical (e.g., assessment, individualized child and family treatment) services to offenders and their families, given limited resources available for clinical evaluation, treatment, and research with this population.

The collaboration was established to enhance service efficiency and efficacy (i.e., no waiting list, comprehensive assessments, clinical consultation, intervention extended to community settings, evaluation data), and to encourage the Balanced and Restorative Justice (BARJ) objectives using measures related to public safety, accountability, competency development, and recidivism. The program was designed for less serious (often first-time) juvenile offenders who pose little threat to the community, and thus, are maintained in community residences rather than being sent to placements. There were no other inclusion or exclusion criteria. The program was initially funded in 1998 by a grant from the Pennsylvania Commission on Crime and Delinquency.

Structure and Process

Upon adjudication of a sex crime, juveniles who are mandated to probation are scheduled to receive program services for approximately 1 year, although there is considerable variation in the duration of participation (most cases range from 7 to 15 months). Briefly, two probation officers and a supervisor from the SSU manage all youth who remain in the community through ongoing monitoring and supervision, administrative sanctions, and the provision of a sex offender education group.

A team of diagnostic and research assessors conducts all evaluations, and two clinicians who occasionally work with advanced trainees provide clinical services to all youth and their families. The clinical components include: (a) an initial diagnostic/psychiatric evaluation, (b) on-site mental health treatment and/or clinical consultation to SSU staff, (c) community treatment services (e.g., home or school visits), and (d) coordination or liaison with local agencies serving the family. A collaborative treatment team meeting is held each week to review program and case progress, and quarterly interdisciplinary program meetings are held with staff from the SSU and SAFE to discuss case progress, obstacles, and plans. Monthly service documentation/status reports are completed by SAFE clinicians who render ratings of service use, clinical impact (e.g., on selected targets), and goal achievement on a monthly basis to supplement the formal progress notes. Finally, SSU staff complete a discharge impressions form on each youth.

Case Characteristics

In terms of the background and clinical problems of our population, the youth are all male, generally young in age ($M = 14.7$; $SD = 2.0$; range = 10-19), and of modest overall intelligence ($M = 89.5$; $SD = 16.1$; range = 74-127). The racial and ethnic characteristics of this group generally reflect the demographics of the juvenile justice system in Pittsburgh (52% Caucasian; 47% African-American; 1% Other).

The adolescents are charged and then adjudicated of a variety of offenses, with the most common being indecent assault (81%, 88%), involuntary deviate sexual intercourse (39%, 11%), indecent exposure (18%, 12%), aggravated indecent assault (13%, 6%), harassment (9%, 6%), and then rape (18%, 5%), respectively. Seventy-one percent have engaged in some act involving penetration; 65% of the victims were younger by at least 4 years of age. Physical coercion is used in 25% of the cases. In terms of their intake clinical characteristics (see Table 1), half of the youth are diagnosed with at least one major psychiatric disorder. A subset exhibits clinically significant impairment and also reports modest rates of sexual and physical abuse.

INITIAL CONTACTS WITH FAMILY

The first contact, either by phone or mail, attempts to engage the family in the assessment and treatment process, and to develop rapport and a working relationship with the parents or legal guardian. Given their involvement with a lengthy and at times confusing legal process that led to their child's adjudication, it is not unusual for the family to exhibit denial, anger, guilt, blame, self-blame, shame, and despair when scheduling the first court-mandated assessment appointment. Dismissing the family's emotional reactions to the allegations may result in more resistance, which may be compounded by adverse reactions from others (neighbors, peers, relatives, etc.) regarding the news of this allegation. Thus, to enhance engagement, we have found it help-

TABLE 1. Intake Characteristics of Adolescent Sexual Offenders and Their Families

Clinical Data	% Above Cutoff/Mean
Parent/Family:	
Poor Monitoring	87
Limited Positive Parenting	60
Low Parental Involvement	47
Inconsistent Parental Discipline	47
Parental Depression	29
Parental History of Childhood Sexual Abuse	37
Youth:	
DSM-IV Axis I Diagnosis	60
Overall Child Impairment	40
Depression	38
Anxiety	33
Psychopathy–Callous/Unemotional Traits	21
Psychopathy–Conduct Problems	14
	% Reporting
Multiple Dating Partners	43
Unprotected Sex	50
History of Sexual Abuse	14
History of Physical Abuse	36
History of Emotional Abuse	50

Note. See Table 2 for these measures: APQ; BDI; CTS-PC; K-SADS; CIS; SCARED; PSD; PSV.

ful to provide a full explanation of various considerations relating to the assessment (e.g., describe benefits of a comprehensive assessment and parental/guardian involvement; validate family's reactions to adjudication and normalize experiences; identify target areas for treatment; encourage parents to be proactive with child; stress the family's strengths and resiliency).

We also use Motivational Interviewing and Enhancement techniques to maximize the juvenile and family's receptivity to any subsequent intervention plans (for further discussion of the use of Motivational Interviewing, see Lambie & McCarthy, this issue). In general, we attempt to highlight the "pros and cons" of addressing any salient clinical problems or concerns about their adjustment, and articulate some of the obstacles to making changes in individual or family functions. Thus, it is important to remain sensitive to the family's emotional situation in order to establish a working alliance with the parents and gain support for the treatment of their child.

ASSESSMENT

Purpose

The purpose of our assessment is: (a) to consider the predisposing and precipitating factors for the sexual offense, (b) to assess the juvenile's strengths and weakness, (c) to gather details about the sexual offense and the particular context in which it has occurred, (d) to determine the juvenile and families' motivation and commitment to treatment, (e) to identify treatment needs and design an intervention strategy, and (f) to determine risk for reoffending. The SAFE Program utilizes an ecological framework wherein the juvenile and his sexual offense are viewed within a system of protective and risk factors interacting across four levels: (a) individual or ontogenic level, (b) family micro-system level, (c) community exo-system, and (d) cultural social macro-system (Brofenbrenner, 1977). Understanding how the juvenile interacts in his environment and viewing the juvenile's identity as a multidimensional construct assists in identifying family, social, and cultural factors that may have contributed to his sexually abusive behavior.

The assessment represents a collaborative process involving the juvenile, the parents or legal guardian, and the probation officer. The planning and preparation of the assessment begins once the referral information from the probation officer is reviewed (i.e., juvenile petition, adjudication summary, police report, victim statement, court order, history of prior court involvement; child protection services reports, prior psychiatric and psychological reports, school records, demographic information). These documents also help the assessor to better understand the family's reactions to the incident (e.g., embarrassment, shame, guilt vs. denial, and minimization), their history with the legal, mental health, and child welfare systems, and any contradictions between what is reported in the report and by the family. The assessment often requires between two to three sessions of two hours each. Once the assessment is completed, the juvenile and his family are assigned to a SAFE treatment clinician.

Content of Assessment

The assessment of juveniles adjudicated of a sexual offense and court mandated to the SAFE Program reflects a comprehensive approach that examines a wide range of domains. The primary domains assessed are: (a) individual history and mental health diagnosis, (b) family composition, history, and functioning, (c) intellectual ability, (d) sexual history and sexual behavior, (e) circumstances and details of the offense, and (f) motivation to change and treatment compliance. The assessment is occasionally complicated due to client and system factors involved in this process, such as the mandated nature of the assessment and treatment, juvenile and family denial, minimization, and embarrassment of the offense, and the lack of motivation to participate. Thus, it is important to consider the individual needs of the juvenile and his family when planning and preparing each assessment.

Process and Procedures

After the assessment is scheduled, the juvenile and his family come to the office for their first assessment session aware of the general length of the assessment. Once in the clinician's office, the engagement process continues with a discussion of the juvenile's awareness of the program's policy and the court mandate for participation, which is acknowledged by only some juveniles. During this discussion, the clinician can observe the juvenile and his parent(s) as they discuss the reasons to conduct an assessment, which helps the clinician to understand their perceptions of the offense and the victim, and commitment and motivation to treatment.

The clinician begins the assessment with an orientation to the program and the expectations for their participation, followed by an explanation of the limits of confidentiality and reporting laws. Once they sign all administrative forms (e.g., release for health protected information), the research component is explained, and informed consent is obtained from the guardian for juveniles or from those youth who are 18 years of age who wish to participate.

The assessor conducts a diagnostic and sexual offender-specific clinical interview with each juvenile and guardian separately, while a clinical assistant administers clinical research measures with the other informant. The juvenile and a parent (mostly the primary caregiver) are assessed on a standardized battery of self-report and interview instruments as shown in Table 2. Assessments are conducted at intake, discharge, and 1- and 2-year follow-up. At discharge, the youth completes all of the same measures from intake, an 8-item consumer satisfaction questionnaire (CSQ-8; Larsen, Attkisson, Hargreaves, & Nguyen, 1979), and a questionnaire addressing barriers to treatment. During the follow-up assessments, the youth completes all the prior measures including a questionnaire designed to determine involvement in various sexual activities or experiences ("My Sexual Experiences") and additional mental health services. This material is reviewed and coded by trained, research assessment staff. Each informant receives a separate payment for information at intake, discharge, and follow-up.

At the end of the assessment sessions the assessment clinician meets with the family to briefly summarize some of the areas identified as areas for treatment, to answer any questions, and discuss initial plans for and interests in treatment. At this point, the assessment is then completed. The information is used to generate a report that includes norms and *T*-scores for each measure that is discussed in the treatment team meeting and then with the juvenile and his family during the first treatment session.

INITIAL TREATMENT CONTACTS: FAMILY ORIENTATION AND SYSTEM COORDINATION

Treating community-based juvenile sex offenders is challenging for both the families and their providers. Families are persuaded by the courts to perceive community-based treatment as a privilege and a better alternative to sanctions and placement away from their families. Initially this transition to life on probation is difficult for most families, as parents often report that they feel as if the entire family has been placed on probation. The adolescent may still reside in their home, go to the same school, and socialize with the same friends, but life as they know it has been drastically altered and restricted.

Challenges for Families: Initial Reactions

Parents state that the upheaval sexual abuse creates is unlike any other family crisis, especially when their son is the perpetrator. Unlike other child problems such as an illness, parents in our program tend to avoid accessing their

TABLE 2. Representative Assessment Measures for Use with Juveniles and Their Parents

K-SADS-PL (Schedule for Affective Disorders and Schizophrenia for School Aged Children 6-18 years–Lifetime Version)	Interview to evaluate the presence of all Axis I child psychiatric disorders, both currently and lifetime (e.g., ADHD, ODD, anxiety, MDD)	(Kaufman, Birmaher, Brent, Rao, & Ryan, 1996)
JSA (Juvenile Sex Abusers Questionnaire)	To examine the details of the offense, denial, admittance, thoughts, feelings, empathy	(Kolko, Baumann, & Bukstein, 1999)
PSV (Physical and Sexual Violence Scale)	Juvenile's history of abuse	(Kolko et al., 1999)
ASBI (Adolescent Sexual Behavior Inventory–Adolescent Version)	The ASBI is a 38-item self-report inventory of sexual behavior	(Friedrich, Luecke, Bielke, & Place, 1992)
BDI (Beck Depression Inventory)	Measures the severity of depressive symptoms	(Beck, Ward, Mendelson, Mock, & Erbaugh, 1961)
TSCC (Trauma Symptom Checklist for Children)	The TSCC is a standardized self-report instrument for children that evaluates various sequelae of abuse (e.g., depression, sexual concerns, posttraumatic stress)	(Briere, 1996)
CBCL (Child Behavior Checklist)	CBCL measures individual factors (e.g., depression, somatic complaints, hyperactivity, sexual behavior, aggressiveness); yields externalizing, internalizing, & total problem scores	(Achenbach, 1991)
SACA (Services Assessment for Children and Adolescents)	Questions about any treatment the juveniles may have received for emotional, behavioral, or drug and alcohol problems	(Hoagwood et al., 2000)
IOWA (Connor's Parenting Rating Scale)	This parent and teacher measure will provide a dimensional assessment of inattention/overactivity and oppositional behaviors at home/school	(Pelham, Milich, Murphy, & Murphy, 1989)
Scale for Anxiety and Related Disorders (SCARED)	Abbreviated version of the Screen for Child Anxiety Related Emotional Disorders	(Birmaher, Khetarpal, Brent, & Cully, 1997)
FRM (Family Relationships Measure)	Parent's perceptions of the dynamics and relationships within the family	(Tolan, Gorman-Smith, Huesmann, & Zelli, 1997)
APQ (Alabama Parenting Questionnaire)	Evaluates six dimensions of parenting practices and activities (e.g., involvement, positive parenting, corporal punishment) related to antisocial behavior	(Shelton, Frick, & Wooten, 1996)

TABLE 2 (continued)

CTS-P (Conflict Tactics Scale–Parent Version)	Assesses three revised factors related to parental discipline (non-violent discipline, psychological aggression, physical assault)	(Straus, Hamby, Finkelhor, Moore, & Runyan, 1998)
PERQ-SO (Family History, Perceived Emotional Reactivity Questionnaire)	(Partner relationship history, Perceived Emotional Reactivity Questionnaire)	(Cohen & Mannarino, 1988)
Family History	Partner relationship history, domestic abuse history, family substance abuse history, family history of psychiatric disorders, and geographic stability of child	(Kolko et al., 1999)
PCL-YV (The Hare Psychopathy Checklist: Youth Version)	To assess the juvenile's interpersonal style, to obtain information about aspects of his life and to assess the credibility of his statements	(Forth, Hart, & Hare, 1990)
ACS (Abel, Becker, & Kaplan, Adolescent Cognition Scale)	A 32-item true/false self report designed to assess juveniles' distorted cognitions regarding sexual behaviors	(Abel & Becker, 1984)
CIS (Columbia Impairment Scale-Adolescent Version)	For the juvenile to identify how much of a problem he has in different areas of his life	(Bird, Shaffer, Fisher, & Gould, 1993).
K-BIT (Kaufman Brief Intelligence Test)	Brief Intelligence Test	(Kaufman & Kaufman, 1990)
My Sexual Experiences	Questions about the juvenile's sexual experiences (follow-up only)	(Kolko et al., 1999).
Client Satisfaction Questionnaire-8 (CSQ8)	To examine their perceptions of the acceptability and helpfulness of treatment at post-treatment	(Attkisson & Greenfield, 1996)
Barriers to Treatment Scale	Parent measure of 44 different barriers to treatment	(Kazdin et al., 1997)

extensive family and peer support systems, and often feel forced to resort to a life of social isolation and secrecy. This is a time when the clinician may attempt to validate their experiences (e.g., anger, frustration, confusion, denial, self-blame, helplessness), but to also begin a discussion of the offense with their child and his role in the incident.

Challenges for Community-Based Clinicians

As with parents, community-based clinicians face difficult circumstances that may jeopardize treatment progress and client engagement, though they have the unique opportunity of treating these adolescents within the context of their families, schools, and communities. They also have access to multiple information sources that can provide the treatment team with insight into the adolescent's world and the family's functioning. And, yet, the clinicians broker different roles in this process that can create conflicts, such as providing supportive services to the famiy while they concurrently act as an extension of the probation officers' monitoring and enforcement system. As a result, they must conscientiously avoid any splitting between the two parties ("good cop, bad cop") and work toward compatible program goals.

A second challenge is the expectation for clinicians to collaborate with other community agencies involved with the family (e.g., Intensive Case Managers, Wrap-Around Services), but this can be a challenge due to the chaotic lifestyles and demands of the families. Especially for those families receiving other services, the clinician needs to ensure that all of the services provided can be coordinated to yield the maximum benefit. Finally, clinicians must carefully orchestrate any efforts to challenge the child's defenses and harmful thoughts, choices, and behaviors so as to avoid triggering any unmonitored deterioration in the community. Since these adolescents are exposed to numerous risks (e.g., potential victims, drugs and alcohol, self-injurious materials), clinicians must enhance the adolescent's support systems as the family continues to practice any new skills and offer psychoeducation (e.g., offender treatment materials) to other providers when requested, especially when serious psychopathology is evident. On average, the SAFE Program provides one year of outpatient sex-offender specific treatment that occurs within this context, securing basic needs and family stability first, and then addressing the offending concerns.

A final challenge is the inaccessibility of some of these adolescents due to their involvement in other activities and corresponding barriers to keeping appointments (e.g., limited transportation resources, parental dysfunction), though the inaccessibility may also reflect avoidant behavior, defiance, and the testing of limits. To engage these clients, we extend services into the home, school, or probation office, occasionally through joint visits with the probation officer to assess home safety and the feasibility of conducting treatment sessions outside the clinic. In general, community sessions allow the clinician to observe the child practicing newly acquired skills, monitor targeted risks, behaviors, and interactions (e.g., sleeping arrangements, Internet use), verify the adolescent's report of his behavior, choices, interactions, and overall functioning, and effectively implement behavior modification plans by being familiar with the multiple systems within which the child is involved. Ultimately, such efforts increase communication between providers and assist in creating and then monitoring safety strategies within the family and neighborhood.

Orientation to Community-Based Treatment

After the assessment phase, families are assigned to a treatment clinician and first receive an orientation regarding treatment for the child and the family, and a review of limited confidentiality, treatment expectations, and safety plans. The rationale for treatment includes several concepts or considerations: (a) their possible reactions (e.g., frustration); (b) how we collaborate with probation; (c) how we address choices/behaviors and teach skills; (d) family support and involvement are important; (e) treatment can be stressful and difficult to attend; (f) respect, honesty, and active participation will make treatment go better and faster; (g) where appropriate, we try to challenge families to think of new ideas and actions; and (h) an effort is made to help them develop more satisfying relationships. The notion of *choice* and the child's strengths are emphasized throughout treatment.

The SAFE Program's utilization of limited confidentiality allows clinicians to update the probation staff on the family's participation, engagement, and progress in treatment, family issues (e.g., abuse, financial problems, health concerns, living arrangements), and potential violations of probation (e.g., drug use, truancy, additional sex offenses). As stated earlier, clients are informed of the obligation to contact probation regarding these violations.

We also discuss the clinic's reputation with the adolescent during the first session (SAFE Program is part of a psychiatric hospital with inpatient and outpatient mental health programs) and the court mandate to receive mental health treatment at a psychiatric research hospital, given assumptions that our clinic, "is for crazy people." While about half of our adolescents meet criteria for a psychiatric diagnosis, we do not want them to maintain the belief that they were mandated to our program because they are perceived to be "crazy" or "mentally ill." We also need to address the family's concerns regarding research in general and potential side effects of participation in a research study, which are often clarified with both parties. Finally, we discuss the reasons why children offend (e.g., sadness, frustration, excitement, anger) and our treatment targets ("we help kids, teenagers, and adults with their thoughts, feelings, and behaviors").

As mentioned previously, *choice* should be emphasized throughout treatment and should begin during the first session. Clinicians can create numerous opportunities for the adolescent to make choices that foster a sense of control and contribution for the youth. They need to be mindful that the adolescent has recently been faced with experiences that have stripped him of his ability to make his own choices. Whenever possible, clinicians need to create opportunities for youth to practice this basic, yet necessary, skill (e.g., "we are going to talk about making healthy choices that help you feel like you are in control of your life, but you can decide what you would like to discuss first–what to expect during treatment, what the SAFE Program is all about, and ways to get to know each other better. What would you like to start with?").

Relationship building exercises are also a necessary component of the first session. These exercises should target discussions about the adolescent's strengths, relationships, interests, hobbies, and extra-curricular activities. Exercises that can be used for relationship building and completed by both the client and clinician include board games, card games, creating play-dough sculptures, completing worksheets, designing and decorating a journal that begins with the youth's positive attributes, or creating a collage from magazine pages and art materials that visually depicts the child's strengths and areas of interest. Upon completion, these activities can be processed with dialogue regarding the youth's thoughts and feelings about his strengths and positive attributes. Areas of interest, hobbies, and extra-curricular activities that are identified by the adolescent may offer insight into rewards that can be utilized throughout treatment to praise, encourage engagement, and facilitate treatment progress. Following this orientation, the clinician provides parents with a very similar orientation to and rationale for treatment, and addresses any questions they may have about the program and treatment course.

Certainly, we are mindful that our parents start treatment after several assessment sessions when measures are completed regarding their own childhood, upbringing, and personal victimization. These intrusive questions may elicit memories of their own abuse and victimization, which has been reported by several of the mothers, especially sexual abuse. Some have received prior treatment to help cope with their traumatic experiences or mental health diagnoses (e.g., depression, anxiety, and PTSD), but others have not. We attend to these issues and monitor their mood and functioning, offering psychiatric consultation and treatment as needed. Processing these experiences, monitoring their current functioning, and gathering information about those who are aware of their victimization are reviewed in this initial phase.

COGNITIVE-BEHAVIORAL TREATMENT: INTERVENTION PROCEDURES AND TARGETS

Background and Orientation to CBT

The SAFE Program draws heavily upon the cognitive-behavioral therapy (CBT) model and its emphasis of the interplay among the cognitive, affective, and behavioral systems. Thus, we focus on examination and restructuring of cognitions based on rationality and validity (see Beck, 1970), teaching strategies to develop specific problem-solving skills (D'Zurilla & Goldfried, 1971), and practicing various interpersonal and self-control skills. CBT applications relevant to working with adolescent sexual offenders are also incorporated (Becker & Kaplan, 1993; Greenberger & Pedesky, 1995; Linehan, 1993; Mackey, Donovan, & Marlatt, 1991).

The practice of CBT varies, but there are distinguishing features that set CBT interventions apart from other approaches (Granvold, 1997). These include the following: (a) establishing the client's problems and their etiology through private meetings with the therapist, (b) a collaborative effort between the client and therapist to resolve the problems, (c) therapists convey that all humans are worthy to promote the adoption of this philosophy by the client, (d) structured and directive sessions in which the therapist manages issues such as noncompliance, power struggles, and treatment termination, (e) the client takes an active role in resolving the problem through homework and self-report, (f) methods are interactive, (g) the use of Socratic questioning to encourage self-discovery, (h) an empirical focus is used to provide evidence of change, impairment, and/or process, (i) structure allows for time-limited therapy, and (j) relapse prevention to address maintenance after treatment termination.

These 10 operating features of CBT permit this approach to work effectively with adolescents who have sexually offended. The sexual abuse cycle (Lane, 1997) operates under the assumptions that: (a) sexually abusive acts are not impulsive, (b) sexual behaviors feel good and are ways of self-soothing, (c) all offenders have some level of cognitive distortions, (d) antecedent(s) preclude the behavior, and (e) the sexual behavior has a compensatory aspect to off-set negative emotions. To address the problem of sexually abusive behavior, CBT can be used to structure the treatment course and goals, minimize feelings of shame by demonstrating that all humans are worthy, address noncompliance and power struggles in sessions and other relationships, encourage the client to take responsibility for the abusive behavior, conceptualize the behavior using functional analysis methods, and create a relapse prevention plan to promote appropriate relationships after termination.

Adolescents and their families are explained the SAFE Program's CBT-based theoretical orientation during the initial phase of treatment. Usually, this involves describing the three response channels (thoughts, feelings, actions) and how these responses will be examined and developed to help the adolescent make appropriate and effective choices. We utilize a CBT card game activity to orient the adolescent to this model. (See Appendix A for a sample CBT card game and some examples of how to facilitate several sessions of the activity.) The activity introduces multiplex patterns and lends itself to client self-expression.

Session Structure

During the initial phase of treatment, adolescents are oriented to the session structure within our CBT model. Sessions should be predictable for the youth and foster an environment and sequence that allows them to make sense of their experiences and the issues addressed in treatment. We teach the adolescent to gain control of his thoughts, choices, and behaviors as he responds to challenging probation regulations and family circumstances. Although structured, choices are presented to the adolescent throughout the session to allow him to apply the problem solving skills he has learned.

Our treatment sessions are structured with the following components: (a) a mood check, (b) review of the week's events and any prior homework, (c) setting the session agenda, (d) skill-building, (e) homework assignment, and (f) eliciting feedback from the youth. The mood check and review of the adolescent's weekly events allow the clinician to monitor the youth's mood, assist the adolescent in ongoing affect identification and intensity gauging, and identify significant events and progress that has occurred since the previous session. Homework is a vital part of the development of skills learned in treatment and assists the youth to integrate them in their home, school, and community environments. We also elicit ongoing feedback regarding the youth's comprehension of the material presented, their homework assignments, and their emotional and cognitive reactions to the treatment content (Friedberg & McClure, 2002)

Treatment Planning and Goal Setting

We review all of the assessment findings with the family, such as any formal diagnoses, the endorsement of individual symptoms that merit monitoring, the adolescent's functioning at home, school, and in the community, parental and family functioning, and their current health and mental health services. When supplemented with a discussion of the family's current strengths, this review provides the impetus for identifying any perceived problems worthy of intervention. For adolescents with a psychiatric diagnosis, psychoeducation and literature are provided regarding symptoms and treatment options. Clinicians process any reactions to the information and the label of a diagnosis. Consultations with the program psychiatrist are scheduled during this initial phase for those families interested in gaining additional knowledge on medication supplements that work in conjunction with therapy.

Parents may have acute health or mental health treatment needs that hinder their healthy functioning and parental practices. Clinicians may conduct an individual session with a parent in this initial phase of treatment to gain insight into the parent's mental health issues and functioning. Referrals to community providers are made by the clinician to connect families and address basic needs. It is imperative to provide support to parents and gain their trust in order to promote success and healthy functioning in the family.

Parents may need additional information to understand their child's offense cycle and gain control of the emotional reactions caused by this familial upheaval. During assessment, parents are provided with literature explaining sexual behavior problems in children and adolescents (*From Trauma to Understanding*; Pithers, Gray, Cunningham, & Lane, 1993). Parents are encouraged to review this material before the first treatment session that clinicians can use to facilitate discussion of sexual abuse and trauma, the ramifications of sexual assault, treatment options for offenders, and treatment outcome data.

Treatment Domains and Representative Clinical Techniques

After the clinician has reviewed the assessment findings with the family, there is a dialogue regarding treatment domains. Probation staff will also provide feedback regarding their observations of the child's behavior in the weekly probation group, at school, and in the home. Our most common treatment domains are the following: sexual offending behavior, sex and sexuality, victimization, self-esteem and emotional self-understanding, thinking patterns, healthy relationships, anger control, school consequences, safety planning, obstacles to success, and diagnosis-specific treatment.

Sexual offending behavior. This treatment domain focuses on assisting the adolescent and family in understanding the youth's offense cycle including the motivations and circumstances that led to the child acting out through sexually offensive means. Barriers to offending are identified as well as arousal patterns that involve the youth's victim or potential victims. Exploring the youth's arousal patterns and fantasies works well within the CBT model. (See Appendix B, Exercises 2-4 for example exercises used to address the treatment domain of sexual offending behavior through journaling, rating, and charting.)

Sex and sexuality. Psychoeducation fosters a dialogue regarding sexuality, reproduction, STDs, contraception, sexual orientation, gender identity issues, and the general risks of sexuality, both personal and legal. Clinicians provide accurate information regarding these issues and bridge the gap in the youth's knowledge base that may be most significantly influenced by his peer group. Values, morals, and spiritual influences regarding sexuality are presented within the context of the family's values, morals, and spiritual beliefs. Fantasies, masturbation patterns, and deviant arousals and interests are identified and addressed throughout this treatment domain. (See Appendix B, Exercise 1 for an example of how to elicit the youth's sexual experiences as well as process patterns, fantasies, and sexual beliefs.)

Victimization. Throughout this treatment objective the clinician assists the youth and family in understanding the effects of abuse on the victim and the victim's family, and fosters the development of victim empathy. Personal victimization, trauma, and bullying are processed and treated as needed. Youth and parents that meet criteria for Posttraumatic Stress Disorder (PTSD) are treated through the use of in-vivo and prolonged exposure (Foa & Rothbaum, 1998). When appropriate and legally available, community-based clinicians have sought to coordinate clarification sessions (e.g., apology and safety plan reviews) and mediation between the offending youth and the victim. These procedures have been especially useful for intra-familial offenses.

Self-esteem and emotional self. Affect identification skills are developed through this treatment domain. Issues of self-esteem and creating a positive self-image are addressed as well. Emotions involved in the offense cycle and the adolescent's experiences with personal trauma are explored. Youth are able to identify the connection between their thoughts, feeling, choices, and behavioral reactions. Healthy, safe, and legal behaviors are identified and practiced through skills building.

Understanding thinking patterns. Adolescents continue to explore the connections between their thoughts, feelings, choices, and behaviors through dialogue, role-play, CBT exercises, worksheets, journaling, and homework assignments. An increase in insight into their thoughts, choices, and behaviors is fostered. The basic tenants of CBT are applied throughout this treatment domain. Choice and problem-solving skills are emphasized regarding the youth's attitude, opinions, perspectives, and behaviors.

Healthy relationships. Through this treatment objective the youth and family analyze the adolescent's relationships in all environments and systems through dialogue, role play, CBT exercises, worksheets, and homework assignments. Familial relationship issues and boundaries are addressed through family sessions. Peer relationships, friendships, intimacy, and social group affiliations are explored regarding healthy relationship choices and patterns. Dating relationships and sexual behavior are addressed within this context as well. Boundaries, honest and effective communication skills, problem-solving skills, and healthy and age appropriate social skills are identified and practiced in reference to all relationships.

Anger control. This treatment domain is addressed with youth and families that have histories and current displays of unhealthy behaviors motivated by anger. Affect identification skills are developed and practiced individually with the adolescent and within family sessions through dialogue, role-play, CBT exercises, worksheets, journaling, and homework assignments. Relaxation techniques using diaphragmatic breathing, guided imagery, and deep muscle relaxation are also used throughout individual and family sessions (Kolko & Swenson, 2002). Application of these skills in the community and at home with parents is assigned as homework. Healthy and legal behavioral alternatives, impulsivity, and the analysis of cause and effect patterns related to anger are also explored.

School. This treatment domain focuses on the adolescent's relationships in the school community, academic capabilities and performance, academic motivation and organization, and behaviors and choices within the school environment. Additional academic resources such as Special Education, GED programs, and life skills training are secured and monitored by the community-based clinician and probation officer. School visits with administration and classroom observations of behavior and performance are completed throughout the treatment course for youth struggling with school success and bullying. Clinicians can request teachers to complete evaluations of the student's behavior and academic performance throughout the academic year.

Consequences. Assisting the youth and family in understanding the internal and external effects of abuse on the victim, the victim's family, the offending adolescent, his family, and the community at large are explored throughout this treatment goal. Long-term consequences that will continue to occur throughout the course of the child's life in regard to having a criminal record are identified and processed with the adolescent and family.

Safety planning. This treatment domain includes creating safety plans for the abuse cycles of the adolescent and the family as needed. Adolescents maintained in the community may potentially have contact with their victim, the victim's family, or the victim's friends. Additional safety-plans for such contacts are also explored. Contracts for safety are created and monitored for self-injurious and suicidal youth as needed.

Obstacles to success. Any aspect of the youth's life that keeps him from being successful is addressed through this treatment domain. Adolescents involved in the SAFE Program have addressed issues including but not limited to drug and alcohol abuse, the absence of a father figure in the family and parental abandonment, the abuse history of a parent, parenting their own children, exposure to violence and organized crime within their community and neighborhood, parental health issues such as AIDS and Multiple Sclerosis, the adolescent's physical disabilities, poor hygiene, and securing employment.

General Comments

The treatment course for community-based sex specific treatment at the SAFE Program typically lasts 12 months in duration with weekly sessions.

This length of time creates an advantage for providing thorough treatment that addresses both the individual issues of the adolescent and the family issues inherent in unhealthy functioning. As mentioned previously in this article, roughly half of our clients meet criteria for a psychiatric diagnosis. In addition to the treatment domains mentioned above, SAFE clinicians have access to a variety of treatment protocols for common diagnoses among our youth that can be intertwined with sex offender-specific treatment objectives, though both are often altered to incorporate evolving treatment needs for the adolescent and his family. Flexibility is also employed within the treatment domains to incorporate variations of CBT treatment modalities for youth functioning at a lower cognitive level due to mental retardation and developmental delays. Creative and concrete treatment methods are implemented whenever necessary to assist the adolescent in understanding abstract concepts involved in sex specific treatment that are incorporated into skills building and safety planning. The use of creativity is not limited to lower functioning clients, but increasingly implemented with all youth as a means to foster healthy, safe, and alternative expression that reveals their innermost thoughts, feelings, and motivations for behavior.

CBT WITH PARENTS AND FAMILIES OF ADOLESCENT SEXUAL OFFENDERS

Overview and Background

As treatment for this population evolves, professionals, and researchers have conceptualized the behavior embedded within multiple levels (Hiinton, Sheperis, & Sims, 2003), notably, family, school, peers, culture, and socioeconomic status. Reviews of the treatment outcome literature document the efficacy of family therapy with adolescents who exhibit behavior problems (Kazdin, 1993; Liddle & Dakof, 1995; for further support, see Zankman & Bonomo, this issue). In a comparative study of adolescent sex offenders and youth with conduct disorders, families of the offenders told more lies, had more family myths, and were more likely to be involved in taboo behavior (Baker, Tabacoff, Tornusciolo, & Eisenstadt, 2003). A cognitive-behavioral family therapy approach assesses the cognitive dimensions that influence behavior among family members and may assist in determining offending contributors (Hanna & Brown, 1999). Given the multidimensional determinants of sexual offending behavior, family therapy (FT) may serve as a comprehensive method to treat adolescent sexual offenders.

The combination of CBT and FT approaches has been applied in other interventions for adolescent sexual offenders. Multisystemic therapy (MST) is a family-based approach that utilizes the social ecological theory and flexibility of CBT in application to an individual's family, school, peers, and community (Borduin, Henggeler, Blaske, & Stein, 1990). The component of FT brought to adolescent sex offender treatment through MST has addressed some of the core issues contributing to delinquent behavior

Family Applications and Methods

General family targets. The SAFE Program utilizes the CBT model and techniques in conjunction with FT to create a balance of treatment for each individual client. The role of FT in adolescent sexual offender treatment is to: (a) validate the family's life experiences and that of the juvenile justice system, (b) recognize family strengths for building relapse prevention, (c) address appropriate parent practices and skills, and (d) address family abuse history.

Family engagement. As mentioned previously, the feelings of guilt, shame, and helplessness that parents may experience due to the offense can turn into denial, self-blame, and child blame. These emotional responses can be a barrier to their child's treatment. To enhance engagement, Motivational Interviewing (MI) is used to validate the family's emotional experience, respect their experience, and encourage ownership of the desired change (Miller & Rollnick, 2002). MI works with resistance by abandoning confrontation, persuasion, and warning techniques; in turn, it utilizes reflective, strategic, and specific response techniques. This requires continuous self-monitoring which may not always be easy to maintain (for more details, see Lambie & McCarthy, this issue). In the SAFE Program, MI is used to address potential denial/minimization of the offense, emotional reactions, and treatment engagement.

Compounded by a busy schedule, the fact that many parents view themselves as ancillary to treatment highlights the necessity to promote engagement in their adolescent's treatment. The utilization of such strategies at the start of treatment may help to minimize any treatment barriers caused by their rising levels of emotional distress. The following are guidelines that we use to encourage parental involvement with children/adolescents: (a) recognize "change talk" used by parents ("I heard you say that you didn't like how things were going at home, what is it that you would like to see change?"); (b) validate their experiences and emotions ("It must be extremely difficult to look after your child every moment of the day."); (c) support the parent's choice of appropriate discipline/rewards ("That must have been a tough choice, but given what you've said it seems you feel, it was the most beneficial choice for the entire family."); (d) provide a resource for parents to consult ("When you get an idea, give me a call, I'd like to hear about your creativity."); (e) regularly seek the parents' feedback on treatment ("Since it's been difficult for you to join us for sessions, I wanted to see what you thought about the latest treatment goal we've been working on."); and (f) promote their role as valuable and necessary for change ("It's obvious when you help out with the homework assignments, your son is much more confident in expressing his thoughts and feelings.").

Relapse prevention plans. Relapse prevention planning becomes central to the second role of FT in treatment with adolescent sexual offenders, which is identifying family strengths. Once the adolescent is no longer on probation or mandated to treatment, the family once again becomes the primary interventionist. It is the responsibility of the adolescent and family to cope with triggers, seek help when need is identified, and keep potential victims safe. Reframing what the client and family are identifying as the problem(s) is an effective strategy to start the process of strength identification and relapse prevention (Budman & Gurman, 1988). For instance, if a family reports a history of alcohol abuse and child protection services but currently reports no such struggles in the past 5 years, the therapist may point out the "resiliency" and "strength" required in overcoming these hardships. Subsequent work can be completed to address the methods they have utilized and apply these strategies to the relapse prevention plan.

Parenting practices. Parenting practices refer to discipline and reward choices, clarifying expectations, using authority, and family rituals. Structural FT operates under the theory that transactions between family members impacts or regulates individual behavior (Minuchin, 1974). According to this theory, parents have the greatest power of influence on their offspring given their development.

Addressing how one parents is a sensitive issue, since virtually all parents feels they may have "messed up" at least once in rearing their children. The parents of adolescent sexual offenders may internalize blame for the offending behavior; therefore it is imperative for the therapist to utilize a sensitive approach or risk treatment disengagement. The SAFE team attempts to disarm families with an explanation of the parent as the expert on their child. Thus, parents become the teachers and more amenable to discussing parenting practices. Once the parent is engaged, it is easy to explore successful versus unsuccessful discipline, the approved and unapproved routines of the children, and the handling of important rituals (e.g., religious events, birthdays, deaths, anniversaries).

Most programs targeting parenting skills training operate under one of three approaches: behavioral parent training, family skills training, and family therapy (Kumpfer & Rose, 2003). The SAFE Program combines elements of each approach by utilizing varied session structures when necessary for each individual family. SAFE team clinicians commonly use the family skills training session structure to address how and why the sexual offending behavior occurred. Parents address their response to the offending behavior individually and the adolescent addresses his sexual abuse cycle individually. The joint sessions become a sharing of individual understanding and an opportunity to express remorse and support.

The parenting practices important to teach are placing responsibility for an individual's behavior on that individual, rewarding positive behavior, having clear and realistic expectations for their children, and creating family rituals that everyone can contribute to. Misplaced blame influences many of these parenting choices. Teaching parents to reward positive behaviors may reveal a new parent perception of the good their children do rather than just the bad. Realistic expectations improve the function of each role. Rituals increase monitoring and moments for effective communication and are therefore quite important in relapse prevention and family functioning.

The process of changing parent practices is not exact and may not always be welcomed by a family. Inadequacy and blame are not feelings that parents easily report. To minimize these feelings and other impairments, several steps for dealing with parental dysfunction with adolescents can be followed as illustrated here: (a) rebuild parental confidence (e.g., explore the parent's confidence of being a "good" parent; find successes to draw upon to illustrate functional parenting; address feelings of shame, guilt, and blame); (b) rebuild a sense of parental responsibility (e.g., review the responsibility they had when their adolescent was an infant, illustrate how the adolescent life cycle requires parenting via limitations and privileges; distinguish between feelings of responsibility versus self-blame); (c) reestablish worth of being needed (e.g., review the parent's own adolescent experience, what was it they "needed" most; explore how their adolescent "needs" them emotionally; assist parents in creating a behavior modification plan); and (d) have parents challenge the effectiveness of their choices (e.g., encourage parents to explore alternatives even if they say it won't work, roll with resistance).

Victimization/abuse history. Abuse history in a family can be influential in the parenting choices as well as family interactions and cohesion. Addressing a family's abuse history is well documented as an important step in resolving family conflict, increasing cohesion, and improving overall functioning (Kolko & Swenson, 2002; Pithers, Gray, Busconi, & Houchens, 1998). This exploration fosters an understanding of the offending behavior context, begins to break down family secrecy, and possibly builds or repairs family relationships (Baker et al., 2003).

Addressing the victimization of a parent also impacts their ability to cope with the abusive behavior of their child. A treatment model presented by Kolko and Swenson (Kolko, 2002) combines basic techniques of individualized CBT with family therapy to enable the family to move from individual impact of abuse to clarification. This clarification could attend to the disengagement or enmeshment of relationships and bring into light appropriate family cohesion. Presenting the CBT model to demonstrate an understanding for how individuals respond to situations will assist parents in addressing abuse history.

Methods used by the SAFE Program to address abuse histories include the family genogram, "life" book/scrapbook creation, and behavior modification plans as well as targeting parental perspectives on violence, stress management, and expectations for children (Kolko & Swenson, 2002). In severe cases of abuse where daily life is impaired, exposure treatment has been effective in reducing PTSD symptoms (Foa & Rothbaum, 1998). The methods mentioned here usually require intensive work and numerous sessions. It is also important for clinicians engaging in such treatment interventions to be mindful of their own abuse histories and ideas of abuse patterns.

Views on sexuality. Sex-offender treatment works within the context of the family by maintaining respect and validating the family's unique situation, including their view of sexuality. Parents should be comfortable with the therapist speaking to their child about sexuality. In order to establish this comfort level, clinicians should keep parents involved in treatment through their approval or disapproval of session sexual content. Also, addressing family boundaries and relationships through family homework assignments can challenge inappropriateness and reinforce appropriateness. A useful assessment and therapeutic tool is the cost/benefit analysis chart. Ask the adolescent and parent to contemplate abstinence versus sexual activity by creating four quadrants addressing all advantages and disadvantages to each option. This discussion can reveal much in terms of family values and judgment.

Communication skills. FT is a useful format to teach communication skills between parents and adolescents. Some obstacles to effective communication include calling one another names, use of sarcasm, giving lectures, exaggerating complaints, and avoiding topics (Robin & Foster, 1989). Four steps illustrated by Kolko and Swenson (Kolko, 2002) guide the therapist in assisting families to adopt alternative patterns of communication: (a) point out the communication obstacle and its effect(s), (b) provide alternative communication patterns or skills, (c) demonstrate the new alternative, and then (d) instruct the family to practice it. The alternative presented will depend on the specific communication problem, but the focus remains on improving the communication. Some helpful communication skills to pass on to families include paying attention not only to words but to body language, being clear and direct, speaking only for oneself, asking questions for clarity, checking to make sure that what one has said has been understood, and avoiding the above mentioned communication obstacles.

Comments. Adolescent sexual offender treatment has the intention of preventing further victims and rehabilitating a young life. Including FT in the repertoire of treatments can target more of the core elements for change. A family-based approach can assist in decreasing denial or disgust for the adolescent, addressing parent issues to break down barriers of recovery, engaging the parents in effective parenting skills to increase family functioning, unifying the family in treatment, and encouraging the family to be a positive resource for one another.

CONCLUSION

Our collaborative outpatient program integrates mental health and probationary services designed to manage and treat adolescent sexual offenders and their families. One advantage to this program structure is the ability to capitalize upon the respective strengths of these two systems, notably, the administration of monitoring and sanctions (probation) and the delivery of assessment and treatment services (mental health). The use of limited confidentiality waivers and research consent documents also provides protections for subjects while making explicit the importance of communication regarding program goals, progress, and plans. The approach emphasizes the use of assessment information to individualize treatment for these youth and their families within the mental health system. Although there are many programs targeting juvenile sex offenders, few integrate juvenile justice and mental health resources with the same clients, especially with outpatients maintained in the community.

The SAFE Program emphasizes an array of goals that extends beyond primary attention to youths' sexual offense disclosures and a review of relapse prevention or safety plans. The broad scope of the program is needed given that one-half of these youth do not appear to suffer from any formal psychiatric disorder. In general, our overall assessment information and clinical experience highlight the importance of targeting four general domains: (a) the sexual offense, (b) individual psychopathology and family dysfunction, (c) general adaptive behavior and competencies/skills, and (d) relationships with peers, teachers, and family members. Where applicable, specialized interventions have been directed to the youth's exposure to violence and victimization, his experience of grief/loss and intimacy needs, and both parent effectiveness and family functions/structure.

Even with this supportive clinical context and diverse clinical programming, providing services to this population is not easy to accomplish, can require considerable expenses, may conflict with the content of other ongoing family services, and/or is guided by few empirically-based principles or outcomes. We are in the process of collecting program evaluation data with follow-up evaluations from the youth and their parents in an effort to examine our outcomes and predictors of recidivism. However, such information is difficult to collect and the conduct of sound, methodologically rigorous outcome studies remains a challenge. Clearly, studies of the impact and cost-effectiveness of treatment are needed to evaluate the relative benefits of these and other outpatient programs for this important population. Moreover, policies that emphasize the coordination of mental health assessment and treatment are necessary to increase the likelihood that these cases receive services designed to enhance personal competence and family functioning, and to promote public safety. Ultimately, the judicious application and evaluation of such specialized resources may provide useful guidelines for the contemporary and effec- tive community management of young sexual offenders and their families.

REFERENCES

Abel, G., & Becker, J. V. (1984). *Adult cognition scale.* Atlanta, GA: Abel Behavioral Medicine Laboratory.

Achenbach, T. M. (1991). *Integrative guide for the 1991 CBCL/4-18, YSR, and TRF profiles.* Burlington, VT: University of Vermont, Department of Psychiatry.

Attkisson, C. C., & Greenfield, T. K. (1999). The UCSF Client Satisfaction Scales: I. The Client Satisfaction Questionnaire-8. In M. Maruish (Ed.), *The use of psychological testing for treatment planning and outcomes assessment* (pp. 1333-1346). Manwah, NJ: Lawrence Erlbaum Associates.

Baker, A. J. L., Tabacoff, R., Tornusciolo, G., & Eisenstadt, M. (2003). Family secrecy: A comparative study of juvenile sex offenders and youth with conduct disorders. *Family Process, 42,* 105-116.

Barbaree, H. E., Marshall, W. L., & McCormick, J. (1998). The development of deviant sexual behaviour among adolescents and its implications for prevention and treatment. *The Irish Journal of Psychology, 19*(1), 1-31.

Beck, A. T. (1970). Cognitive therapy: Nature and relation to behavior therapy. *Behavior Therapy, 1,* 184-200.

Beck, A. T., Ward, C. H., Mendelson, M., Mock, J., & Erbaugh, J. (1961). An inventory for measuring depression. *Archives of General Psychiatry, 4,* 561-571.

Becker, J. V., & Kaplan, M. S. (1993). Cognitive behavioral treatment of the juvenile sex offender. In H. Barbaree, W. L. Marshall, & S. M. Hudson (Eds.), *The juvenile sex offender* (pp. 264-277). New York: Guilford Press.

Bird, H., Shaffer, D., Fisher, P., & Gould, M. S. (1993). The Columbia Impairment Scale (CIS): Pilot findings on a measure of global impairment for children and adolescents. *International Journal of Methods in Psychiatric Research, 3*(3), 167-176.

Birmaher, B., Khetarpal, S., Brent, D., & Cully, M. (1997). The screen for child anxiety related emotional disorders (SCARED): Scale construction and psychometric characteristics. *Journal of the American Academy of Child & Adolescent Psychiatry, 36*(4), 545-553.

Borduin, C. M., Henggeler, S. W., Blaske, D. M., & Stein, R. (1990). Multisystemic treatment of adolescent sexual offenders. *International Journal of Offender Therapy and Comparative Criminology, 34,* 105-113.

Borduin, C. M., & Schaeffer, C. M. (1998). Violent offending in adolescence: Epidemiology, correlates, outcomes, and treatment. In R. Monetmayor (Ed.), *Delinquent violent youth: Theory and interventions* (pp. 144-174). Newbury Park, CA: Sage.

Briere, J. (1996). *Trauma Symptom Checklist for Children: Professional manual.* Odessa, FL: Psychological Assessment Resources, Inc.

Brofenbrenner, U. (1977). Toward an experimental ecology of human development. *American Psychologist, 32,* 513-531.

Budman, S. H., & Gurman, A. S. (1988). *Theory and practice of brief therapy.* New York: Guilford Press.

Center for Sex Offender Management [CSOM]. (1999). *Compendium of OJP-sponsored projects relating to sex offenders.* Unpublished manuscript.

Cohen, J. A., & Mannarino, A. P. (1988). Psychological symptoms in sexually abused girls. *Child Abuse & Neglect, 12,* 571-577.

D'Zurilla, T. J., & Goldfried, M. R. (1971). Problem solving and behavior modification. *Journal of Abnormal Psychology, 78,* 107-126.

Foa, E. B., & Rothbaum, B. O. (1998). *Treating the trauma of rape: Cognitive-behavioral therapy for PTSD.* New York: Guilford Press.

Ford, M. E., & Linney, J. A. (1995). Comparative analysis of juvenile sexual offenders, violent nonsexual offenders, and status offenders. *Journal of Interpersonal Violence, 10*(1), 56-70.

Forth, A. E., Hart, S. D., & Hare, R. D. (1990). Assessment of psychopathy in young offenders. *Psychological Assessment, 2,* 342-344.

Friedberg, R. D., & McClure, J. M. (2002). *Clinical practice of cognitive therapy with children and adolescents.* New York: Guilford Press.

Friedrich, W. N., Luecke, W. J., Bielke, R. L., & Place, V. (1992). Psychotherapy outcome of sexually abused boys: An agency study. *Journal of Interpersonal Violence, 7,* 369-409.

Granvold, D. K. (1997). Cognitive-behavioral therapy with adults. In J. R. Brandell (Ed.), *Theory and practice in clinical social work.* New York: Free Press.

Greenberger, D., & Pedesky, C. A. (1995). *Mind over mood: A cognitive therapy treatment manual for clients.* New York: Guilford Press.

Hanna, S. M., & Brown, J. H. (1999). *The practice of family therapy* (2nd ed.). Belmont, CA: Wadsworth.

Hiinton, W. J., Sheperis, C., & Sims, P. (2003). Family-based approaches to juvenile delinquency: A review of literature. *Family Journal: Counseling & Therapy for Couples & Families, 11*(2), 167-173.

Hoagwood, K., Horwitz, S., Stiffman, A., Weisz, J., Bean, D., Rae, D., Compton, W., Cottler, L., Bickman, L., & Leaf, P. (2000). Concordance between parent reports of children's mental health services and records: The Services Assessment for Children and Adolescents (SACA). *Journal of Child & Family Studies, 9,* 315-331.

Hunter, J. A., Figueredo, A., Malamuth, N. M., & Becker, J. V. (2003). Juvenile sex offenders: Toward the development of a typology. *Sexual Abuse: A Journal of Research and Treatment, 15*(1), 27-48.

Hunter, J. A., Hazelwood, R. R., & Slesinger, D. (2000). Juvenile-perpetrated sex crimes: Patterns of offending and predictors of violence. *Journal of Family Violence, 15*(1), 81-93.

Kaufman, A. S., & Kaufman, N. L. (1990). *Kaufman Brief Intelligence Test.* Circle Pines, MN: American Guidance Service, Inc.

Kaufman, J., Birmaher, B., Brent, D. A., Rao, U., & Ryan, N. D. (1996). *KIDDIE-SADS-present and lifetime version (K-SADS-PL).* Unpublished instrument.

Kazdin, A. E. (1993). Psychotherapy for children and adolescents: Current progress and future research directions. *American Psychologist, 48*, 644-657.

Kazdin, A. E., Holland, L. Crowley, M., & Breton, S. (1997). Barriers to treatment participation scale: Evaluation and validation in the context of child outpatient treatment. *Journal of Child Psychology and Psychiatry, 38*, 1051-1062.

Kobayashi, J., Sales, B. D., Becker, J. V., Figueredo, A., & Kaplan, M. S. (1995). Perceived parental deviants, parent-child bonding, child abuse, and child sexual aggression. *Sexual Abuse: A Journal of Research and Treatment, 7*, 25-44.

Kolko, D. J. (2002). Child physical abuse. In T. Reid (Ed.), *APSAC handbook of child maltreatment* (2nd ed.) (pp. 21-54). Thousand Oaks, CA: Sage.

Kolko, D. J., Baumann, B., & Bukstein, O. G. (1999). *Community-based, wraparound mental health services for juvenile sex offenders, grant.* Pittsburgh, PA: Western Psychiatric Institute and Clinic.

Kolko, D. J., & Swenson, C. C. (2002). *Assessing and treating physically abused children and their families: A cognitive behavioral approach.* Thousand Oaks, CA: Sage Publications.

Kumpfer, K. L., & Rose, A. (2003). Family-strengthening approaches for the prevention of youth problem behaviors. *American Psychologist, 58*, 457-465.

Lambie, I., & McCarthy, J. (2004). Interviewing strategies with sexually abusive youth. *Journal of Child Sexual Abuse, 13*(3/4), pp. 107-123.

Lane, S. L. (1997). The sexual abuse cycle. In S. L. Lane (Ed.), *Juvenile sexual offending: Causes, consequences, and correction* (rev. ed.) (pp. 77-121). San Francisco: Jossey-Bass Publishing.

Larsen, D. L., Attkisson, C. C., Hargreaves, W. A., & Nguyen, T. D. (1979). Assessment of client/patient satisfaction: Development of a general scale. *Evaluation and Program Planning, 2*, 197-207.

Liddle, H. A., & Dakof, G. A. (1995). Family based treatment for adolescent drug use: State of the science. In D. Czechowicz (Ed.), *Adolescent drug abuse: Clinical assessment and therapeutic interventions* (pp. 218-254). Rockville, MD: National Institute on Drug Abuse.

Linehan, M. M. (1993). *Skills training manual for treating borderline personality disorder.* New York: Guilford Press.

Mackey, P. W., Donovan, D. M., & Marlatt, G. A. (1991). Cognitive and behavioral approaches to alcohol abuse. In S. I. Miller (Ed.), *Clinical textbook of clinical disorders* (pp. 452-481). New York: Guilford Press.

Marshall, W. L., Anderson, D., & Fernandez, Y. (1999). *Cognitive-behavioral treatment of sexual offenders.* New York: Wiley.

Miller, W. R., & Rollnick, S. (2002). *Motivational interviewing: Preparing people for change* (2nd ed.). New York: Guilford Press.

Minuchin, S. (1974). *Families & family therapy.* Cambridge, MA: Harvard University Press.

Pelham, W. E., Milich, R., Murphy, D. A., & Murphy, H. A. (1989). Normative data on the IOWA Conners Teacher Rating Scale. *Journal of Clinical Child Psychology, 18,* 259-262.

Pithers, W. D., Gray, A. S., Busconi, A., & Houchens, P. (1998). Caregivers of children with sexual behavior problems: Psychological and familial functioning. *Child Abuse & Neglect, 22*(2), 129-141.

Pithers, W. D., Gray, A. S., Cunningham, C. E., & Lane, S. (1993). *From trauma to understanding: A guide for parents of children with sexual behavior problems.* Brandon, VT: Safer Society Press.

Robin, A. L., & Foster, S. L. (1989). *Negotiation parent-adolescent conflict: A behavioral-family systems approach.* New York: Guilford Press.

Shelton, K. K., Frick, P. J., & Wooten, J. (1996). Assessment of parenting practices in families of elementary school-age children. *Journal of Clinical Child Psychology, 25,* 317-329.

Straus, M. A., Hamby, S. L., Finkelhor, D., Moore, D. W., & Runyan, D. (1998). Identification of child maltreatment with the parent-child conflict tactics scales: Development and psychometric data for a national sample of American parents. *Child Abuse & Neglect, 22*(4), 249-270.

Tolan, P. H., Gorman-Smith, D., Huesmann, L. R., & Zelli, A. (1997). Assessment of family relationship characteristics: A measure to explain risk for antisocial behavior and depression among urban youth. *Psychological Assessment, 9*(3), 212-223.

Veneziano, C., & Veneziano, L. (2002). Adolescent sex offenders: A review of the literature. *Trauma Violence & Abuse, 3*(4), 247-260.

Worling, J. (2001). Personality-based typology of adolescent male sexual offenders: Differences in recidivism rates, victim-selection characteristics, and personal victimization histories. *Sexual Abuse: A Journal of Research and Treatment, 13*(3), 149-166.

Zankman, S., & Bonomo, J. (2004). Working with parents to reduce juvenile sex offender recidivism. *Journal of Child Sexual Abuse, 13*(3/4), pp. 139-156

APPENDIX A

CBT Cards

Purpose

Once a client can identify thoughts, feelings, and behaviors, CBT Cards can be introduced. A set of cards with 6 thoughts, 6 feelings, and 6 behaviors is presented to the client in a random order. The cards are used to evaluate knowledge and understanding, determine thought processes, demonstrate personal logic, challenge logic, and life application.

Instructions and Processing

Numerous variations can be made with this exercise. The following are just a few comments on how to begin using the CBT card exercise.

Sample "Thought" Card	Sample "Feeling" Card	Sample "Behavior" Card
Labels:	Labels:	Labels:
I like her	Love	Kissing
I hate her	Upset	Fighting
He's cool	Happy	Talking Back
She's hot	Angry	Touching
I can't stand her	Excited	Masturbate
She doesn't like me	Frustrated	Abuse

- He/she is asked to separate the cards into thought, feeling, and behavior categories. Discuss what makes each a thought, feeling or behavior.
- Ask the client to put 1 card from each category in a logical order. Discuss his choices.
- Ask the client to add 2 or 3 feeling cards to the sequence and explain how the sequence would play out. Or 2 or 3 more thought cards . . . etc.
- Challenge the client to create sequences beginning each with a thought, then a feeling, then a behavior. Which sequence was more difficult to create? Which one was easier?
- The client could be asked to create a sequence that ends negatively or positively.
- Ask the client to create a sequence that begins positively but ends negatively. Explore where in the sequence (was it a thought, feeling, behavior?) and how it changed.

APPENDIX A (continued)

- Have the client create his own thought, feeling, and behavior cards that pertain to his offense. Label each card as a thought, feeling, or behavior and have the client arrange their offense sequence in the order that it occurred. Examine the pattern and the number of thoughts, feelings, and/or behaviors. Where could the sequence have changed to eliminate the offense? Would it be an addition or subtraction of a thought, feeling, or behavior? How would the client have changed the pre-offense pattern? Continue to manipulate the cards to show how.

(Developed by Colleen Noel, MSW, LSW)

APPENDIX B

Samples of Youth Treatment Exercises

Exercise 1: Sexuality Timeline Cards

Purpose

The purpose of this exercise is to gather information regarding how the client has arrived at his definition of sexuality, values and morals regarding sexuality, sexual preferences, sexual orientation, and problem solving skills regarding sexuality. This card game is an alternative to using a standard timeline worksheet.

Rationale

"Today we're going to talk about the things that influence our opinions about sexuality in general. We're also going to look at what has influenced the way we make choices about sexuality and sexual behavior, like our values and morals, our opinions about right and wrong, and our sexual orientation. We made cards of all the things that influence kids and adults. We're going to try and think of specific examples for each topic. This may help us understand the way you think about your sexuality. It may also help us figure out some of the motivations behind your offense. In addition to knowing what has influenced you, we also want to figure out how strongly these experiences have impacted you. Then we're going to put the cards in chronological order, like a timeline, and look for patterns."

Instructions and Processing

Complete this activity for a variety of time points: from birth until the offense, from the offense until today, from the offense through the client's future/ adult life.

Time-Line Card Topics

(Create multiple cards of each topic)

- Abuse
- My Experiences
- Video games
- TV
- Internet
- Conversations with peers
- Health class
- My parents' experiences
- Religion

- My offense
- Dating
- Books
- Music
- School
- My friend's experiences
- Home
- My sibling's experiences
- Other

Instruct the client to divide the cards into two piles, "Topics that are easy to discuss," and "Topics that are difficult to discuss."

- Emphasizing *choice*, allow client to choose which pile to process first. Process both piles.
- Assist the client in identifying specific examples of how these topics have influenced his sexuality in general or focus on specific aspects of sexuality, i.e., sexual orientation.

Examples of Specific Experiences Associated with Each Topic

- Abuse: From my dad
- My offense: 8-year-old sister
- My experiences: Hand holding, kissing
- Dating: Former girlfriends, girls that rejected my advances
- Video games: Violent content
- Books
- TV: TV shows, pornography
- Music: Music videos, song lyrics, CD covers and photos that are sexual
- Internet: Caught by Mom looking at pornography
- School: Rules at school and dress code for females, dances at school ("humping" on the dance floor), groping girls in the hallway

APPENDIX B. Exercise 1 (continued)

- Conversations with peers about sexuality: At the lunch table talking about their dating and sexual experiences, talking with friend about his gay experiences, being bullied and called names like "fag" and "queer"
- My friends' experiences: Dating, sexual behavior, being gay
- Health class: Sex education on sexuality, sexual behavior, reproduction, contraception, and STDs, Health class view of sexuality versus religion
- Home: What I've heard and seen
- My parents' experiences: Mom's affairs/cheating, multiple husbands
- My siblings' experiences: Brother's girlfriends sleeping over, brother getting girlfriend pregnant
- Religion: Sex before marriage is sinful
- Other: Examples that don't fit into the other categories
- Process the client's thoughts and feelings regarding each specific example (i.e., When you heard that your brother got his girlfriend pregnant, what was your reaction? What were the thoughts that were going through your head? How did that make you feel?).
- Then have the client rate how significant this influence is on a scale of 1-10, 1= not at all, 10 = very strong influence.
- After processing specific examples of each topic, ask the client to organize the cards chronologically in the structure of a time-line for the various time points. Process possible patterns and behavioral responses within the time-line (i.e., It sounds like when your friends talked about their sexual experiences at the lunch table you would try to do the same sexual things with your girlfriend soon after. Would you say this is true? Is it safe to say those conversations have influenced you? What other patterns do you notice?).

(Developed by Gretchen M. Thomas, MSW, LSW)

Exercise 2: Arousal Journal Homework

Purpose

The purpose of this homework assignment is to gather information regarding the client's arousal patterns, frequency of arousals, intensity of arousals, and masturbation patterns.

Instructions and Processing

This assignment can be completed for homework when focusing on the treatment domains of sexual offending behavior, sex and sexuality, healthy relationships, and safety planning. It should be emphasized that clients complete the journal each day. This assignment can then be processed during the treatment session. The adolescent should be asked to identify his thoughts, feelings, and behaviors regarding each arousal. Process questions should focus on assisting the youth to identify arousal patterns in arousal targets, frequency, intensity, and masturbation.

	Sun	Mon	Tues	Wed	Thurs	Fri	Sat
Who was arousing to you today? (first name, age)							
What aspect of that person was arousing? (smile, body part, interaction, your conversation, their personality, clothing)							
How arousing was this experience? 1 = makes you take a second look, 2 = physically stimulating, 3 = urge to masturbate	1 2 3	1 2 3	1 2 3	1 2 3	1 2 3	1 2 3	1 2 3
Did you masturbate to this experience?	Yes No	Yes No	Yes No	Yes No	Yes No	Yes No	Yes No

(Developed by Gretchen M. Thomas, MSW, LSW)

Exercise 3: Arousal Patterns Homework

Purpose

The purpose of this homework assignment is to gather information about the client's arousal patterns and intensity, and masturbation patterns as they relate to various age and gender groups.

Instructions and Processing

This assignment can be completed when focusing on the treatment domains of sexual offending behavior, sex and sexuality, healthy relationships, and safety planning. This assignment can then be processed during the treatment session. Assist the youth to identify arousal patterns, intensity of arousals, and masturbation patterns as they relate to various age groups and gender.

APPENDIX B. Exercise 3 (continued)

	Peers	Adults 18 & older	Adolescents 12-14 years	Kids 9-11 years	Kids 6-8 years	Kids 3-5 years
Describe characteristics of this age group.						
When you look at a person in this age group that you find attractive, what is your gut reaction?						
What are your thoughts?						
What emotions are you feeling?						
What does your body feel like? (heart races; hands feel clammy; start sweating)						
What would you do next?						
What kinds of sex feelings do you have in your body (an erection; do you masturbate or have urges to masturbate?)						
How would you approach this person?						
What are the consequences for being sexually active with her/ him?						

Comparisons

When do you feel most aroused? (By whom? What's the setting? What's the activity?)

What is most arousing for you? (How they walk, talk, body, interactions with you, personality?)

Which age group is most arousing to you? Why? Due to what characteristics?

How do you feel about your attractions to others?

What are other's reactions to your attractions?

(Developed by Gretchen M. Thomas, MSW, LSW)

Exercise 4: Fantasy Charting Homework

Purpose

The purpose of this homework assignment is to gather information regarding the client's sexual fantasy patterns, arousal patterns, intensity of fantasies and arousals, content of sexual fantasies, and masturbation patterns.

Instructions and Processing

This assignment can be completed for homework when focusing on the treatment domains of sexual offending behavior, sex and sexuality, healthy relationships, and safety planning. This assignment can then be processed during the treatment session. Process questions should focus on assisting the youth to identify sexual fantasy patterns, arousal patterns, intensity of fantasies and arousals, and masturbation patterns.

	Date:	Date:
Your "real life" location at the time of the fantasy:		
The location within your fantasy:		
"Real life" events that took place before your fantasy:		
Thoughts before your fantasy:		
Feelings before your fantasy:		
People identified in your fantasy (i.e., your sexual partner):		
Their feelings and reactions to you:		
Your behaviors and actions towards them or with them:		
Your fantasy behavior described by a stranger (as if someone was watching a movie of your fantasy):		
Your fantasy behavior described by your best friend (What would s/he think? Would this be out of character for you?):		
Did you masturbate to your fantasy or have the urge to masturbate?		
Thoughts after your fantasy:		
Feelings after your fantasy:		
What does this fantasy mean to you?		
Have you had this fantasy before?		
Your fantasy behavior described by a stranger (as if someone was watching a movie of your fantasy):		
Your fantasy behavior described by your best friend (What would s/he think? Would this be out of character for you?):		
Your fantasy behavior described by a stranger (as if someone was watching a movie of your fantasy):		

APPENDIX B. Exercise 4 (continued)

	Date:	Date:
Did you masturbate to your fantasy or have the urge to masturbate?		
Thoughts after your fantasy:		
Feelings after your fantasy:		
What does this fantasy mean to you?		
Have you had this fantasy before?		

(Developed by Gretchen M. Thomas, MSW, LSW)

An Integrated Experiential Approach to Treating Young People Who Sexually Abuse

Robert E. Longo

SUMMARY. This article promotes the use of an integrated (holistic) approach to treating juvenile sexual offenders. An integrated model takes into account the fact that: (a) youth are resilient, (b) youth progress through various stages of development, (c) these stages are often arrested as a result of trauma, child abuse and neglect, and attachment disorders, (d) humanistic approaches and the therapeutic relationship are essential to the healing and recovery process, (e) youth learn and work with a variety of learning styles and multiple intelligences, (f) many traditional assessment and treatment approaches can be modified and blended with an integrated approach, and (g) the use of experiential treatments can have a positive and profound impact in treating youth with sexual behavior problems. *[Article copies available for a fee from The Haworth Document Delivery Service: 1-800-HAWORTH. E-mail address: <docdelivery@haworthpress.com> Website: <http://www.HaworthPress.com> © 2004 by The Haworth Press, Inc. All rights reserved.]*

Address correspondence to: Robert E. Longo, MRC, LPC, New Hope Treatment Centers, 7515 Northside Drive, North Charleston, SC 29420 (E-mail: robl@ newhopetreatment.com).

[Haworth co-indexing entry note]: "An Integrated Experimental Approach to Treating Young People Who Sexually Abuse." Longo, Robert E. Co-published simultaneously in *Journal of Child Sexual Abuse* (The Haworth Maltreatment and Trauma Press, an imprint of The Haworth Press, Inc.) Vol. 13, No. 3/4, 2004, pp. 193-213; and: *Identifying and Treating Youth Who Sexually Offend: Current Approaches, Techniques, and Research* (ed: Robert Geffner et al.) The Haworth Maltreatment and Trauma Press, an imprint of The Haworth Press, Inc., 2004, pp. 193-213. Single or multiple copies of this article are available for a fee from The Haworth Document Delivery Service [1-800-HAWORTH, 9:00 a.m. - 5:00 p.m. (EST). E-mail address: docdelivery@haworthpress.com].

Digital Object Identifier: 10.1300/J070v13n03_10

KEYWORDS. Juvenile, youth, sex offender, sexual abuse, experiential treatment, ecological, integrated, holistic

The field of assessing and treating juvenile sexual offenders (JSOs), although not new, is still in a developmental stage. As of the writing of this paper, there is no literature that defines the 'best practice' in treating youth with sexual behavior problems (Chaffin, 2002; Development Services Group, 2000). In fact, the field still operates with the understanding that much of what is done in assessing and treating youth with sexual behavior problems is based on many assumptions (National Task Force, 1993).

There are few studies that address the outcome and recidivism rates for JSOs, and of those few published studies, only a few have control groups. Although the assessment and treatment of youth with sexual behavior problems have been developing and growing over the course of the past 25 years (Burton, Freeman-Longo, Fiske, Levins, & Smith-Darden, 2000), this growth has been influenced primarily by the field of treating adult sexual abusers and prison-based models. More often than not there has been a trickle-down effect in the assessment and treatment of JSOs without looking at youth who sexually abuse as a separate and distinct group of patients with individual differences and treatment needs. In many cases developmental and contextual issues have been ignored in working with this population (Ryan et al., 1999).

In many programs this trickle-down process has resulted in the following: (a) the misuse of technology; (b) the lack of addressing youth and their treatment needs by taking into account their developmental stage; (c) the use of language and materials that may not be easily understood by youth who have learning disabilities; (d) highly confrontational approaches that may trigger trauma in youth with histories of child abuse and neglect; (e) a failure to address cultural needs and differences; and (f) a failure to recognize the resiliency in youth (Bell, 2002).

The majority of JSO treatment programs have generally adhered to traditional sex offender treatment models and strategies for treating adolescents with sexual behavior problems. These standard treatments usually include cognitive-behavioral/relapse prevention models, and a variety of treatment modalities including teaching the sexual abuse cycle, empathy training, anger management, social and interpersonal skills training, cognitive restructuring, emotional development, teaching coping responses and interventions, assertiveness training, journaling, sex education, and communication skills (Burton et al., 2000; Freeman-Longo, Bird, Stevenson, & Fiske, 1995; Knopp, Freeman-Longo, & Stevenson, 1993).

Recently, some of the more traditional approaches to treating sexual abusers have come under criticism, including relapse prevention (RP), the most widely used treatment model by programs treating both juvenile and adult sexual abusers (Laws, Hudson, & Ward, 2000; Ward, 2002; Ward & Hudson, 1996). First, the model offers limited ways to account for offense behavior, is rigid, and is inflexible. Second, the presentation of the offense chain is rigid, leaving no room for individual differences in behavior (there is no flexibility in the chain of behaviors and events leading to sexual assault). Third, RP is very academic (it intellectualizes sex offending) with abstract concepts and complex language, and fourth, it relies on coping strategies that are not positive goal oriented (i.e., avoidance and escape). RP has many strengths as well as limitations, but it is a viable model that when modified can be used in conjunction with an integrated approach.

INTEGRATED (HOLISTIC) TREATMENT AND WELL-BEING

An integrated (holistic) approach to treatment is a blend of traditional and non-traditional approaches with a focus on healing and well-being. In working with youth with sexual behavior problems, an integrated approach incorporates and modifies, yet moves beyond the traditional cognitive-behavioral and relapse prevention models most commonly used by the majority of such programs. It uses a balance of theoretical and humanistic knowledge that embraces the concept that the therapeutic relationship is the focal point of treatment and essential to the treatment process. There is an overall focus on patient well-being (Ward & Stewart, 2002).

A Return to Basics

An integrated treatment approach in its simplest form is a return to basics. First, it addresses the four universal needs for: (a) generosity, (b) belonging, (c) mastery, and (d) independence (Brendtro, Brokenleg, & Van Bockern, 1990). The need for generosity is the need for people to engage in personal sharing. This is not a giving of materialistic goods, but rather a giving and sharing of time, one's feelings, and one's self. The need for belonging transcends all cultures and societies. Human beings are social animals with a need to belong to a family, a community, a society, and the need to feel connected to the universe. The lack of belonging leaves one feeling isolated and lonely, and intimacy suffers. The need for mastery is essential for personal growth and learning. Every person needs to feel self-sufficient and assured that they can master the tasks that will take them through life. Finally, the need for independence is the need to live in a fashion that is free from unhealthy co-dependence upon others. Healthy independence means being responsible for one's self and using healthy assertiveness to get needs met.

Second, there is a focus on the four aspects of self: (a) the emotional self, (b) the mental self, (c) the physical self, and (d) the spiritual self (Longo, 2001). The combination of these aspects leads to an overall focus on core values and beliefs. Overall, a holistic, ecological approach encourages professionals to assess and work with youth in a comprehensive manner.

No Labeling

Of importance when looking at a holistic model is that treatment helps engage clients by being sensitive to the individual's culture, race, and spirituality. A holistic model addresses and includes all life issues and strives for balance and harmony. Holistic treatment sees each person as unique, yet does not label. In the field of treating sexual abusers, clients are often called and labelled as 'sex offenders.' Many programs often require clients to open group by taking turns saying, "My name is . . . and I'm a sex offender" similar to addictions models such as Alcoholics Anonymous. Negative labels do not help people heal but rather reinforce their staying in the unhealthy state of 'sex offender' for life. A holistic model does not view people by labels or their behavior, but sees people as humans first and then persons with a particular problem.

The Therapeutic Relationship

Holistic treatment sees a healthy therapeutic relationship as the foundation of good treatment and essential to the healing process. It supports a mutual relationship of learning and of give and take. According to Blanchard (1998), a healthy therapeutic relationship consists of the following components: trust, compassion, self-disclosure, humor, respect, congruence, equality, authenticity, vulnerability, warmth, and a willingness to attempt to understand the client's emotional condition and life situation with a concern for his/her growth and happiness.

It is common in society to only view people according to their behavior, and it is easy as mental health practitioners to make this same mistake. It is sometimes difficult to maintain respect for clients who are violent and who have harmed others. However, it is crucial that professionals monitor their own values, beliefs, biases, and angry thoughts. While the client's behavior might be despicable, it is important to view the person beyond the behavior and offer him/her understanding. In order to facilitate the therapeutic relationship and maximize the potential for both therapist and client to learn and grow, there must be an element of trust, compassion, and respect for the client. The client must experience the professional as genuine and supportive yet challenging of unhealthy ways. This can still be done while still holding the client accountable for unacceptable behavior.

Multiple Learning Styles

Integrated experiential models of treatment seek to bring a variety of theories and models into the treatment process to enhance a person's potential. For example Howard Gardner (1983), noted for his work on multiple intelligences, teaches that youth have a variety of learning styles and abilities. He suggests that there are seven learning styles common to youth: (a) intrapersonal intelligence, (b) interpersonal intelligence, (c) visual/spatial intelligence, (d) verbal/linguistic intelligence, (e) logical mathematical intelligence, (f) musical/rhythmic intelligence, and (g) body/kinesthetic intelligence.

Intrapersonal intelligence involves knowledge of the internal aspects of the self, such as feelings, the range of emotional responses, thinking processes, self-reflection, and meta-cognition (a sense of our intuition and awareness of spiritual realities). In working with youth with behavioral problems, it is not likely that this intelligence has been developed. Thus, one facet of treatment is to develop this intelligence in order to promote the client's ability to form relationships, develop empathy, and work with unhealthy thinking patterns. If this intelligence is not developed as a part of treatment, there is less likelihood that cognitive restructuring and emotional development will realize its fullest potential as part of the treatment process. Examples of methods to develop this intelligence include silent meditation/reflection, thinking strategies, emotional processing, focusing/concentration skills, and complex guided imagery.

Interpersonal intelligence involves the ability to work cooperatively with others in a group as well as the ability to communicate verbally and non-verbally with other people. It also involves the capacity to notice distinctions among others; for example, contrasts in moods and temperament. Examples of methods to develop this intelligence include giving and receiving feedback, intuiting other's feelings, teaching cooperative learning strategies, practicing empathy, building collaboration skills, and group projects.

Visual/spatial intelligence involves skills in visual arts (including painting, drawing, and sculpture) and games that require the ability to visualize objects from different perspectives and angles, such as chess. For youth who do not work well with verbal/linguistic intelligences, this intelligence can be a primary mode of learning and assimilating information. Experiential therapies are useful in working with those who use this form of intelligence. Examples of methods to develop this intelligence include guided imagery, working with color schemes and designs, human sculptures, human still photos, mime, art therapies, and working with pictures.

Verbal/linguistic intelligence is related to the use of words and language, both written and spoken. This is the intelligence most treatment programs for youth with sexual behavior problems rely upon, as they incorporate a variety of reading and writing assignments. Use of this intelligence is also used in sit down individual and group therapies, psycho-educational classes, and the like. For youth who do not learn well with this intelligence it is likely the client will not do well in treatment or may even drop out of or fail in treatment. Examples of methods to develop this intelligence include reading, vocabulary development, journal/diary keeping, creative writing, use of humor, impromptu speaking, storytelling, and role-plays.

Logical mathematical intelligence is most often associated with what is known as "scientific thinking," or inductive reasoning. It requires the capacity to recognize patterns, work with abstract symbols, and see connections between separate and distinct pieces of information. Many clients who suffer developmental delays and learning disabilities will often not rely upon this form of intelligence for learning. Examples of methods to develop this intelligence include outlining, number sequences, calculation, problem solving, and pattern games.

Musical/rhythmic intelligence includes such capacities as the recognition of rhythmic and tonal patterns, including sensitivity to various environmental sounds, the human voice, and musical instruments. Of all forms of intelligence, the "consciousness altering" effect of music and rhythm on the brain is probably the greatest. Examples of methods to develop this intelligence include teaching rhythmic patterns, vocal sounds and tones, music composition, percussion vibrations, humming, singing, music performance, and music therapy.

Body/kinesthetic intelligence is related to physical movement and the knowledge/wisdom of the body, including the brain's motor cortex that controls bodily motion. This intelligence relies on the ability to use the body to express emotions, to play a game, and to create new products. It is "learning by doing." Examples of methods to develop this intelligence include folk/creative dance, martial arts, physical exercise, mime, and experiential therapies such as drama therapy and role-playing.

A NOTE ON REACTIVE ATTACHMENT DISORDER

Juvenile sexual offenders in treatment are often given diagnoses such as Attachment Disorder and Oppositional Defiant Disorder, and often have severe behavioral problems. Insecure attachment and Attachment Disorder (AD), also known as Reactive Attachment Disorder (RAD), is a relatively new diagnosis in the DSM-IV-TR (American Psychiatric Association, 2000) and is often misunderstood. Insecure attachment (which is not diagnosable) and AD (which is diagnosable) are conditions in which individuals have difficulty forming loving, caring, lasting, intimate, relationships. Attachment and bonding are generally used interchangeably. AD youth usually do not learn how to trust, and often fail to develop a conscience. They learn that the world is not a safe place.

RAD, as defined by the DSM-IV-TR (American Psychiatric Association, 2000), requires etiological factors such as gross deprivation of care or successive multiple caregivers for diagnosis. Attachment disordered youth may present in two ways.

In inhibited RAD, the child does not initiate or respond to social interactions in a developmentally appropriate manner. When caregivers are unreliable, inconsistent, or respond in an unpredictable and uncertain way, the child may not be able to establish a pattern of confident expectation. One result is insecure attachment, a less than optimal internal sense of confidence and trust in others. The child uses psychological defenses to avoid disappointments, which may contribute to a negative working model of relationships and insecurity.

In disinhibited RAD, the child has diffuse attachments, indiscriminate sociability, and excessive familiarity with strangers. These children repeatedly lose attachment figures or have multiple caregivers, and thus they have never had the chance to develop a continuous and consistent attachment to any one person. The usual anxiety and concern with strangers is not present. AD youth are often masters at manipulating their environment and people within them. They may demonstrate learning problems in school and often lack a conscience because they lack real trust in anyone.

Overall symptoms of Attachment Disorder may include the following: (a) poor peer relations, (b) a lack of cause and effect thinking, (c) superficial charm, (d) indiscriminate affection with strangers, (e) stealing or lying, (f) destruction of self, others, and/or things, (g) a lack of conscience, (h) developmental lags, (i) poor impulse control, (j) lack of eye contact, (k) pre-occupation with fire, blood, and/or gore, (l) fighting for control over everything, (m) cruelty to animals and/or siblings, (n) hoarding or gorging food, and (o) inappropriate demanding or clinging behavior.

On the flip side, healthy attachment helps promote the following: (a) the development of a conscience, (b) the ability to think logically, (c) the ability to cope with stress and frustration, (d) the development of relationships, (e) the ability to handle perceived threats to self, (f) the ability to become self-reliant, and (g) the ability to handle fear and worry.

Successful therapy with youth facing attachment problems depends upon the therapist's willingness to use unconventional strategies. Some of these strategies are to find and to face the depth of the feelings that these youth keep hidden, and to revisit traumas together with the child. Therapists need to be prepared to face the horrors that many of these youth have experienced if they ever hope to help them heal. Critical goals of treatment may include but are not limited to the following: (a) resolution of early losses, (b) development of trust, (c) modulation of affect, (d) development of internal control, (e) correcting distorted thinking patterns, (f) development of reciprocal relationships, (g) learning appropriate responses to external structure and societal rules, and (h) development of self-respect.

GUIDELINES AND PRINCIPLES FOR USING EXPERIENTIAL TREATMENTS

There are several basic guidelines and principles to take into account when using integrated experiential treatments. As exciting as this work can be, one must use caution and keep in mind the well-being of the patient. Experiential treatment can move the patient more quickly and in different ways than traditional "talk" therapies. An experienced clinician using experiential therapies can enhance treatment by helping provide opportunities for insights to patient learning, and making the overall treatment experience more attractive and interesting. The challenge for experiential treatment providers is to offer the opportunity for patients to learn without telling patients what to do and how to do it, what to think, and what to feel.

Currently, verbal/linguistic-based cognitive-behavioral treatment methods dominate the world of programs treating youth and adolescents. However, experiential treatments can be used in conjunction with most cognitive-behavioral treatment models that address empathy, anger management, perspective taking, cognitive restructuring, decision-making, education, life skills development, and interventions for problems experienced by the patient. Methods include psycho-education, social and life skills development, competency skills building, and coping skills. All programming should try to match the cognitive skills of the patient and be delivered by competent staff members that are committed to the program, program philosophy, and process. Treatment should also be based upon the stages of development through which youth are likely to progress.

The patients' behavioral responses to situations are typically learned and strengthened through frequent repetition. Learned behavior is closely connected to doing experiential work. Both are composed of definitions of performance and imply a learning of roles. Experiential treatments do not exclude the basic cognitive-behavioral treatments used in most residential and community-based programs, but rather work in conjunction with them to enhance them.

Two important concepts within cognitive-behavioral treatment that are closely linked to experiential learning processes are role reversal and perspective taking. The emphasis on role reversal is familiar to most therapists who see the value in having a patient switch roles with another person, usually a significant person in the patient's life, such as a father, mother, sibling, close friend, or teacher with whom they have an unresolved conflict. Playing relevant roles facilitates the patient's learning and skills development while engaging him/her in perspective taking and, in some cases, empathic roles. The active representation and exploration of his/her own life is essential to good treatment (J. Bergman, personal communication, September 7, 2001).

New behavior is not taught by describing it or telling someone about it. It becomes incorporated into one's life by re-enactment and rehearsal (practice), which is a vital part of the process. One of the critical points in this work is to have the patient look critically at his/her own behavior. Behavior does not occur in a vacuum. Where there is behavior, there are thoughts (cognitions), and feelings (emotions) guiding it (Longo, 2001).

Programs and patients need to develop cognitive dexterity. Cognitive dexterity is the ability of individuals to look at all possibilities and situations, and to be able to read multiple rather than singular meanings. Patients need the ability to be able to respond to situations in a variety of ways, and to explore different ways of learning and thinking. Cognitive dexterity also refers to a mental ability that is open, flexible, and able to generate realistic solutions to complex problems; it defies rigid thinking and prioritizes flexibility and spontaneity. Insisting on one right way (singular) limits this ability and inhibits the development of a mentally dextrous approach to social interactions and life problems. Learning to weigh all of the possible perspectives encourages standing in another's shoes before actions are taken (perspective taking and empathy). Experiential treatments provide opportunities for patients to learn through one or more of the multiple intelligences they typically use.

Using Experiential Exercises

There are several basic principles one is encouraged to follow in using experiential treatments with youth. This work does not require anything more than time and a willingness to experiment and be creative. The basic principles for this work are summarized below.

Be creative. The first basic principle is that the facilitator (leader, clinician, trainer) of experiential exercises must feel comfortable being creative. Not everyone is comfortable standing up before a group and engaging in the exercises that follow. Some people may have a discomfort about the use of touch, some may have physical limitations, and others may simply be embarrassed to engage is this type of work. The facilitator must be sensitive to his/her level of comfort with these activities and be willing to actively participate.

Do not go into this work with expectations of successful outcomes. Practitioners often have expectations that what they do must be perfect. This is not the case with experiential exercises. If you are using a creative process you must be prepared that sometimes you will experience failure or the exercises will simply flop. When doing this work, focus on the process and not particular outcomes. Sometimes an anticipated outcome will occur, while at other times a very different yet positive outcome will emerge. Don't create unrealistic expectations for yourself or for the clients.

It is okay to make mistakes and experience exercise failures. One cannot predict human behavior, especially with youth. It may take time and several groups using only warm-up exercises to move the clients into a serious mode versus a "silly" mode. Kids will ham things up just to have fun and be silly. This is okay. Let them have the time to discover, explore, and learn.

Practice exercises first before using them in clinical or teaching situations. It is strongly suggested that you do each exercise yourself before you engage patients in doing them. One way of understanding the exercises and ensuring their success is to practice them alone or with other colleagues or friends. Become familiar with them and the potential outcomes.

Spontaneity and creativity are foundations of the work. Being creative requires the facilitator to be comfortable with being spontaneous. In the middle of an exercise it is totally permissible to shift gears and move in a different direction depending upon the process of the group. Try to avoid rigid thinking and fixed outcomes. Spontaneity and creativity go hand in hand.

Involve all staff and patients. Experiential exercises require that everyone participate unless physical limitations or other disabilities prevent them from doing so. Warm-up exercises are designed to help build comfort in doing this work. It is a time to learn to work with basic props and kinesis. It is also a time to have fun as the patients learn and become more comfortable with experiential work. Again, this may take some time. Don't rush the process. It is more important that everyone is involved and learns to develop a personal level of comfort in doing the work.

All patients are given the opportunity to work. Most practitioners have had the experience of working with patients who are "wallflowers" and who are quite comfortable not saying or doing anything in the group. One of the beauties of experiential work is that it involves everyone. If the patient refuses to participate, the patient can observe and give feedback to others. Certainly, onlookers have their own experience in just watching experiential work.

All material is authentic in the work. As long as you do not tell patients what to say or what to do, and what to think and feel, the work that results is real and authentic. Even if the patient responds in a nervous way (nervous laughter) or silly fashion (distracting or avoidant behavior), what is seen in the patient is real and authentic, and therefore worthy of the effort. Such reactions can and should be explored with the patient.

Don't tell patients what to think and feel. One of the essential points in this type of work is to have the patient look critically at his/her own behavior. Programs and their staff need to develop cognitive dexterity by honoring the patient's ability to identify the meaning of their own thoughts and feelings. This leads to patient self-discovery and patients memory of past events that in turn lead to self-expression and associated thoughts and feelings.

Be careful about telling patients what to do. Obviously, facilitators have to take charge over a variety of issues including the patients' safety, the safety of others, and maintaining a safe environment. These exercises require that participants be given directions and told how to follow them. It is how they are told that matters. Aggressive and/or controlling patients do not like being told what to do. Encourage and support them without being overbearing and overly controlling/ directive. We do not want participants to react or act out in response to this work, but rather to respond to the situations we create in doing experiential work. This work is about behavioral change and not behavioral control. The goal is for patients to understand the whys, hows, and benefits of visual/spatial, kinetic, and language-based treatment.

As a final note, in working with youth there is a tendency (conscious or subconscious) to push them into traditional gender roles (J. Bergman, personal communication, September 7, 2001; Robinson, 2002). For example, male roles include being strong, silent, in control, independent, and not giving the appearance of looking weak. For females, the traditional roles are being dependent, not questioning, focus on beauty and appearance, and not appearing to be smart. In order to effect change in these young people, it is important to break down the gender roles they may use to avoid doing in-depth work.

Engaging Patients in Experiential Treatments and Exercises

When beginning this work with patients it is important to start with warm-up exercises. Patients need to become comfortable with these most basic, fun activities before moving into introductory and then more advanced exercises. Warm-up exercises should include activities that help patients explore and gradually learn to be comfortable with thoughts, words, movement, and touch while having fun. These exercise are also important in building group cohesion, cooperation, trust between patients, and trust between patients and staff. The process for engaging patients in experiential treatments requires the following principles.

Explain the exercises to the patients. It is important to explain the exercises to patients. Get their permission (use informed consent if necessary) to participate and immediately address any concerns or reluctance.

The patient must have the physical and emotional skills to understand the exercise. It is essential that the patients have the physical and emotional skills to understand what is going on and what the work is about. When working with younger children, make sure the exercises are modified to work with their level of understanding and psychomotor ability. Keep in mind the patients' learning style.

Work in the here and now. It is important to work in the present–the "here and now." Even when addressing past events, the work the patient does should be focused on intrapersonal processes in the here and now. For example, when working on past events suggest to the patient that she/he experience it now with leading statements such as, "imagine you are in that situation now; describe the environment, naming who is present, and *what* you are doing now." Avoid having participants describe the past. Rather, have them describe what they want and need in the present.

The patient must have ultimate control. The patient must able to make a safe place in his/her head in case he/she needs to go there (J. Bergman, personal communication, September 7, 2001). A safe place can be any place or anything in terms of a mental image that gives the patient a sense of safety and comfort. The patient has total control of his or her safe place and determines who can be there with him or her and who cannot. If the patient wants to stop the exercise, honor the patient's request to do so.

The patient understands that he/she can stop the exercise at any time. It is critical that the patient understands that he/she can stop the exercise at any time;

that he/she is in control, not the leader. There should never be a consequence to a patient for not participating in or stopping an exercise once it has begun.

TYPES OF EXERCISES

There are several types of exercises one can use to incorporate experiential work into the treatment process with JSOs (Longo, 2002). They include but are not limited to the following:

The Three T's

The "three T's" stands for team building, trust, and touch. Many of the exercises that focus on any one of these skills usually incorporate the others (e.g., team building requires trust, and touch is often a part of many team and trust building exercises).

Words and Language

These are exercises that involve (a) self-expression, (b) self-exploration, and (c) self-disclosure. Many exercises that build the patients comfort in talking and relating to others additionally focus on self-expression, self-exploration, and self-disclosure. These exercises also focus on cognitive restructuring.

Cognitive Restructuring

These exercises involve self-awareness, interpersonal skills, intra-personal skills, and self-esteem building. Cognitive distortions usually impact interpersonal relationships in a negative way. Exercises that focus on cognitive restructuring also help facilitate stronger relationships. Cognitive distortions directly affect the patient's ability to recognize and express emotions.

Emotional Development and Expression

These are exercises that involve identification and recognition of feelings and the development of empathy. These exercises also focus on personal victimization and personal abuse work that are often linked to the patient's anger and problematic behaviors.

Behavioral Issues

These are exercises that involve anger management and assertiveness training. Exercises that focus on managing behavior also use cognitive restructuring, which in turn address the patient's core values and beliefs.

Values Clarification and Personal Beliefs

As the patient works with his/her core values and beliefs, their social skills and competency skills are usually enhanced.

Skills Building

These exercises focus on building social competencies, social skills, and peer relations.

SAMPLE EXERCISES

The following are examples of experiential exercises based on Longo (2002).

The Three T's: Trust, Teamwork, and Touch

Monster legs exercise. The purpose of this exercise is to build group trust and learn teamwork (see Table 1). Participants are dependent upon each other to complete the exercise. This exercise is a spin-off of the three-legged race.

In a large open space or outdoors participants are asked to stand in a straight line. Each participant has his/her left leg tied to the person's right leg (next to him/her) and the participant's right leg tied to the person's left leg (next to him/her). Only the participants on each end of the line have a free (unbound)

TABLE 1. Monster Legs Exercise

Purpose	To build trust and teamwork
Level	Warm-up
Group size	8-10
Time (in minutes)	5
Materials needed	Bandanas or 3 foot long cloth strips
Cautions	Use an open space free of obstacles to bump into or fall on. Best done outside or on carpeted surface. PAL[a] = H
Variations	Yes
Process questions	Yes[b]

Note. [a]PAL is Physical Activity Level. Ratings are L (low; minimal or none), M (medium; requires some physical activity), and H (high; requires a lot of physical activity). [b]Basic process questions for any exercise include: What was the experience like for you? What were you thinking? What were you feeling?

leg. The leader ties each pair of legs together with a strip of cloth or two ban-
dannas tied together. The participants are given instructions for movement.
For example they are told to walk like a clock hand forward around a tree or
stationary object. To walk backwards, to walk to one side or the other side, to
form a circle and move in a certain direction, etc.

The following are possible variations:

1. Repeat the same exercise asking some or all participants to close their
   eyes and keep them closed, or use blindfolds for all or some members.
   They are instructed to follow the voice and instructions of the leader.
2. One of the participants is given the task to be the leader and instruct the
   group where and how to move.

Words and Language

Media expert exercise. The purpose of this exercise is to facilitate comfort
with using language and words and to facilitate self-disclosure (see Table 2).

The leader picks four participants. One is selected as the "expert" and the
others are interviewers from the media. The leader assigns a topic to the "expert" and the media interviewers take turns asking him/her three or four questions. Then the expert becomes an interviewer, and a new expert is selected
and is now the expert of a new topic.

The following is a possible variation: As the experts change, a new topic is
selected that ups the anti and the effect. Examples of expert topics could include: (a) "Corsini trouser fleas" (a fictitious insect), (b) "invisible dental
floss," or (c) "sole-less shoes." More intense topics could include "standing on

TABLE 2. Media Expert Exercise

Purpose	To facilitate self-disclosure
Level	Warm-up, Introductory
Group size	Groups of 4
Time (in minutes)	5-10 per group
Materials needed	None
Cautions	Can trigger issues that need therapeutic follow-up/attention. PAL[a] = L
Variations	Yes
Process questions	Yes

Note. [a]PAL is Physical Activity Level. Ratings are L (low; minimal or none), M (medium; requires some physical activity), and H (high; requires a lot of physical activity).

your head to manage anger," or "bubble gum as a contraceptive device." Most intense topics could include the impact of sexual abuse on victims, handling the death of a friend, or the loss of a parent.

Values and Beliefs

My beliefs exercise. The purpose of this exercise is to develop trust, explore movement, and understand differences between people (see Table 3).

Group participants sit in circle. Five signs are taped to the wall around the room. Signs say: (a) Strongly Agree, (b) Mildly Agree, (c) Mildly Disagree, (d) Strongly Disagree, and (e) No Opinion. The group leader reads statements and participants go to the sign that represents their beliefs.

Examples of statements include the following:

1. It's okay to copy someone else's homework if they say you can do so.
2. Boys and girls are equal in all respects.
3. There is only one true religion in the world.
4. Most athletes are self-centered.
5. Bad kids come from bad families.
6. Criminals are born as criminals.
7. The press has the right to print whatever it chooses.
8. School should be year round with only a two-week summer break.
9. Every child should have his/her own phone and phone number.
10. Every family should be limited to two children.

TABLE 3. My Beliefs Exercise

Purpose	To develop trust, explore movement, and explore differences between people
Level	Warm-up
Group size	All
Time (in minutes)	10-15
Materials needed	Large empty room
Cautions	None; PAL[a] = L
Variations	Yes
Process questions	Yes

Note. [a]PAL is Physical Activity Level. Ratings are L (low; minimal or none), M (medium; requires some physical activity), and H (high; requires a lot of physical activity).

A possible variation could be to use statements about treatment, families, or other issues. Following the exercise, discuss the following process questions:

1. What is it like (what do you think and how do you feel) when others have similar beliefs?
2. What is it like (what do you think and how do you feel) when others have different beliefs?

Cognitive Restructuring

Role throw-away exercise. The purpose of this exercise is to facilitate self-disclosure and personal insight (see Table 4).

Participants sit in a circle. Each has paper and pencil. The paper is folded in half and then in half again so it has four quarters. Participants are to write four roles they assume in their lives that are important, such as patient, child, student, friend, athlete, etc.

Each person takes a turn briefly discussing his/her roles with the group. After a group discussion each participant tears off one role and throws it in the box in the center of circle. Then each participant takes a turn to discuss how it would feel if he/she could really throw away one role in his/her life. A possible variation might be to repeat the exercise with all four roles. Following the exercise, discuss the following process questions:

1. What would be the impact of throwing away a life role?
2. What would be difficult about throwing away a life role?
3. What would be different about not having the associated responsibilities and demands of the role?

TABLE 4. Role Throw-Away Exercise

Purpose	To facilitate self-disclosure and personal insight
Level	Intermediate
Group size	8-12
Time (in minutes)	8-10 per person
Materials needed	Paper, pen or pencil, small box (i.e., shoe box)
Cautions	Can open up personal issues, problems, and emotions. PAL[a] = L
Variations	Yes
Process questions	Yes

Note. [a]PAL is Physical Activity Level. Ratings are L (low; minimal or none), M (medium; requires some physical activity), and H (high; requires a lot of physical activity).

Emotional

Personas exercise. The purpose of this exercise is to facilitate self-disclosure, trust, and personal sharing (see Table 5).

In order to do this exercise the facilitator must have a variety of masks, preferably professionally made, that represent a variety of feelings and emotions (i.e., silly, sad, happy, angry, anxious, depressed, confused, concerned, content, etc.).

The facilitator explains to participants that most people have at least three personas: a public/current persona (the person they are in public around others), a private or secret persona (the part of them that few if any people know about), and a future persona (the person they see themselves being in the future). Each persona has many feelings or emotions attached to these. Masks are placed in the middle of the floor and participants are instructed to pick one mask that best represents their private/secret persona. After each person selects a mask, the facilitator encourages volunteers to share why they chose that mask and the feeling(s) it represents. Following the exercise, discuss the following process questions:

1. Why did you choose the particular mask?
2. What feeling is most closely associated with the mask you chose?

Behavioral

Arguments exercise. The purpose of this exercise is to facilitate self-expression and work on anger control (see Table 6).

Group participants sit in a circle. The trainer initiates a group discussion about the various ways in which people tend to argue with each other. For example, how does arguing tie into anger and personal ways of expressing anger? How do the patients deal with disagreements and arguments with other staff/patients? Two participants at a time are selected and stand in the center of the circle. They are instructed to have an argument. They select a topic or the trainer/group leader gives them an argument topic. They are instructed to argue with one of the following stipulations: (a) argue with no restrictions, (b) argue without being allowed to use swear words, or (c) argue with hands in pockets.

The following are possible variations:

1. Where do you draw the line? Many of us have a point beyond which we may tell the truth and deny a particular action or behavior. Explore with the group who would deny to a parent or spouse that they, (a) got a park-

ing ticket, (b) got a speeding ticket for $200, (c) had a car accident and in fact is was your fault, and (d) had an affair or got a woman pregnant.
2. Two participants stand in the center of the circle and have an argument; one person is instructed to use one of the following types of denial. A subject for the argument is given by the leader/trainer. Examples of subjects include the following: (a) complete outright denial, (b) denial of denial (denial that you are denying the problem), (c) denial of responsibility for your behavior, (d) denial of intention to do a particular act or behavior, (e) denial of facts about what you have done, (f) denial of harm to the person you acted out against, (g) denial of violence or aggression, (h) denial of planning your behavior, and (i) denial of the frequency you have engaged in a particular behavior.

TABLE 5. Personas Exercise

Purpose	To facilitate self-disclosure, trust, and personal sharing
Level	Intermediate/Advanced
Group size	8-12
Time (in minutes)	5-10 per person
Materials needed	Masks
Cautions	Can open up emotions, personal issues and problems. PAL[a] = L
Variations	Yes
Process questions	Yes

Note. [a]PAL is Physical Activity Level. Ratings are L (low; minimal or none), M (medium; requires some physical activity), and H (high; requires a lot of physical activity).

TABLE 6. Arguments Exercise

Purpose	Facilitate interpersonal skills, anger expression, self-disclosure, trust
Level	Intermediate
Group size	Two per team/pair
Time (in minutes)	10 per pair
Materials needed	None
Cautions	Can open up personal issues and emotions. PAL[a] = M
Variations	Yes
Process questions	Yes

Note. [a]PAL is Physical Activity Level. Ratings are L (low; minimal or none), M (medium; requires some physical activity), and H (high; requires a lot of physical activity).

Following the exercise, discuss the following process questions:

1. What was hard about this exercise?
2. What did you learn about yourself?
3. What did you learn about others?

CLOSING COMMENTS

Experiential treatment with youth is rapidly growing in its acceptance within the field. It is becoming more recognized that the trickle-down of adult sex-offender treatment methods and models have serious shortcomings and potentially negative implications in regard to their application to youth with sexual behavior problems. Youth are resilient and have a tremendous capacity to recover from trauma and childhood experiences that have resulted in serious behavioral problems. In working with youth it is important to take into account that they are *not* miniature adults, and work with them must take into account developmental and contextual issues as well as learning differences and learning disabilities.

Holistic treatment means treating the whole person and not just a particular problem. All too often programs treating youth with sexual behavior problems view the client in the context of the referring problem. They see the child as a sex offender instead of as a child with many parts of which sexually abusive behavior is only one aspect. The other parts include the many other parts of the client's life such as family, peers, community, school, hobbies and interests, sports, dating, and so forth. When practitioners see a person with many facets, many of which are damaged parts, then they are better able to understand the complex nature of what must be treated. Each part that is damaged needs to be repaired and given the time and opportunity to heal. A holistic approach works toward healing the whole person.

The use of experiential treatments can help make treatment more easily understood and meaningful to patients. Additionally, they can facilitate personal growth in a variety of treatment arenas including emotional development, use of language and words, cognitive restructuring, behavioral management, values and personal beliefs, and social skills building. This can be especially useful when traditional sit-down talk therapy may not be as effective or have the necessary impact to facilitate client motivation, insight, and change.

REFERENCES

American Psychiatric Association. (2000). *Diagnostic and statistical manual of mental Disorders* (text revision). Washington, DC: Author.

Bell, C.C. (2002). *Cultivating resiliency in youth: Gift from within.* Retrieved October 16, 2002, from: http://www.sourcemaine.com/gift/Html/cultivat.html

Blanchard, G. (1998). *The difficult connection.* Brandon, VT: Safer Society Press.

Brendtro, L., Brokenleg, M., & Van Bockern, S. (1990). *Reclaiming youth at risk: Our hope for the future.* Bloomington, IN: National Education Service.

Burton, D., Freeman-Longo, R., Fiske, J., Levins, J., & Smith-Darden, J. (2000). *1996 nationwide survey of treatment programs and models: Serving abuse reactive youth and adolescent and adult sexual offenders.* Brandon, VT: Safer Society Press.

Chaffin, M. (2002, February). Paper presented at the South Carolina Colloquium on Child Sexual Abuse, Charleston, SC.

Development Services Group. (2000). *Understanding treatment and accountability in juvenile sex offending: Results and recommendations from an OJJDP focus group.* Prepared for: Office of Juvenile Justice and Delinquency Prevention Training and Technical Assistance Division. Inc. 7315 Wisconsin Avenue, Suite 700E, Bethesda, MD 20814.

Freeman-Longo, R.E., Bird, S., Stevenson, W.F., & Fiske, J.A. (1995). *1994 Nationwide survey of treatment programs and models: Serving abuse reactive youth and adolescent and adult sexual offenders.* Brandon, VT: Safer Society Press.

Gardner, H. (1983). *Frames of mind: The theory of multiple intelligences.* New York: Basic Books.

Knopp, F.H., Freeman-Longo, R.E., & Stevenson, W. F. (1993). *Nationwide survey of juvenile and adult sex offender treatment programs and models, 1992.* Orwell, VT: Safer Society Press.

Laws, D.R., Hudson, S.M., & Ward, T. (2002). *Remaking relapse prevention with sex offenders: A sourcebook.* Thousand Oaks, CA: Sage Publications.

Longo, R.E. (2001). *Paths to wellness: A holistic approach and guide for personal recovery.* Holyoke, MA: NEARI Press.

Longo, R.E. (2002). *New hope exercises for youth.* Unpublished manuscript.

National Task Force on Juvenile Sexual Offending. (1993). The revised report from the national task force on juvenile sexual offending, 1993 of the national adolescent perpetrator network. *Juvenile and Family Court Journal, 44*(4).

Robinson, S.L. (2002). *Growing beyond.* Holyoke, MA: NEARI Press.

Ryan, G. et al. (1999). *Web of meaning: A developmental-contextual approach in sexual abuse treatment.* Brandon, VT: Safer Society Press.

Ward, T. (2002). Good lives and the rehabilitation of offenders: Promises and problems. *Aggression and Violent Behavior, 7,* 1-17.

Ward, T., & Hudson, S.M. (1996). Relapse prevention: A critical analysis. *Sexual Abuse: A Journal of Research and Treatment, 8* (3), 177-200.

Ward, T., & Stewart, C.A. (2002). Good lives and the rehabilitation of sexual offenders. In T. Ward, D.R. Laws, & S.M. Hudson (Eds.), *Sexual deviance: Theoretical issues and controversies* (pp. 21-44). Thousand Oaks, CA: Sage Press.

Multi-Family Group Therapy
for Sexually Abusive Youth

David Nahum
Marci Mandel Brewer

SUMMARY. Although Multi-Family Group Therapy (MFGT) has been a researched intervention for nearly 40 years, clinicians working with sexually abusive youth and their families have only more recently begun to utilize the intervention. We believe MFGT for a sexual offense-specific treatment population is a sophisticated and powerful clin-

---

Address correspondence to: David Nahum, EdD, 599 Topeka Way, Suite 300, Castle Rock, CO 80104 (E-mail: barndoctors@juno.com); or Marci Mandel Brewer, LCSW, 2755 South Locust Street, Suite 101, Denver, CO 80222 (E-mail: mmbrewer@msn.com).

The authors would like to thank the Colorado Front Range sexual offense-specific treatment community including clinical colleagues, victim therapists and advocates, probation and social service departments, schools, the Colorado Sex Offender Management Board (SOMB), and especially the families of high risk youth who continue to teach and inspire them with renewed hope in their efforts to create a safer and more humane community.

[Haworth co-indexing entry note]: "Multi-Family Group Therapy for Sexually Abusive Youth." Nahum, David, and Marci Mandel Brewer. Co-published simultaneously in *Journal of Child Sexual Abuse* (The Haworth Maltreatment and Trauma Press, an imprint of The Haworth Press, Inc.) Vol. 13, No. 3/4, 2004, pp. 215-243; and: *Identifying and Treating Youth Who Sexually Offend: Current Approaches, Techniques, and Research* (ed: Robert Geffner et al.) The Haworth Maltreatment and Trauma Press, an imprint of The Haworth Press, Inc., 2004, pp. 215-243. Single or multiple copies of this article are available for a fee from The Haworth Document Delivery Service [1-800-HAWORTH, 9:00 a.m. - 5:00 p.m. (EST). E-mail address: docdelivery@haworthpress.com].

Digital Object Identifier: 10.1300/J070v13n03_11

ical intervention with unique advantages including economical use of clinician resources, family-to-family transfer of knowledge and mentoring, community-based resourcefulness, and accelerated catalyzing of emotions. This article will provide direction on establishing the MFGT format as well as discuss its goals, curriculum, facilitation priorities, and strategies. *[Article copies available for a fee from The Haworth Document Delivery Service: 1-800-HAWORTH. E-mail address: <docdelivery@haworthpress.com> Website: <http://www.HaworthPress.com> © 2004 by The Haworth Press, Inc. All rights reserved.]*

KEYWORDS. Multi-family group therapy, sexual offense-specific treatment, juvenile sexual offender, group therapy, family therapy

MULTI-FAMILY GROUP THERAPY

Clinicians engaged in the treatment of difficult populations must rely upon the most progressive and intensive interventions in the pursuit of client behavioral change, health, and insight. Multi-Family Group Therapy (MFGT) was first presented in the professional literature in the 1960s as a useful adjunct to traditional therapy formats (Leichter & Schulman, 1968). MFGT has also been referred to in the literature as a multi-family psychoeducation group (MFPG), with the latter emphasizing a more educational curriculum over a psychotherapeutic, process-oriented agenda.

MFGT, as it is referred to in this article, is a clinician-facilitated treatment group comprised of several youth, their parents, and adjunct caregivers. MFGT becomes a microcosm of society where families can interact with and influence one another, and multigenerational family process can be observed and changed. MFGT process parallels family systems theory, where change in individual members impacts the entire group and more global group change is infectious to individuals.

MFGT has been shown to enhance knowledge, skills, support, and treatment attitudes in families of children with Bipolar Disorder, Major Depressive Disorder, or Dysthymic Disorder (Fristad, Goldberg-Arnold, & Gavazzi, 2002) and reduce levels of expressed emotion (EE) in relatives of adults suffering from Bipolar Disorder (Honig, Hofman, Rozendaal, & Dingemans, 1997). In the latter study, a reduction in the number of hospital admissions was also noted. The MFGT intervention has also shown promising results in work with high-risk schizophrenics and their families (Falloon, Liberman, Lillie, & Vaughn, 1981), and beneficial to Kosovar refugees by increasing social support and willingness to access community psychiatric services (Weine et al., 2003). The intervention has proven as well to be of value to non-psychiatric populations such as gifted American Indian adolescents and their parents (Robbins, Tonemah, & Robbins, 2002).

In addition to proven efficacy with a variety of clinical populations, multi-family group therapy (MFGT) offers several distinct advantages over more traditional treatment modalities.

Economical. A dozen or more families can be served by a small team of clinicians.

Family-to-family transfer of knowledge. Newer families can have direct access to the wisdom more experienced families have gleaned over the course of the treatment experience, thereby creating a transferable fund of knowledge.

Family-to-family modeling and mentoring. More seasoned parents can model pro-treatment attitudes, parenting, communication, and supervision skills to new participants, thereby jump-starting their entry into the treatment process.

Accelerated learning about the family's role and behavior in society. MFGT becomes a microcosm of societal roles, values, and motivations, providing a valuable window into the family's interface with society. These are insights that can be passed onto the youth's individual therapist for use in future therapy sessions.

Building community-based resourcefulness. Families can begin the process of supporting and relying upon one other as neighbors and experiential peers, and not just on the transient treatment team professionals.

Catalyzing emotions. The emotional intensity generated by this group format aids in bringing feelings, motivations, and perspectives to the surface, thereby allowing opportunities to confront denial and more quickly push families in the direction of curative emotional experiences.

Accelerating honesty and genuineness. Families have greater difficulty hiding counter-treatment attitudes, distortions, and secrecy amongst a roomful of their peers. The group aids in providing a more accurate representation of the family and youth participants.

Thus, clinicians have been turning to the MFGT intervention in an effort to accelerate change and bring health to a diverse population of families.

MULTI-FAMILY GROUP THERAPY
WITH SEXUALLY ABUSIVE YOUTH

Treatment of youthful sex offenders, often referred to as sexual offense-specific treatment, is a challenging endeavor due to the multi-problem profile of both youth and families, trans-generational patterns of abuse, frequent presence of denial, and the historically lengthy treatment process. Youth-oriented goals for this intensive treatment process include improving community safety, improving supervision of high-risk youth, assessing and reducing risk of recidivism, profiling offense patterns, and teaching offenders to improve self-control and decision-making skills.

For all treatment bound youth, effective family and/or caregiver participation is both necessary and critical to the execution of treatment plan objectives (for further support, see Zankman & Bonomo, this issue). The emotionally balanced, informed, and committed parent can provide important leadership within the treatment team and persuade non-compliant youth to break through denial and make strides in accountability and responsibility. Positive family participation can also model empathic regard for others and perseverance in the face of adversity. Additionally, it is the families of high-risk youth who will assume the full spectrum of supervision responsibilities once the treatment team eventually transitions out of involvement in the case. Typical family treatment goals include gaining a clearer understanding of not only what happened during the offense (disclosure), but how and why it happened (motivation and planning), and working to prevent continued abusive behavior (relapse prevention).

As families are often court-ordered to participate in sexual offense-specific treatment and known to bring with them distrust for the court and social service systems, influencing positive participation and building trust can be a challenge. The traditional family interventions for this population–individual family therapy sessions and psychoeducational groups for parents–have met important treatment needs but struggle to help families overcome shame and isolation, receive validation for their role as a parent in the throws of a major life disruption, and create the context for corrective social experiences.

While several authors have written about the goals of family therapy with sexually abusive youth, the dynamics present in incestuous families, and the proposed curriculum for psychoeducational family and parent groups, direction on the actual facilitation of the MFGT intervention has not been made available. The clinical team preparing to facilitate MFGT with youthful offenders and their families will face several unique challenges not present in other therapeutic groups.

Managing a very large group. With increased group size, especially as the number of participants approaches 50 or more, comes the challenge of managing more complex group process, heightened intensity, and responsibility for meeting the clinical needs of diverse individuals. Due to its size alone, this group is at risk of getting out of control and lacking safety and productivity.

Managing and tracking three distinct levels of clinical process: Individual members, family systems, and the larger group meta-process. The facilitating clinicians face the unique challenge of monitoring and integrating these three distinct levels of clinical process into a smooth flowing format that is clinically relevant and beneficial to the audience.

Tracking and intervening in multi-generational processes. Present within a single-family system might be three distinct generations of participants and even an adjunct caregiver such as a foster parent. Involving these individuals and speaking to their unique relationship to one another as well as the youthful offender requires a higher level of clinical awareness and expertise.

Talking with a diverse audience about sex. Facilitating a large, heterogeneous, and trans-generational group discussion about sex and sexual offending can feel daunting and intimidating. The effective facilitator will capture a language and pace that is receptive to such a diverse audience.

Managing the dynamics within a multi-therapist team. Coordinating the efforts of multiple therapists within an emotionally intense and often chaotic setting requires insightful teamwork, planning, and integrated interventions.

ESTABLISHING THE GROUP

What follows is a template for establishing MFGT for sexually abusive youth and their families in either an outpatient or residential setting. This article does not intend to provide detailed instruction on how to conduct general sexual offense-specific family therapy per se, but how to bring the MFGT component to a practice already versed in the intricacies of work with sexually abusive youth and their families.

Size and Space Requirements

MFGT is most productive with an audience of 10-15 families. Smaller numbers set the stage for stagnation and a vacuum of family texture, stories, and shared experience. Conversely, when the group is too large, it becomes difficult to engage each individual in a quality manner and allow space for their stories to be told. As the group size approaches 45 or more members, those who seek refuge in silence are also more successful at remaining in hiding.

It goes without saying that a comfortable, spacious, and well-lit room helps to set the tone for a successful group. Large gatherings of families require space and privacy. It is critical that each participant have a chair to sit in and that these chairs be arranged in a circle or rounded rectangle whereby each participants can make eye contact with the entire group. A double-circle or two concentric circles is inappropriate for this group, as it prevents eye-to-eye contact and sets the stage for avoidant back row participants. It is not advisable that tables be placed in the middle of the circle, though this may be unavoidable given room configurations and size restrictions. Availability of several large dry erase or black boards is also recommended.

It may be useful to have several side tables outside of the group circle for placement of nametags, food, or beverages. Regarding food and beverages, it has been observed that a small offering of food and possibly coffee puts people at ease and provides a bit of nourishment during stressful social discourse. Families may also be willing to put in place a rotating "potluck" schedule whereby they take turns bringing food to the group. Ideally, the families themselves will take charge of the food schedule. It can be interesting to see who takes charge of organizing the group's energy around a snack schedule, who forgets to bring their contribution, and who puts their heart into feeding the "family" of participants. In residential treatment settings, families can be invited to arrive an hour prior to group to participate in a picnic or barbecue and accelerate the process of getting comfortable with one another.

Intake and Participant Selection

It is important that youth and families joining MFGT are participants in the same treatment program with a unifying treatment curriculum, mission, and philosophy. Any effort to pool families from several local but independent programs into a collective Multi-Family Group event is discouraged due to the absence of this common philosophical thread and the difficulty establishing seamless communication between facilitators and the frontline clinicians.

As new families enter an outpatient sexual offense-specific treatment program, it is suggested that they undergo at least a 1-month period of orientation to treatment language, goals, process, and philosophy prior to joining MFGT. It is the youth's individual therapist or family therapist, often one in the same, who assumes the task of orienting families and ultimately referring them to MFGT. In residential treatment settings, given the importance of building homogeneous milieu goals and process, it is generally understood that all families will join MFGT.

Family factors which might preclude MFGT participation include: (a) extremely rigid and closed family systems with extremely reactive and hostile responses to challenge, (b) parents who present with clinically narcissistic or borderline features that disrupt the group process and distract from others' needs being met, (c) active substance abusing systems, (d) criminalistic or antisocial family systems, (e) parents under suspicion of sexual offending, (f) parents in full denial regarding their child's offending behaviors, and (g) those who present as overtly disengaged or prone to sabotaging treatment efforts. The presence of antisocial beliefs, while not a complete rule-out for family participation, is certainly a flag for closer scrutiny.

Increasingly, 8- through 11-year-olds are being admitted into outpatient sexual offense-specific treatment programs, and as their age may be similar to that of peer victims, it is not advised that they join a large heterogeneous multi-family group. Surprisingly, it has not been especially problematic mixing sexually abusive male and female teens.

Adult or late teenaged siblings of offending youth may participate in the group, so long as they are not suspected as having their own perpetrator profile. Younger siblings who are secondary, but not primary victims of the abuse, are considered inappropriate for participation due to the group's sexually provocative content and intensity. Sibling therapy, however, is valid and necessary in the course of each family's treatment, and is conducted in private family sessions outside of the MFGT model.

Grandparents, aunts, uncles, and other adult-aged extended family members who serve a supervisory role are also welcomed, once again, so long as they are not contributors to trans-generation patterns of abuse. Their presence provides a powerful opportunity to both increase the quality of adult supervisors surrounding a youth and add fuel to efforts to decrease family denial and minimization. Foster parents or other primary caregivers are also welcomed and viewed as easy to integrate into the group's agenda. For youth who attend group with both parents and an adjunct caregiver such as a foster parent, some coordination of purpose is necessary to ensure they are not pitted against one another by manipulative or provocative youth.

Special Populations to Consider

Parents and caregivers who themselves are survivors of abuse can struggle in this group format as they are more susceptible to becoming either emotionally reactive or emotionally blunted amidst the provocative dialogue. It is important to identify these individuals early on and consider whether they are capable of weathering the group dynamics and benefiting from participation. It is not unusual at this juncture to refer untreated survivors of abuse or trauma out for their own adjunct course of individual therapy.

The inclusion of divorced or separated parents presents a different sort of challenge. If their relationship is adversarial, the group is likely to only exacerbate tensions, with the end result being a further split in the quality of supervision and a child who may use this opportunity to further his or her manipulative ends. In situations of insurmountable conflict, a schedule of rotating participation should be proposed, though this is clearly not ideal.

A third population likely to challenge group facilitators is lower IQ or special needs youth and/or parents. It has been our experience that this subgroup is quickly lost in the fray of heated conversation and raw emotional exchange.

Individuals with an IQ below 70 are best served in private family therapy sessions with a curriculum and pace that best matches their cognitive abilities.

Finally, youth engaged in treatment for hands-off offenses such as frottage, exhibitionism, or voyeurism, or youth charged for lower lever offenses with same aged peers are best not mixed with youth in treatment for multiple hands-on offenses against younger children. The differing offense profiles create an absence of common ground and a barrier to inter-family relationship building as families compare notes on their children's offenses and legal predicaments.

Group Length and Time

A group with an open door to new participants and an ongoing versus time-limited format is recommended and considered most conducive to creating a dynamic, learning-intensive, process-rich experience for participants. Time-limited groups risk becoming heavy on psychoeducational curriculum with an over-structured content and calendar and a tendency for participants to "watch the clock" and not fully commit themselves to the group process. Newly admitted participants add life to the group, and take their place in the family-to-family teaching and transfer of wisdom so central to the group's mission. Should one be limited to an 8- or 12-week window of group activity, the arrangement can still be beneficial to participants so long as the curriculum and expectations are within reason.

Regarding the frequency of MFGT meetings, a format that has proven useful reserves the first week of the month for an "adults only" parents' group, with the second and third weeks of the month set aside for MFGT, and the forth week left unscheduled and available for private family sessions as needed. An ideal group length is 90 minutes with participants gathering at 6:00 p.m.

Attendance Requirements

Families who begin to develop a pattern of poor attendance to the group are likely to fall behind on group process and learning and ultimately limit the growth of their peers. Since the activities of a comprehensive sexual offense-specific treatment program are time consuming, one should not necessarily conclude that attendance shortfalls are due to family oppositionality or avoidance. Such families should be timed-out of group participation and referred back to either their multi-disciplinary team or individual family therapist to generate solutions to the attendance problem. It may also be possible to invite such families to bring this attendance issue to the group and enlist the support and feedback of peers who have struggled with similar scheduling and time management issues.

Funding Considerations

In a climate of state, city, and county cutbacks to social service and probation budgets, adjunct therapies are less likely to be approved for funding. Financially strapped parents who are already assuming court costs and the expense of weekly individual and group therapy for their offending teen, are also poor candidates for footing the MFGT bill. Insurance companies have never covered the cost of court-ordered treatment protocols. Thus, treatment providers who value and support the utility of the MFGT intervention may have to resolve themselves to providing the intervention free of charge and in exchange for accelerated treatment progress.

GROUP CONTENT

Group Confidentiality

Given the very personal nature of sexual offense-specific treatment and the need to quickly establish safety parameters, especially with a mix of multiple families, it is advisable to have group members sign a confidentiality disclosure form specific to the group. Youth are especially prone to break confidentiality by reporting vignettes from MFGT to members of their adolescent psychotherapy group not engaged in the MFGT intervention.

Group Goals

Group goals provide the compass that guides group content, process, and facilitation. MFGT for sexually abusive youth was born out of the realization that the families of youth in treatment were voicing significant shame, experiencing isolation, and searching for validation in their role of a struggling parent. Thus, one initial goal is to provide families with a vehicle for increased competence and holistic well-being, as well as an "emotional anchor" to see them through the lengthy treatment process. Parents who are welcomed, cared for, and understood from the onset are more likely to be emotionally available to their children, and the children, likewise, are better positioned to endure the rigors of intensive treatment. As briefly reviewed earlier, there are a myriad of goals for MFGT, consisting of the following overlapping youth, family, and sexual offense-specific treatment goals.

Improving community safety. Community safety is the group's overriding first priority, with individual wants coming second. Although initially difficult for families to understand, the community is the group's first client. Determining a youth's community privileges, establishing visitation with parents or siblings, and monitoring school or employment functioning are all examples of the difficult treatment decisions inherent in balancing community safety with individual requests. The MFGT format is an excellent arena for families to compare their changed lifestyle with those of peers and hopefully come to terms with the priority of community safety. Community safety is also enhanced through the group's constant emphasis on peer feedback and accountability for daily decisions and behaviors.

Improving supervision of high-risk youth. The more eyes available to focus on a client's thoughts, feelings, and behaviors, the better the supervision and the more effective the overall treatment plan. MFGT provides such a context, as all families bond and become each other's support system. Weekly check-ins provide a powerful open forum for reviewing behavioral lapses, with MFGT-centered accountability proving to be far more powerful than the leverage available through a traditional peer milieu or lone clinician authoritarian influence. MFGT also provides caregivers with shocking reminders to maintain a position of "healthy suspicion" with high-risk youth who have a proven capacity for deception and dishonesty.

Disclosure and understanding motivation for the abuse. This curriculum module is central to sexual offense-specific treatment and a critical piece of family learning. Fundamental to safety is the need to understand how the abuse occurred. Offense patterns cannot remain a mystery; secrecy and deception must be replaced by honesty and accountability. As families cycle through this discovery process, MFGT is an ideal forum for sharing insights, deepening awareness, and shedding light upon each other's blind spots.

Teaching offenders to delay gratification, improve decision-making skills, and interrupt their cycle of abuse. While these goals are commonplace in the treatment of sexually abusive youth, MFGT once again provides the learning laboratory and expanded database of family experiences that accelerates learning and holds youth more accountable for their actions.

Developing empathy. While a formal definition of empathy is still up for debate, and measuring this construct has proven to be difficult, it is generally agreed that sexual offense-specific treatment strives to increase a young person's ability to experience and respect the feelings of others, particularly victims, and to use this knowledge as a deterrent to future abusive behavior. In MFGT, frequent opportunities exist for youth to experience in a live and very direct manner, both the positive and negative ways in which they have impacted others. Helping sexually abusive youth to "stand in another's shoes" and appreciate the trauma experienced by secondary and tertiary victims, as well as their primary victim(s), is at the heart of treatment goals. MFGT is unique in that participating youth are positioned to not only develop empathy for their family members, but to absorb powerful emotional moments as empathy is modeled by peers.

Establish a supportive and psychologically safe environment that facilitates diverse views, conversation, and learning. This is a central principle of all group facilitation and a true necessity if parents are to stay put and work through the intense shock, denial, grief, and shame so prevalent in the early stages of treatment. MFGT provides an experiential opportunity to state strong opinions, be humbled by the wisdom of peers, model and exercise respect, and step out of counterproductive power and control dynamics.

Instill values of hope and hard work. Without a vision of hope and access to proactive interventions that direct energy in a positive direction, families are at risk to become passive, emotionally frozen, or helpless in the face of efforts to understand the problem of sexual abuse. MFGT creates a unique forum where success stories, emotional healing, and proof of treatment effectiveness provide evidence that hard work and determination are worth the investment for both parents and youth.

Usual internal and external barriers include denial of offenses, minimization of harm, emotional disconnect from the victim's experience, defensiveness, poor attendance, transportation problems, enabling behaviors, family chaos and disorganization, misdirected hostility, secrets, covert agendas, distrust of "the system," and undiagnosed mental health issues. MFGT participants are constantly uncovering and confronting such barriers, with more seasoned parents helping newer families with this process. Compared to traditional family therapy with a single family and therapist, MFGT provides a milieu where it is considerably more difficult to hide counter-treatment attitudes or practices.

Provide a laboratory for social, emotional, and parent skill building. Assertiveness, anger management, social skills, self-observation, decision making, self-regulation, parenting competency, boundary identification and management, and communication of needs/wants are the skill sets commonly addressed and built upon during group discourse. Since the MFGT laboratory is rich in information, educational social interactions, and diversity, group members absorb information quickly and position themselves to pass this learning on to subsequent families.

Support and engender pro-social change. MFGT, in its best and most persuasive form, instills in participants a desire to change, the momentum to transform initial tentative signs of change (first order) into more permanent lifestyle changes (second order), and the support to sustain transformation of attitude and behavior.

Creating the Group Curriculum

Establishing a curriculum for MFGT is considerably easier than managing the ensuing group process. Several authors have written about recommended content areas for MFGT (Gil, 1993b; Thomas, 1991) and many of their ideas have been incorporated into the curriculum that will follow. Clinicians who struggle with the task of assembling a sexual offense-specific curriculum for the group are probably ill prepared to manage a room full of emotionally charged families. Regardless, it is critical that the language and content of the MFGT curriculum match the materials being presented in individual family therapy sessions, as well as in the youth's individual and group therapy sessions. It is also useful to present parents with a "Welcome Guide to Treatment" or brief booklet outlining stages of treatment, philosophical approaches, program rules, and prominent treatment language or concepts. This welcome guide can become a unifying document that creates the perception of all participants being "on the same page" with regard to treatment goals and objectives.

Group Rituals

Each group session should begin with a ritual of three successive events.

Facilitators welcome participants to the group. Facilitators review old business related to scheduling and present updates on the resolution of client crises from prior meetings. New group members are invited to introduce themselves, presenting as little or as much personal background as they wish. When new members are present, all youth are asked to state their name, age, number of months in the program, and a general summary of their offending behaviors. It can be instructive to watch for group members who use this brief personal introduction as a springboard for launching into a longwinded monologue. Facilitators must encourage group members to be brief with their introduction and move on to the next participant. For the newly formed group it will be important that facilitators take time to explain to families the purpose of the group, reviewing goals and the principles of support along with community safety.

Review of group rules. Group rules should be referenced at the beginning of each group session, particularly when the group is in early developmental stages, when a new member is being introduced, or when the group members are creating an excess of chaos or disruption. It is valuable to post them on the wall of the meeting room. As it becomes necessary to add new rules, group time is set aside specifically for this purpose. For the newly formed multi-family group, the establishment of group rules proves to be an important exercise in building group culture and commitment. The process begins by asking a youth or parent volunteer to begin fielding and listing rules generated by the group. This exercise sets the stage for interesting moral and ethical debates amongst group members and an exploration of treatment needs and values. As new members are integrated into the group, an existing member can be called upon to bring them up to speed on the rule definitions and purpose.

Introducing topics. Group facilitators are now positioned to give an overview of the curriculum to be taught that evening or have the option of fielding topics from group participants. Following presentation of a particular topic area, it is the task of facilitators to direct participants towards a meaningful, personal, and emotionally rich discussion.

Group Curriculum

Should the group facilitators decide to present a topic area, they may choose either a specific curriculum module or experiential exercise. Curriculum modules are best for the less evolved group, with group exercises serving the purpose of putting knowledge into action and increasing the contact between participants. Recommended curriculum and exercises follow, not necessarily in the order of presentation.

Introduction to sexual offense-specific (SOS) treatment. Describe how this treatment modality differs from traditional psychotherapy and why it requires such intensive family participation. Some particular differences include: (a) the dynamic of being court-ordered into treatment versus voluntary participation, (b) involvement in a therapeutic relationship marked by less trust and increased therapist control, (c) therapist-driven goal setting versus client initiated seeking of help, personal growth, or relief, (d) explicitly stated values regarding sexual abuse versus a non-judgmental stance, (e) the role and necessity of setting limits, (f) limited confidentiality, (g) the unreliable nature of trusting the client, (h) the tendency of clients to be manipulative and please their therapist versus being sincerely invested in change, and (i) the use of confrontation (Salter, 1988).

Next, present national recidivism rates with and without treatment. Outline the treatment process including anticipated length of treatment, treatment goals, program philosophy, and treatment language. Discuss why full sexual history disclosure and polygraph are central to the treatment process.

The family's role in treatment. Review typical family reactions to having a child charged with a sexual offense. Clarify the family's role in the treatment team and how they can best support the child during the treatment process. For those families with both a youthful offender in treatment and a victimized sibling at home, it will be important to appreciate this parenting challenge. Encourage an open sharing of experiences from both new admitted and more committed and treatment savvy parents. Parents are encouraged to take responsibility for their role in setting the stage for abuse to occur, but not for the abusive acts themselves.

Understanding and accepting this distinction is critical to parents who may arrive in treatment paralyzed by guilt, carrying their child's responsibility for the abusive acts, but at the same time needing to take a hard and fast look at family of origin factors that precipitated or kindled the abuse. Freeing parents of guilt and allowing responsibility to land squarely in the hands of offending youth can be an especially healing and empowering experience for traumatized parents.

Informed supervision and safety planning. Parents are instructed on how to responsibly supervise youth at home, school, and other community settings and how to safety plan effectively. Parents are encouraged to adopt a perspective of "healthy suspicion" in the day-to-day scrutiny of their child. The components of a thoroughly written safety plan are reviewed. Families are introduced to the model of Containment Treatment (Tedeschi & Smith, 1999) that popularizes the notion that one best manages high risk youth, especially sexually abusive ones, by surrounding them by a closely knit, highly communicative, an interdependent group of responsible adult supervisors.

Principles of Containment Treatment include: (a) the importance of balancing authority and nurturance, (b) the notion that it is inhumane to allow offenders to continue to damage themselves or others, (c) valuing a healthy level of anxiety for offenders over the treatment process, (d) recognition that sexually abusive youth will not readily seek accountability, (e) acceptance of the need to be intrusive with high risk youth as an act of caring, (f) identification of probation and treatment as a community privilege for offenders, and (g) use of daily safety planning (planful forethought) as one accepts that troubled youth will encounter high risk situations on a daily basis.

Introduction to cognitive tool cards. "Tool Cards" (Smith, 1999) are a set of 40 visual flash cards that help youth, especially those presenting with ADHD, learning disabilities, cognitive deficits, or lower intelligence, to learn and internalize treatment concepts central to success in sexual offense-specific treatment. Each card contains a treatment concept and accompanying picture to portray that concept. Tool Cards represent concepts such as Stop and Think, Think About the Consequences, Share Your Secrets, Share the Power, and Ask My Body How It Feels.

Family dynamics and issues associated with abuse. The content for this module is drawn from Jerry Thomas' (1991) list of classic family treatment issues and Eliana Gil's (1993a) outline of the dynamics present in incestuous families. Thomas' issues include denial, minimization and projection of blame, lack of empathy, abuse of power, powerlessness, empowerment, anger management, inter-generational abuse, family secrets, blurred role boundaries, confusion about healthy human sexuality, and divided loyalty (in the cases of incest). Gil's work focuses on the difference between overt and covert abuse, incest transmission patterns, and four distinct family profiles: (a) sexualized families, (b) sociopathic families, (c) repressed families, and (d) emotionally-barren families. Inevitably, this module challenges each family to take an objective, non-defensive look at their role in setting the stage for their child to develop abusive behavior patterns.

Defining sexual abuse and abusive interactions. Sexual abuse involves sexual contact with: (a) lack of consent, (b) lack of equality, and/or (c) use of coercion (Ryan & Lane, 1997). Consent includes each participant understanding the proposed sexual behavior, an awareness of its potential consequences, the ability to refuse without repercussion, and the ability to give permission (i.e., sobriety and intact mental status). Equality refers to the type of relationship between individuals (i.e., being in a position of trust), intellectual level, size, and age. The act of coercion can include grooming behaviors, pressure, bribery, threats, intimidation, and force. It is also necessary to define all types of abuse, including physical, emotional, verbal, and psychological.

Why youth sexually offend. Here the practitioners can present Finkelhor's (1984) model of Four Preconditions of Sexual Abuse: (a) motivation, (b) internal barriers, (c) external barriers, and (d) victim resistance. Common motivations for the abuse can be reviewed, including: (a) power and control, (b) revenge, (c) sexual gratification, (d) intimacy seeking, (e) curiosity, (f) peer pressure, or (g) an effort to work through one's own abuse. Next, describe the heterogeneous nature of sexually abusive youth (i.e., different family histories, family constellations, socioeconomic status, ethnic backgrounds, reasons for offending, etc.) and present several typologies for sexually abusive youth including the model recently published by Hunter, Figueredo, Malamuth, and Becker (2003) (for in-depth descriptions of typologies for sexually abusive youth, see Rasmussen, this issue).

Defining healthy sexual development in children and adolescents. Include a description of the difference between a sexualized child and sexually abusive youth. Define the term "culpability" and explain how it may play a role in determining "victim" versus "victimizer" status. Describe the continuum of normal and "red flag" sexual behaviors in both children and adolescents (Ryan & Lane, 1997; for an in-depth discussion of differentiating sexual behaviors in children and adolescents, see Rasmussen, this issue).

Defining deviant sexual behaviors. Define "deviant sexual behaviors" as those occurring outside of cultural norms and laws. List the more common categories of deviant sexual preference, being sure to differentiate between "hands on" and "hand off" offenses. It will be important to clarify that homosexuality does not fit the definition of deviant. Within this module it may prove tempting to branch into a discussion of risk assessment-static and dynamic variables shown to be associated with an increased risk of reoffense. However, it may be best to refrain from this discussion, as parents have a tendency to keep a running list of variables their child does not present with, and consciously or sub-consciously minimize their level of risk.

Introduction of the cycle of abuse. The Cycle of Abuse (Ryan & Lane, 1995) inevitably becomes a central concept in the early stages of the treatment process. Its visual and intellectually tangible nature helps parents to face the reality that their child's abusive behavior did not "just happen," but was preceded by clear attitudinal and behavioral change. Additionally, the Cycle of Abuse model offers parents an opportunity to proactively identify precipitants to reoffense and intervene before a youth resorts to reoffense or other abusive behavior (for further discussion of the cycle of abuse, see Zankman & Bonomo, this issue).

How victims are impacted by sexual abuse. Group participants are generally unaware of the extent to which victims are impacted by sexual abuse, both in the short-term and longitudinally. This module is an eye-opener for parents and youth who might minimize the effects of a young person's abusive behaviors. Primary victims (immediate or central) are differentiated from secondary victims (parents and non-abused siblings). This discussion becomes emotional as parents are finally able to demonstrate to offending youth how they too were impacted by the sexual offense.

The use of a guest speaker is suggested during this learning module–a survivor of sexual abuse who has successfully completed his/her own treatment and wishes to speak on the impact of abuse. An adult survivor is suggested, as youth may be simply too vulnerable amongst a group of other juveniles. Preparing the guest speaker for this event is critical, and having their own therapist present with them is often helpful. A therapist treating victims in the community can also serve as a powerful guest in lieu of a direct client survivor.

The victim clarification process and criteria for family reunification. The term "victim clarification process" refers to a series of carefully planned and orchestrated therapeutic meetings between offender, survivor (victim), supporting therapists, and sometimes parents of the survivor, during which the perpetrator takes full responsibility for their abusive behaviors and answers any of the survivor's questions. The clarification process should primarily benefit the survivor, though the perpetrator should experientially evidence improved empathy skills, understanding the harm and impact they have done, with healthy levels of guilt and remorse that serve as motivators to prevent relapse. Give a general description of this process, criteria for beginning the clarification process, and criteria for family reunification (i.e., the offender's return to home). Encourage participants to identify victims by first name and not refer to them as "John's victim."

Introduction to the polygraph exam. Describe what the polygraph measures and why is it is an important treatment tool in the pursuit of full sexual history disclosure and ongoing monitoring of behaviors. Since polygraph results are not admissible as evidence in court, this can be a challenging and potentially heated discussion. As it is less usual for youth to be administered the Penile Plethysmograph (a measure of sexual arousal) or Abel Assessment (a measure of sexual interest), these discussions are best reserved for individual family sessions.

Introduction to thinking errors. Present group members with a list of thinking errors–also known as cognitive distortions–and describe each in detail, and have them identify those most commonly used by family members. At a minimum, group members should be able to identify denial, justifications, minimization, negative anticipation, "should" statements, externalization of blame, mind reading, black-and-white thinking, filtering, and being right. Once participants grasp the concept of a thinking error, move on to outlining the causal progression of thoughts to feelings to behaviors. Faulty thinking puts one at risk for distorted emotions and compromising behavior, which is thus the incentive to examine the thinking patterns of sexually abusive youth. It is useful to highlight the protective role that thinking errors, particularly denial, play in helping a young person cope with the emotional fallout resulting from their destructive behavior.

Inviting outside speakers. Sometimes the presence of a polygraph examiner, caseworker, court appointed Guardian Ad Litem (GAL), probation officer, police officer, therapist who specializes in the treatment of victims, or victim's advocate from the District Attorney's office can enlighten the group with new information or offer new perspectives that help treatment participants to see their role in the expanded treatment community.

Experiential Exercises

The family genogram exercise. Each family is given a large sheet of paper and an assortment of colored markers. Following a brief demonstration of family genogram construction, they are asked to take 20 minutes to complete a three-generation genogram highlighting: victims of abuse, perpetrators of abuse, emotional cut-offs, individuals who have engaged in criminal behavior, individuals with mental health issues, individuals with substance abuse issues, and individuals they view as functioning well. Each family is then given the opportunity to present their extended family to the group with the goal of identifying "patterns" of behavior or historical links to their child's abusive behavior. This exercise accelerates the process of getting acquainted and is a test of family honesty and willingness to be vulnerable amongst peers. At best, the exercise forces families to unveil secrets, view the big picture of family dysfunction, and remove barriers to becoming emotionally connected with other group members. Inevitably, youth learn something new about their family of origin.

The expert panel. Choose three or four parents or youth who are veterans of the group, seat them together, and announce that they will comprise a panel of "experts" made available to answer questions for the group. Solicit questions from other parents and kids regarding the application of treatment concepts, insights/learning from the treatment process, and "advice" regarding specific treatment issues. The exercise takes on an intriguing dynamic when individuals harboring counter-treatment attitudes or behaviors are either placed on the panel by strategic facilitators or naively self-select themselves as "experts." The group is then positioned to discover these individuals, confront their denial or superficiality, and then offer direction and supportive feedback.

Safety lineup. During this exercise, youth are asked to arrange themselves (seated or standing) in order from "least safe" to "most safe." Allow youth to struggle with the task of deciding "who stands where" in the lineup. Do the senior youth automatically place themselves at the top of the safety continuum or does the peer group choose to place the most intimidating individuals at the top? Once arranged, ask youth, parents, and then group facilitators to comment on where youth have chosen to place themselves in the lineup. Does the placement of each youth fit with their presentation or skill level?

Safety planning scenarios. Create about six written scenarios describing high-risk youth in a variety of community activities. Divide the group into six subgroups and rotate the written scenarios through the subgroups allowing each group approximately 5 minutes to identify safety concerns. Following a review of the scenarios, facilitate a discussion of group member concerns and recommended safety plans for each scenario.

Learning review. Go around the circle of participants and have each group member state one important piece of learning they have absorbed over the course of MFGT. Have a group member write these points on a large sheet of paper to be archived for reflection in later group meetings. Facilitate a discussion of these items, allowing participants to teach the information to one another.

Lapse review. Separate the youth and adults into different corners of the room and have them generate a master list of possible youth and parent lapses over the course of treatment. The adult list typically includes not providing adequate supervision, modeling hostile or abusive interactions to children, keeping family secrets, denying the severity of family problems, and rescuing youth from accountability for their behaviors. Youth lapses include viewing pornography, faking cooperation, not putting effort into treatment assignments, fantasizing about victims, using drugs or alcohol, sexually objectifying others, and lying about time spent with antisocial peers. One the lists are assembled, encourage group members to present their findings and facilitate a discussion of these items, highlighting the difference between youth and adult perceptions of risk.

Focus on a specific youth or family issue. It is often useful to capitalize on a current youth, family, or parent crisis and utilize this as a "teaching moment" for the entire group. For example, a youth who has failed his third polygraph and continues to deny the presence of additional victims, may be asked to "present his case" to the group and make himself open to group feedback.

The learning book. The Learning Book is an open and anonymous journal for use by any member of the group to log important learning, insights, or opinion. The book circulates freely throughout the group and group members are encouraged to bring the journal home but return it for the subsequent group.

The silent facilitators. An interesting way to encourage group participation and leadership is to render the facilitators unable to speak. Born out of a group training curriculum in which facilitators remain silent for an entire 3-day training seminar, this exercise consists of the facilitators silently arriving to group and presenting the group with the following note: "We are pleased to be here tonight at your group and will not be speaking for the next 60 minutes. It is your task to take your broad base of knowledge and develop a meaningful use of this time. We are here to assist you in the event of an emergency." Clearly, this exercise is most appropriate for advanced groups.

Before and after paintings. In this exercise individual families are asked to collaborate on two separate paintings symbolizing the family's experience before and after involvement in treatment. Leaving instructions as unstructured as possible is advised as it pushes family members to converse and settle upon their particular interpretation of the task. Paintings can then be shared with the greater group. This exercise is useful in that paintings succeed in expressing emotions that participants struggle to verbalize.

The transition book. The Transition Book, much like the Learning Book, is an open journal for use by group members. The Transition Book, however, may only be written in by group members or facilitators who are successfully transitioning out of the group. This becomes an interesting account of individual perceptions just prior to leaving the group and can serve as document of inspiration for families just beginning the treatment process.

Experiential outdoor activities. Relocating the group outdoors for a portion of MFGT can provide new data about family functioning and inject new energy into the four walls of group routine. Residential treatment settings are most amenable to outdoor activities, as they are more likely to support expanses of grass or open space. Trust building and teamwork generating exercises have proven useful with this population.

FACILITATING THE GROUP

The skilled facilitator of MFGT for sexually abusive youth and their families will present with a strong background in family systems theory (Minuchin, 1974), sexual offense-specific treatment (Gil, 1993b; Ryan & Lane, 1997), and general group theory (Prochaska, Diclemente, & Norcross, 1992; Yalom, 1985). Additional positive qualities include a dynamic personality, reserves of energy, a sense of humor, a difficult-to-rattle demeanor, stress tolerance, the ability to generate meaningful clinical process out of disjointed social discourse, the ability to persevere despite evidence failure, and a genuine fondness for the families and youthful offenders. Thomas (1997) likens the experience to conducting an orchestra. At times it can feel like navigating a minefield or refereeing a back alley brawl. This clinical arena, more than most others, seems to attract the unexpected.

There are a dozen principles of group facilitation that if kept in focus, will aid in the successful management of MFGT. And while this list of general "do's and don'ts" is applicable to the facilitation of most any therapeutic group, this select list has its roots in the unique culture of sexual offense-specific family treatment.

General Principles

Everyone participates. Though certainly not unique to the MFGT format, this item is critical, as family secrets, counter-treatment attitudes, and thinking errors often reside in the withdrawn or constricted individual. Reclusive individuals should be addressed directly and drawn out of hiding, even at the price of hostility or annoyance. Primary counselors in the residential milieu, mental health workers, and the occasional visiting treatment team professional are also not allowed to join in as silent observers. This distracts from feelings of solidarity, hatches feelings of distrust, and creates an "us versus them" dynamic. All professional staff are informed up front, "If you choose to visit the kitchen, you must both cook and accept the risk of getting your hands dirty." Likewise, should group facilitators get themselves into trouble as a result of a callous or insensitive comment or other miscue, they, like all group members, must face the group and get to the business of repairing damage.

Facilitators model pro-social, assertive, and accountable behaviors with direct, accurate communication. Facilitator modeling takes place continuously throughout the group as an important vehicle for educating group members.

Amplify family strengths and evidence of positive change. The families of sexually abusive youth will have already endured an abundance of mixed emotions and stress by the time they arrive in the treatment arena. It will be important to appreciate their strengths and resiliency and not overlook opportunities to comment out loud about their assets. The experience of attitudinal or behavioral change is less likely to be integrated (and thereby solidified) if the client is uninformed of another's positive perceptions of them.

Maximize intensity and emotional impact. Even positive change can be difficult to embrace. In order to reduce a young person's risk of sexual reoffense, significant emotional, cognitive, and behavioral change will be necessary in both youth and parents. Group intensity and facilitator precision are the driving force behind efforts to break old habits and construct new healthier ones. The "bend but don't break" metaphor is useful here. Intensity is also a useful tool for maintaining participant attention in a population that may wish to forget the grave circumstances of their legal mandates or family turmoil.

Balance content and process. This is another basic tenet of all group facilitation. Achieving this balance is especially challenging in a large group setting where meeting the needs of all participants will not be possible at each bend in the road. At times it will be necessary to shut down or redirect group process that seems to be benefiting just a few participants, in favor of topics that capture the interest of the group majority. Dozens of times each session, group facilitators must be prepared to navigate the leap between content learning and the examination of group process.

Infuse each interaction with treatment language and concepts. There is a treatment language germane to sexual offense-specific treatment that strives to educate, punctuate and prioritize safety, and describe high-risk behaviors. Terms such as abusive, accountability, safety plan, treatment tool, lapse, victimization, cycle, and sexual arousal become understood, practiced, and familiar concepts. As community safety is an outgrowth of "living the program," group participants must demonstrate the ability to "live the language" and have their behaviors match their words. The successful multi-family group has at its helm a team of facilitators able use accurate treatment language and weave topic continuity and purpose throughout successive groups. Caution needs to be taken, however, so as not to accept treatment jargon that is a manipulative effort to fake treatment compliance.

Prioritize family-to-family learning over therapist-to-family teaching. Knowing when to get out of the way is an important skill for facilitators of this group. When families begin to interact and exchange learning with one another, even if the discourse is heated, it is generally advisable for the clinical team to blend into the woodwork and allow families the experience of self-sufficiency. Accomplishing this feat may involve breaking eye contact with family members, thereby encouraging them to talk it through or navigate their way through difficult conversation. This family-to-family interface is critical to the evolution of a productive multi-family group.

Prioritize the creation of a safe place. This is yet another mainstay of group facilitation. Without an umbrella of safety, group members cannot begin to let go of prescribed roles, superficiality, defensiveness, and distrust of peers or authority figures. Possibly the best means of prioritizing a culture of group safety is to set firm limits on those individuals who repeatedly speak with hostility or criticism, externalize blame, or shut down the learning of others.

Alternate between focus on individual family issues and the group meta-process. This item is one of the more challenging tasks of group facilitation, though necessary to achieve dynamic conversation and examples to learn by. How much time does one allow a single family to occupy the spotlight of group process before returning focus to broader group experience or themes? Facilitators might reflect to themselves, "How beneficial is the content of this conversation as a teaching moment for the group?" Much like a ping-pong match, facilitators must track the dialogue as it bounces from focus on a single individual, to a particular family system, to a more global group issue, and back again to a different individual. No wonder group facilitation can be exhausting. The "gold mining" metaphor is fitting here–facilitators invest group time in the pursuit of a small vein of conversation, banking their dollar that it will lead to a fortune in learning and personal insight. It is also fitting that the more years one works the mines, the more efficient one gets at extracting the gold.

Interface with and don't lose sight of concurrent treatment modalities. MFGT is most often an adjunct to the more traditional modalities of adolescent individual and group therapy, as well as single family therapy sessions. MFGT facilitators have an obligation to stay connected to the other therapists on the treatment team and abreast of youth progress, family functioning, and the emotional texture experienced in those sessions. The opportunity for strategic collaboration is immense, but generally underutilized in the day-to-day flow of a busy outpatient or residential program.

Strive to create a sense of group ownership. An interesting paradigm shift in group functioning is evident as group members attach to the group's mission, find their place of belonging, and begin to demonstrate commitment to the group process. Signs of progress include group members tolerating confrontation with one another, parents finding a direct and assertive voice in addressing their children, group members not hesitating to make themselves vulnerable, and new families being welcomed and embraced by more senior families. Facilitator interventions that speed the development of ownership include consistently referencing the group as "your group," insistence that participants contribute feedback whenever the group is focused on a particular family's crisis, convincing parents throughout the ebb and flow of crisis and resolution that group is of value, and proactively pulling back when family-to-family process is self-generating and meaningful.

Managing the Facilitation Team

As if the facilitation of a dozen diverse families doesn't present enough of a challenge, organizing the actions and priorities of two to four clinicians comes with its own hazards. A sure way to lose the respect of the parent audience is to appear disorganized, disjointed, or in the worst of cases, in opposition to one another in facilitating MFGT. The ideal team works like a troupe of jugglers–one player is always positioned to catch the other's pins and there is flexibility as to who will perform that evening. Pre-planning and post-review are just the beginning. Nonverbal communication routines need to be highly developed and functional. For example, the chin thrust of one facilitator may direct a second facilitator to the covert whispering or tears of a parent beyond the first facilitator's vantage point. Or the eye contact and raised eyebrows of that same colleague may communicate a need to redirect conversation away from a repetitive monologue.

The simplest format is that of having one clinician assume the role of leader, with the remainder of the facilitation team taking a back seat and not initiating major shifts in conversation or group process. This arrangement is not advised however, as such rigid and prescribed structure resembles the traditional role rigidity present in many of the family systems, creating a parallel process that risks assigning facilitators to polarized roles of good/bad, active/passive, or helpful/hurtful. Facilitators should "play off" one another, passing the director's baton in a smooth, seamless fashion. Predictably, a male/female team provides the best clinical formula and vehicle for capturing transference reactions from the group. The inclusion of a male/female facilitation team also makes possible opportunities to model healthy, constructive, and direct communication between the sexes, a quality lacking in many of the family systems.

As a final note, it is most advantageous for facilitators to sit apart, spread evenly throughout the room, so as to maximize opportunities for data gathering and reduce feelings of intimidation that can be projected by a gathering of authority figures.

Pitfalls, Roadblocks, and Detours

Adequate insight into what can go wrong over the course of facilitating MFGT can be as valuable as guidelines for positive group facilitation. Knowing the terrain and pulse of one's neighborhood can be a lifesaver indeed. And for a large, emotionally charged group with a reputation for diverse opinions and shifting landscapes, structure and purpose can rapidly go astray. Not all clinical disasters however, uphold their reputation with the passage of time. Unproductive groups can offer lessons to all. However, efficient use of client time is certainly an ethical obligation for all clinicians, especially if the stakes are as high as the prevention of additional victims of sexual abuse. The following list provides a useful "cheat sheet" to provide guidance when group process is waning. In diagnosing a functional problem in MFGT, it can be useful for the facilitators to review the following questions:

1. Is this a problem that we have brought upon ourselves or is a group member doing this to us?
2. Who is most bothered by the identified shortfalls in the group functioning? Why them?
3. Are there ways in which this shortfall could provide beneficial learning for the group?
4. Are we prioritizing group goals, learning objectives, and honest engagement of participants?
5. Are we working harder than the parents and kids?
6. Are we talking out loud about observations and concerns?
7. Are we having fun tonight?

The following list of problems and potential remedies is by no means comprehensive, though most common over the course of the group.

Parents don't interact with one another and direct all dialogue through the facilitators. Break eye contact with participants who continue to direct conversation through the facilitators. This will increase their likelihood of conversing with peers. For questions routed through the facilitators, redirect the question to the group, "Who has some thoughts about this question?"

The group lacks energy or participants are bored. This can be an anxiety-provoking phenomenon for facilitators of such a large group. Consider whether participants are overwhelmed by the topic under discussion, communicating boredom with the content of the curriculum, communicating dislike or distrust of the facilitators, or communicating concern about safety parameters in the group.

The group facilitators feel bored or disinterested. Consider whether counter-transference is taking its toll on the team, facilitators have failed to inject novel content or energy into the group, facilitators feel as though they are being held hostage by a group member, or facilitators are at odds with one another and therefore lacking emotional commitment to the group process or mission.

Group members are playing it too safe, risking little, or steering clear of the experience of vulnerability. Wonder whether the group is just too young or un-evolved to venture into these tenuous areas, group members are not experiencing safety or commitment to the group agenda, or a leadership vacuum is present amongst participants. Typically, it is the modeling of an outspoken and confident parent that paves the way for other to disclose their fears, angst, or worries. Should this problem persist, it may be necessary to approach several parents prior to group and request that they undertake this leap forward in disclosure. Once the ice is broken, others are likely to follow suit.

The same group members do all the talking each week. State at the beginning of group, "I've been looking forward to this evening's group because I was certain that some of our quieter members would be ready to step forward and take charge." Consider whether talkative individuals are "rescuing" others from having to "get down to business." If the problem persists, approach the chatty individuals privately and request that they practice more "listening" next group or only speak if they have something new to disclose about themselves.

Group members demonstrate a pattern of complaining to and arguing with facilitators. Wonder whether the friction is a display of "power and control" behaviors typical of that parent subgroup, the antagonist is communicating dissatisfaction for the entire group, the complaining serves as a distraction from more painful treatment issues, or the participant is projecting onto the facilitators anger intended for other members of the treatment team.

Parents repeatedly speak for their child. This phenomenon is common in the early stages of treatment and not necessarily indicative of pathological enmeshment or rescuing. In general, parents respond well to being interrupted mid-sentence and asked to allow their child to find their own words.

Parents repeatedly rescue their child from accountability for his/her sexual offending. This behavior is typically more concerning than the preceding example, as it is likely to run parallel with deeper-seated denial, minimization, avoidance, and enabling. It will be important to point this observation out to the parent, if other group members don't take the initiative, and certainly report this concern to the remainder of the treatment team. The issue may need further scrutiny in individual family therapy sessions.

Youths are rude to their parents or other participants. Ideally, other participants will step in and label this disrespect of others, noting the parallel to the youth's offending patterns. There is no better arena for youths to receive swift feedback regarding their display of abusive or antisocial behavior.

Caregivers and/or youth establish a pattern of giving advice to others while not being open to new learning themselves. This problem can be difficult to identify, as the client can appear to be helpful, enthusiastic, interested in the welfare of others, and teeming with useful advice. However, as the past few sessions are reviewed, it is undeniable that their progress is lacking. One might wonder whether their over-involvement in the facilitation of peer problem solving is not a distraction away from their own intractable treatment issues.

Parent is repeatedly melodramatic. Is this behavior indicative of an emotionally destabilized individual, deeper-seated Axis II features, or attention-seeking behavior? Early on, it is worthwhile to flag parents with this profile, as their presentation creates a group spectacle that drains energy and stunts the participation of others.

A group member repeatedly monopolizes group time. Consider whether this is a particularly needy individual without other social outlets for dialogue, a self-centered individual who is pathologically unaware of his/her need to take center stage, or an anxious parent in need of constant reassurance. Check in with the other facilitators.

Parents collude or form unhealthy alliances. It is not uncommon for dysfunctional families to replicate relationship patterns consisting of poor boundaries, enmeshment, or collusion with other struggling parents. These counterproductive unions are generally not difficult to spot and are associated with controlling or putting down others, deficits in role flexibility, and a vacuum in recent insights or learning. This concern is best addressed with the families in question outside of the formal group process.

CONCLUSIONS

Multi-family group therapy (MFGT) has been utilized for years as a means of gaining clinical leverage with difficult to treat populations. It is not surprising that it has been adapted to address the complex and longitudinal treatment of sexually abusive youth and their families. The intervention brings with it several distinct advantages, has the potential to accelerate treatment progress, and has goals, objectives, and procedures that reinforce one another and support the mission of reducing recidivism. Facilitating the group can be both intimidating and extremely rewarding to the aspiring clinician, and should be considered an advanced therapeutic intervention requiring a sound background in family, group, and sexual offense-specific theory in addition to advanced supervision and expertise. The participating clinician must be comfortable with the most heated and dynamic clinical process and be available to engage emotionally with multi-problem, distressed, and disillusioned parents. The group, with its wide array of interventions, clinical interactions, and fast paced process, also makes for a unique training experience for interns and developing clinicians.

The group format persuades participants to "speak out loud" about sexual abuse and adopt an assertive, action-oriented demeanor. The group emulates community unity, diversity, and networking, and brings with it the potential for novel solutions, peaceful conflict resolution, compromise, and understanding. A circle of teaching emerges, whereby facilitators teach parents, parents share with one another, and parents in turn, impress the facilitators with their resilience and capacity to challenge and overcome fears. With persistence, patience, sound leadership, and learning, the group has the potential to produce parents with well-developed supervision skills, awareness of their role in the etiology of sexual abuse, an improved understanding of normal child sexual behavior, and the determination to make their community a safer place.

While MFGT is often considered an adjunct to the more familiar sexual offense-specific individual therapy and adolescent group formats, it deserves greater recognition as a centerpiece in efforts to create a committed culture of support, accountability, and safety. As such, the absence of a funding source for the group should not preclude its formation. For sexual offense-specific clinicians who through fate or choice have found themselves engaged to the battle to prevent sexual reoffense and a generation of new victims, ending the day in witness to the power of the MFGT intervention can elicit hopefulness and optimism.

REFERENCES

Falloon, I.R., Liberman, R.P., Lillie, F.J., & Vaughn, C.E. (1981). Family therapy of schizophrenics with high risk of relapse. *Family Process, 20* (2), 211-21.

Finkelhor, D. (1984). *Child sexual abuse: New theory & research.* New York: Free Press.

Fristad, M.A., Goldberg-Arnold, J.S., & Gavazzi, S.M. (2002). Multifamily psychoeducation groups (MFPG) for families of children with bipolar disorder. *Bipolar Disorder, 4*(4), 254-62.

Gil, E. (1993a). Family dynamics. In E. Gil, & T.C. Johnson (Eds.), *Sexualized children: Assessment and treatment of sexualized children and children who molest* (pp. 102-120). Rockville, MD: Launch Press.

Gil, E. (1993b). Family treatment. In E. Gil, & T.C. Johnson (Eds.), *Sexualized children: Assessment and treatment of sexualized children and children who molest* (pp. 276-302). Rockville, MD: Launch Press.

Honig, A., Hofman, A., Rozendaal, N., & Dingemans, P. (1997). Psycho-education in bipolar disorder: Effect on expressed emotion. *Psychiatry Research, 72*(1), 17-22.

Hunter, J.A., Figueredo, A.J., Malamuth, N.M., & Becker, J.V. (2003). Juvenile sex offenders: Towards the development of a typology. *Sexual Abuse, 15*(1), 27-48.

Leichter, E., & Schulman, G.L. (1968). Emerging phenomena in multi-family group treatment. *International Journal of Group Psychotherapy, 18*(1), 59-69.

Minuchin, S. (1974). *Families and family therapy.* Cambridge, MA: Harvard University Press.

Prochaska, J.O., Diclemente, C.C., & Norcross, J.C. (1992). In search of how people change: Applications to addictive behavior. *American Psychologist, 47*(9), 1102-1114.

Rasmussen, L.A. (2004). Differentiating youth who sexually abuse: Applying a multi-dimensional framework when assessing and treating subtypes. *Journal of Child Sexual Abuse, 13*(3/4), pp. 57-82.

Robbins, R., Tonemah, S., & Robbins, S. (2002). Project eagle: Techniques for multi-family psycho-educational group therapy with gifted American Indian adolescents and their parents. *American Indian Alaskan Native Mental Health Research, 10*(3), 56-74.

Ryan, G., & Lane, S. (1995). *Cycle of abuse diagram.* Kempe Center training documents. Denver, CO.

Ryan, G., & Lane, S. (1997). *Juvenile sexual offending: Causes, consequences, and Correction* (2nd ed.). San Francisco: Jossey-Bass Publishers.

Salter, A. (1988). *Treating child sexual offenders and victims: A practical guide.* Thousand Oaks, CA: Sage Publications.

Search Institute. (1997). *40 developmental assets.* Retrieved from: http://www.search institute.org

Smith, J. (1999). *Cognitive tool cards.* Retrieved from http://www.thinkittools.com

Smith, J., & Tedeschi, P. (1998). *Point-of-order treatment model.* Unpublished treatment handout. Denver, CO: Resource Center for High Risk Youth.

Tedeschi, P. (1999). *Principles of containment treatment.* Unpublished treatment handout. Denver, CO: Resource Center for High Risk Youth.

Thomas, J. (1991). The adolescent sex offender's family in treatment. In G. Ryan & S.L. Lane (Eds.), *Juvenile sexual offending: Causes, consequences, and corrections* (pp. 333-376). Lexington, MA: Lexington Books.

Thomas, J. (1997). The family in treatment. In G. Ryan, & S.L. Lane (Eds.), *Juvenile sexual offending: Causes, consequences, and corrections* (pp. 360-403). San Francisco: Jossey-Boss Publishers.

Weine, S.M., Raina, D., Zhubi, M., Delesi, M., Huseni, D., Feetham, S., Kulauzovic, Y., Mermelstein, R., Campbell, R.T., Rolland, J., & Pavkovic, I. (2003). The

TAFES multi-family group intervention for Kosovar refugees: A feasibility study. *Journal of Nervous and Mental Disease, 191*(2), 100-7.

Yalom, I.D. (1985). *The theory and practice of group psychotherapy.* New York: Basic Books.

Zankman, S., & Bonomo, J. (2004). Working with parents to reduce juvenile sex offender recidivism. *Journal of Child Sexual Abuse, 13*(3/4), pp. 139-156

Current Practices in Residential Treatment for Adolescent Sex Offenders: A Survey

C. Eugene Walker
David McCormick

SUMMARY. A list of all treatment facilities for adolescent sex offenders that described themselves as inpatient or residential was requested from the Safer Society Foundation in Brandon, Vermont. A total of 203 such facilities were identified in this manner. Each was sent a questionnaire regarding their policies and practices. Of the 50 questionnaires that were returned, 49 were usable. Items on the questionnaire dealt with major phases of operating a residential program, including number of beds, average daily census, number of males and females in treatment, testing and assessment procedures, most frequent diagnoses, average IQ of patients, abuse history, therapeutic approaches used, number and types of

Address correspondence to: C. Eugene Walker, PhD, 1133 North Bank Side Circle, Edmond, OK 73003 (E-mail: genewalker@iname.com).

The authors wish to thank Thomas Donica, MD, Nola Harrison, LSW-C, Terry Masters LSW-C, Barbara Walker, RN, and Barton Turner, PhD, for their assistance in completing this project.

[Haworth co-indexing entry note]: "Current Practices in Residential Treatment for Adolescent Sex Offenders: A Survey." Walker, C. Eugene, and David McCormick. Co-published simultaneously in *Journal of Child Sexual Abuse* (The Haworth Maltreatment and Trauma Press, an imprint of The Haworth Press, Inc.) Vol. 13, No. 3/4, 2004, pp. 245-255; and: *Identifying and Treating Youth Who Sexually Offend: Current Approaches, Techniques, and Research* (ed: Robert Geffner et al.) The Haworth Maltreatment and Trauma Press, an imprint of The Haworth Press, Inc., 2004, pp. 245-255. Single or multiple copies of this article are available for a fee from The Haworth Document Delivery Service [1-800-HAWORTH, 9:00 a.m. - 5:00 p.m. (EST). E-mail address: docdelivery@haworthpress.com].

Digital Object Identifier: 10.1300/J070v13n03_12

individual/group treatment sessions per week, qualifications of thera-
pists, average length of treatment, and follow-up research on treatment.
*[Article copies available for a fee from The Haworth Document Delivery Ser-
vice: 1-800-HAWORTH. E-mail address: <docdelivery@haworthpress.com>
Website: <http://www.HaworthPress.com>* © 2004 by The Haworth Press, Inc.
All rights reserved.]

KEYWORDS. Residential treatment, adolescents, sex offenders, assessment

Data indicates that adolescents commit approximately 30 to 50% of all child
molestations in the United States (Becker, Kaplan, Cunningham-Rathner, &
Kavoussi, 1986) and 20% of rapes (Brown, Flannagan, & McLeod, 1984;
Deisher, Wenet, Paperny, Clark, & Fehrenback, 1982; Groth, Longo, &
McFadin, 1982). Research also indicates that many adult offenders began
their offending careers as adolescents (Hoghughi & Richardson, 1990). Available data suggests a significant reduction in recidivism for adolescent offenders who are given effective psychological intervention (e.g., Rasmussen,
1999).

Dealing with sex offenses poses a significant problem for law enforcement
and the judicial system. Most observers agree on two points. First, a punitive,
corrections-based model that employs primarily incarceration for relatively
brief periods of time is ineffective. Second, the earlier intervention begins, the
better.

While the vast majority of adolescent offenders function well enough and
are in sufficient enough control that they can be treated with intensive outpatient psychotherapy, certain sub populations pose significant problems and require a different approach. Notably among these are intellectually impaired
offenders and seriously emotionally disturbed offenders. Several reports have
appeared in the literature describing residential and inpatient treatment centers
for adolescent offenders and discussing problems in ensuring safety and effective treatment in such centers (Epps, 1994; Mathews, 1997; Ross & de Villier,
1993).

Examination of the literature reveals consensus that treatment is best provided when it emphasizes group psychotherapy from a cognitive-behavioral
theoretical point of view and when it is offense specific. Emphasis is given to
open disclosure of the offense, sex education, empathy, understanding consequences of offending behavior, values clarification, attitude change, impulse
control, anger management, social skills training, relapse prevention, and gen-

eralization of the treatment principles to other behaviors. This developed from follow-up studies indicating that graduates of sex offender treatment programs had a low rate of additional sex offenses but tended to commit other non-sexual offenses at a high rate. Skepticism is discussed with respect to sex drive reduction medication, aversive treatments including electric shocks and shame, physiological measurement of sexual arousal, and polygraph testing (e.g., Ryan & Lane, 1997). Safety issues are a two-edged sword with concerns about community safety and the safety of the offender if placed in a residential program.

Programs to treat adolescent offenders have proliferated and continued to increase beginning with a handful in the mid 1980s and currently comprising over 600, of which over 200 are residential or inpatient. Recently a set of Standards of Care for Youth in Sex Offense-Specific Residential Programs was published (Bengis et al., 1999). Although these guidelines have not been adopted by any official accrediting organization, they are intended to provide guidance for those wishing to provide the best care possible for this patient population. There are four major sections to the guidelines including issues related to program characteristics, staff, safety, and intervention. These standards will be discussed in connection with the data of this survey later in the article.

There is, however, little data providing details of exactly how young adolescents who require residential treatment are actually cared for. For example, do policies and techniques for supervision of these young people, safety precautions, assessment procedures, and components of treatment conform to the published literature and standards, or is the real world different from the ideal presented in print? To answer these questions, the present article describes findings from a survey completed by residential adolescent sex offender treatment programs. The purpose of the survey was to determine current policies and practices in order to describe the "state of the art" for management and treatment of adolescent offenders in inpatient and residential settings. Other general surveys of sex offender programs have been sponsored over the years by the Safer Society Foundation, a non-profit research, advocacy, and referral center on the prevention and treatment of sexual abuse. The most recent one was published in 2000 (Burton & Smith-Darden, 2001). However, the current survey goes into more depth with respect to adolescents. We will compare our data with the Safer Society's data as appropriate.

METHOD

A list of all registered facilities that described themselves as inpatient or residential was requested from the Safer Society Foundation of Brandon, Vermont. A total of 203 such facilities were identified in this manner. Each was sent a questionnaire regarding their policies and practices. Two follow-up mailings were made to increase participation. A total of 50 questionnaires were returned. Of these, 49 were usable. It should be noted that this is a modest rate of return, but it was the best possible based on an initial contact and two follow-up requests.

Items on the questionnaire dealt with virtually all phases of operating a residential program including number of beds, average daily census, number of males and females in treatment, testing and assessment procedures, most frequent diagnoses, average IQ of patients, abuse history, therapeutic approaches used, number and types of individual/group treatment sessions each week, qualifications of therapists, average length of treatment and follow-up research on treatment effectiveness. A copy of the questionnaire can be obtained by contacting the first author of this study.

RESULTS AND DISCUSSION

Examination of the returned questionnaires indicated that they could be divided into two groups: (a) those that were based in mental health facilities ($N = 39$) and (b) those that were in correctional facilities ($N = 10$). Consequently the data was grouped in this manner, and tests of significance were performed to determine whether or not there were significant differences between the two types of treatment facilities. T-tests were employed for continuous data and chi squares for frequency data. This statistical analysis revealed few significant differences. Notably, the mental health facilities were significantly more likely to offer individual psychotherapy; individual psychotherapy sessions were longer; improvement in self-esteem was more likely to be included as a treatment component; there was a higher ratio of registered nurse staff to residents; and a higher percentage of the residents had a diagnosis of ADHD. In the absence of other statistically significant differences between the groups, the data was combined for the remainder of the analyses.

Each facility was requested to provide information about the number of beds available for males and for females at their facility as well as the average daily census for males and females. The mean number of beds for males was 34 and the mean number for females was 1. The average daily census was 33.5 for males and .87 for females. This ratio of male to female residents is what would be expected based on the literature. The average daily census compared to capacity indicates that these units operate essentially at full capacity, which is outstanding in terms of hospital or residential treatment center economics.

In response to a question about the use of psychological testing, 61% of the total sample indicated that psychological testing was a standard part of their intake process. This would appear to be low, because the Standards of Care mentioned earlier (Bengis et al., 1999) encourage the use of psychological testing for admission decisions and treatment planning. These standards also specify that an offense-specific assessment be made of each resident. Table 1 indicates the instruments reported in the present survey as most frequently used. Intelligence testing topped the list with the highest percent, with virtually all programs employing some sort of intellectual assessment. This is reasonable since the intellectual level must be carefully evaluated when cognitive therapy techniques are employed in treatment. Personality assessments such as the MMPI, the Rorschach, and the Multiphasic Sex Inventory were also commonly employed. However, only 16% employed polygraph techniques, 10% used the Hare Psychopathy Checklist, and a mere 6.5% used plethysmograph techniques.

The Safer Society survey (Burton & Smith-Darden, 2001) reported a similarly low rate of 11% for physiological monitoring. The lower use of these techniques is no doubt due in part to the level of training and sophistication as well as equipment and materials necessary to use these approaches. In the case of the polygraph and plethysmograph, questions about the appropriateness of using these with adolescents as well as concerns about reliability and validity no doubt play a part. The Standards of Care (Bengis et al., 1999) specify that the least intrusive methods possible to achieve a positive outcome should be used; intrusive methods should be used only after other methods have failed; and there should be clear safeguards in place to protect the resident against unnecessary or inappropriate use of these methods.

Respondents to the survey indicated the percentage of patients receiving various diagnoses commonly associated with adolescent offenders. Since some pa-

TABLE 1. Assessment Procedures Employed in Residential Treatment Facilities

Procedure	% of Facilities Using Procedure
Wechsler	81
Other I.Q.	19
MMPI	48
Multiphasic Sex Inventory	45
Rorschach	35
Jesness Personality Inventory	19
Polygraph	16
Hare Psychopathy Checklist	10
Plethysmograph	7

tients have multiple diagnoses, the data refer to the frequency with which the diagnosis was employed and not the number of patients. Diagnoses employed, from most to least common were Conduct Disorder (63%), ADHD (36%), learning disabilities (36%), depression (35%), substance abuse (30%), anxiety (15%), pedophilia (15%), psychosis (7%), mental retardation (5%), and seizures (2%).

Respondents also indicated the estimated number of patients in the facilities falling into different categories of intellectual ability. As would be expected, the IQ scores show a wide range with the majority falling in the normal range of intelligence. The percentages for each category of intelligence were as follows: (a) Below 50 (.43%), (b) 50-69 (5%), (c) 70-89 (40%), (d) 90-110 (42%), (e) 111-120 (9%), and (f) 121 or above (3%).

When asked to indicate their best estimation regarding the percentage of their patients who had suffered maltreatment, the results were as follows: (a) sexual abuse (63%), (b) physical abuse (57%), (c) emotional abuse (71%), and (d) neglect (58%). These estimates were based on all sources including documented instances, revelations in therapy, and other reliable sources of information. It is interesting to note that the estimated rate of emotional abuse was even higher than sexual abuse among these young people. Physical neglect and physical abuse, however, were also reported in over 50% of the cases. It should be recalled that these are inpatient treatment centers, and the rates for outpatients are generally lower (e.g., Zakireh, 2000). This is partly because there is a positive interaction between abuse and psychopathology (Cooper, Murphy, & Haynes, 1996), and because the decision to employ residential treatment (particularly hospitalization) is positively related to the presence of psychopathology.

When asked to rank order the therapeutic approaches used in their treatment programs, 79% indicated that a cognitive approach was their primary orientation; 68% indicated that a behavioral approach was the secondary orientation used in their program; 42% indicated that family systems was the third option in their treatment program; and 57% noted that psychodynamic therapy was occasionally used as a fourth option. The Safer Society survey (Burton & Smith-Darden, 2001) reported that 79.3% of their residential adolescent programs used a cognitive behavioral/relapse prevention model as their primary theoretical orientation, while other approaches were seldom reported. The Standards of Care (Bengis et al., 1999) specify that treatment should be multi-modal, multi-disciplinary and offense specific.

When questioned about the nature of their treatment program, 76% considered their program highly structured with 79% indicating that they had a specific protocol guiding their treatment program. Respondents were then asked to indicate for a variety of concepts of treatment whether or not the concept was used extensively. Table 2 provides results of this question. While not stated explicitly, the general thrust of the Standards of Care (Bengis et al., 1999) would appear to require a structured program for compliance.

The programs all concentrated on group therapy as the main method for providing treatment. The average number of focused group therapy sessions per week dealing specifically with sexual offending was 3.7. These groups averaged 80 minutes in length with a range from 45 minutes to 120 and had an average of 8-9 patients in each group session. The programs reported an average of two general group sessions per week averaging 43 minutes per group with between 6 and 7 patients in the group. Finally, many programs offered one or two expressive therapy sessions per week averaging 30 minutes with 4 patients per group. The Safer Society survey (Burton & Smith-Darden, 2001) reported a mean of 3.70 group sessions per week, which is the same as was found in the present survey. The average length of these sessions was reported to be 83.36 minutes, which is also essentially the same as reported in the present survey.

As noted earlier in this article, individual psychotherapy was more common among mental health facilities than correctional facilities. Individual sessions were generally approximately 50 minutes in length. Average number of sessions per week was 1. The Safer Society survey (Burton & Smith-Darden,

TABLE 2. Treatment Concepts Used Extensively in Programs Reporting

Treatment Concepts	% Using Concept Extensively
Full Disclosure of Inappropriate Sex Behavior	95
Relapse Prevention	95
Correction of Cognitive Distortions	93
Sexual Assault Cycle	93
Empathy Training	88
Anger Management	72
Social Skills Training	71
Sex Education	62
Values Clarification	53
Insight	50
Impulse Control Training	50
Self-Esteem Training	38
Re-enactment of Sex Offense	23
Sex Addiction Model	20
Shaming	0

2001) reported very similar data (1.27 sessions per week and 51.24 minutes in length). When asked in the present survey who provided individual psychotherapy, facilities reported the following: (a) social workers (60%), (b) licensed professional counselors (46%), (c) psychologists (35%), (d) un-licensed mental health workers (17%), (e) psychiatrists (8%,) and (f) nurses (2%).

The average length of stay in the residential facilities was 16.29 months with a range from 3 to 48. Examination of the Safer Society data (Burton & Smith-Darden, 2001) indicated that the most common length of stay was 12-24 months with a range of 6 months to 36 or more months. Obviously the length of stay in these facilities is well above average for other facilities. How long this will be possible in terms of third party reimbursement is questionable.

Security is a major issue in residential facilities serving adolescent sex offenders. Surprisingly, not all of the facilities employed hall monitors 24 hours per day (85% did, 15% did not) or used routine room checks (81% did, 19% did not). The absence of these would raise serious concerns about security and safety of the residents. Fifty-six percent reported availability of single occupancy rooms; 33% and 45% respectively reported using double and triple occupancy rooms. When roommates were assigned, this was done on the basis of risk factors in 65% of the facilities. A relatively small number, 27% and 29% respectively, used video cameras in public areas or surveillance devices in the sleeping rooms. Table 3 indicates the ratio of staff to patients for different categories of staff. It can be seen from this table that the bulk of the direct patient contact is provided by mental health technicians, social workers, and master's level therapists.

A matter of concern in all facilities providing residential care for sex offenders has to do with whether or not additional inappropriate sexual behavior is occurring on the unit. Respondents to the questionnaire were asked to indicate the number of non-contact sexual behaviors such as exhibitionism and voyeurism that occurred on their unit per year, the number of minor contact incidents where one patient touched or fondled another, and the number of serious incidents where patients engaged in complete sexual acts. For the minor and serious incidents they were also asked to estimate what percent were mutual or voluntary as opposed to coerced. These are obviously estimates made by the staff and need to be viewed with caution. The average number of non-contact sexual behaviors reported was 5 per year. With respect to minor incidents the mean number reported was 6.4 and it was estimated that three quarters of these were voluntary. Concerning major incidents, 1.67 were reported as the frequency per year and two-thirds of these were considered to be voluntary.

TABLE 3. Patient/Staff Ratios Reported by Residential Facilities for Each Profession and Each Shift

Profession	Ratio	N
Day RN/LPN	27.41:1	30
Evening RN/LPN	31.67:1	15
Night RN/LPN	24.96:1	13
Day MHT	6.48:1	29
Evening MHT	6.38:1	30
Night MHT	10.09:1	31
Psychiatrist	29.13:1	36
Psychologist	23.86:1	28
Social Worker	13.60:1	27
Master or PhD level in MH	14.22:1	37
Bachelor's Degree in MH	12.21:1	19
Recreational Therapist	23.47:1	27

There was a very wide range of reporting of frequencies for incidents. For non-contact and minor incidents the range was from 0-52 per year. For major incidents the range reported was 0-10 per year. Fortunately, since the goal of virtually all residential units is to never have incidents of this sort occur, it appears that relatively few incidents occur in most settings. However, the wide range of reports regarding frequency would suggest that safety and security is still a major issue for some institutions. Several sections of the Standards of Care (Bengis et al., 1999) outline the necessity of preventing consensual and non-consensual sexual contact between residents and procedures for dealing with incidents when such occur.

Seventy-eight of the programs reported that they attempted systematic follow-up of their patients after treatment. They reported success rates of contacting and obtaining information about their patients of 61% after 1 year, 35.5% after 2 years and 26.57% after 3 years. Standards of Care (Bengis et al., 1999) require that programs evaluate the effectiveness of their treatment programs.

CONCLUDING COMMENTS

Maintaining a community of adolescent sex offenders who live together 24 hours per day poses unique risks and management problems. The current survey was conducted in an effort to obtain information on the "state of the art" in providing inpatient/residential care for this population. After examining the findings, it was reassuring that there was reasonably good consensus regarding the areas surveyed. Over half of the programs used psychological testing for assessment of new patients. Intelligence testing was most common, with personality testing not quite as common. There was general consensus about the usefulness of cognitive and behavioral treatment models. Group therapy was the most common form of therapy, although individual therapy was offered, especially in mental health facilities as compared to facilities in correctional settings. While group psychotherapy is considered to have significant advantages for sex offending behavior, it would appear that more use of individual therapy might be a useful addition.

Safety of residents is crucial, and most of the facilities appeared to be doing an adequate job in this area. Some facilities, however, reported unacceptable levels of sexual incidents and assault. Since this is such a crucial concern, it may be necessary to form a task force of professionals to study and make recommendations for patient safety in such facilities. The recommendations at a minimum should include architectural design, electronic surveillance, and staff training. Finally, it should be noted that while 78% of the programs attempted to follow up patients after discharge, the scarcity of published data in this area suggests that this is more wishful thinking than reality. It is strongly recommended that more adequate follow-up data be obtained and that these data be correlated with assessment and treatment characteristics in order to know what works and what does not. This needs to be a priority for future research.

REFERENCES

Becker, J.V., Kaplan, M.S., Cunningham-Rathner, J., & Kavoussi, R. (1986). Characteristics of adolescent incest sexual perpetrators: Preliminary findings. *Journal of Family Violence, 1*, 85-97.

Bengis, S., Brown, A., Freeman-Longo, R., Matsuda, B., Ross, J., Singer, K., & Thomas, J. (1999). *Standards of care for youth in sex offense-specific residential programs.* Holyoke, MA: NEARI Press.

Brown, F.J., Flanagan, T.J., & McLeod, M. (Eds.). (1984). *Sourcebook of criminal justice statistics–1983.*Washington, DC: Bureau of Justice Statistics.

Burton, D.L., & Smith-Darden, J. (2001). *North American survey of sexual abuser treatment and models: Summary data 2000.* Brandon, VT: Safer Society Press.

Cooper, C.L., Murphy, W.D., & Haynes, M.R. (1996). Characteristics of abused and non-abused adolescent sexual offenders. *Sexual Abuse: A Journal of Research and Treatment, 8*, 105-119.

Deisher, R.W., Wenet, G.A., Paperny, D.M., Clark, T.F., & Fehrenback, P.A. (1982). Adolescent sexual offense behavior: The role of the physician. *Journal of Adolescent Health Care, 2*, 279-286.

Epps, K. J. (1994). Treating adolescent sex offenders in secure conditions: The experience at Glenthorne Centre. *Journal of Adolescence, 17*, 105-122.

Groth, A.N., Longo, R.E., & McFadin, J.B. (1982). Undetected recidivism among rapists and child molesters. *Crime and Delinquency, 28*, 450-458.

Hoghughi, M., & Richardson, P. (1990, November). The legal sanction. *Community Care, 1*, 21-23.

Mathews, F. (1997). The adolescent sex offender field in Canada: Old problems, current issues, and emerging controversies. *Journal of Child and Youth Care, 11*(1), 55-62.

Rasmussen, L.A. (1999). Factors related to recidivism among juvenile sexual offenders. *Sexual Abuse: A Journal of Research and Treatment, 11*, 69-85.

Ross, J.E., & de Villier, M.P. (1993). Safety considerations in developing an adolescent sex offender program in residential treatment. *Residential Treatment for Children and Youth, 11*, 37-47.

Ryan, G., & Lane, S. (Eds.). (1997). *Juvenile sexual offending: Causes, consequences, and correction.* San Francisco: Jossey-Bass Publishers.

Zakireh, B. (2000). Residential and outpatient adolescent sexual and nonsexual offenders: History, sexual adjustment, clinical, cognitive, and demographic characteristics. *Dissertation Abstracts International: Section B: The Sciences & Engineering, 61*(2-B), 1102.

RECIDIVISM, RESILIENCE, AND TREATMENT EFFECTIVENESS FOR YOUTH WHO SEXUALLY OFFEND

Recidivism and Resilience in Juvenile Sexual Offenders: An Analysis of the Literature

Jill Efta-Breitbach
Kurt A. Freeman

SUMMARY. The majority of research that exists studying juvenile sex offenders (JSOs) is dominated by the predilection that identifying risk factors associated with recidivism will benefit both the JSOs and treatment providers. Further, the majority of existing treatments are guided by research that has identified what makes JSOs more likely to reoffend. Absent from the majority of the literature is an examination of the strengths and positive characteristics demonstrated by JSOs that may prove useful in both reducing recidivism and increasing the likelihood of achieving positive outcomes (i.e., demonstrating resilience). Research

Address correspondence to: Jill Efta-Breitbach, PsyD, Womack Army Medical Center, Fort Bragg, NC 28310 (E-mail: Jill.Breitbach@na.amedd.army.mil).

[Haworth co-indexing entry note]: "Recidivism and Resilience in Juvenile Sexual Offenders: An Analysis of the Literature." Efta-Brietbach, Jill, and Kurt A. Freeman. Co-published simultaneously in *Journal of Child Sexual Abuse* (The Haworth Maltreatment and Trauma Press, an imprint of The Haworth Press, Inc.) Vol. 13, No. 3/4, 2004, pp. 257-279; and: *Identifying and Treating Youth Who Sexually Offend: Current Approaches, Techniques, and Research* (ed: Robert Geffner et al.) The Haworth Maltreatment and Trauma Press, an imprint of The Haworth Press, Inc., 2004, pp. 257-279. Single or multiple copies of this article are available for a fee from The Haworth Document Delivery Service [1-800-HAWORTH, 9:00 a.m. - 5:00 p.m. (EST). E-mail address: docdelivery@haworthpress.com].

examining known risk factors for sexual and nonsexual recidivism is described. Next, literature on resilience is reviewed, followed by a discussion of this literature in the context of treatment for JSOs. Finally, future directions of research are presented. *[Article copies available for a fee from The Haworth Document Delivery Service: 1-800-HAWORTH. E-mail address: <docdelivery@haworthpress.com> Website: <http://www.HaworthPress.com> © 2004 by The Haworth Press, Inc. All rights reserved.]*

KEYWORDS. Juveniles, sexual offending, recidivism, resilience, treatment

The prevalence of sex offenses committed by juvenile sexual offenders (JSOs) has only recently been explored, and implications of the data are staggering. The National Crime Victimization Survey (NCVS) found that in 1997, individuals under the age of 18 were involved in 27% of all serious violent victimizations, including 14% of sexual assaults and 27% of aggravated assaults (Snyder & Sickmund, as cited in Office of Juvenile Justice and Delinquency, 1999). More specific to the topic of this article, it is estimated that juveniles, particularly males, are responsible for 20% of all rapes and 30 to 50% of all child molestations (Brown, Flanagan, & McLeod, 1984). Moreover, almost 50% of adult sex offenders disclose engaging in some form of sexual offending during adolescence (Able, Mittleman, & Becker, 1985), and the ratio of committed offenses to arrests can be as low as 1:150 (Abel et al., 1987). In addition, juveniles are responsible for approximately 60% of all sexual offenses committed against children younger than 12 years of age (Bourke & Donohue, 1996). Given these statistics, it is not surprising that increasing focus has been given to this population.

In addition to documenting the prevalence of sexual offenses committed by juveniles, researchers have evaluated the course of such offenses by looking at rates of recidivism. Recidivism, or reoffending, is generally defined as the reconviction of a JSO in juvenile court of another criminal offense (Rasmussen, 1999). Research has consistently shown that sexual and nonsexual recidivism rates are dissimilar, with sexual reoffenses occurring at a lower rate. Retrospectively established sexual recidivism rates during follow-up periods of up to 10 years range from 6% to 20% (Becker & Hunter, 1997; Bremer, 1992; Hagan & Gust-Brey, 1999; Kahn & Chambers, 1991; Langstrom & Grann, 2000; Smith & Monastersky, 1986). For example, Rasmussen (1999) found that sexual reoffending was lower (14.1%) than nonsexual reoffending (54.1%). Langstrom and Grann (2000) found that 65% of their sample of 56

JSOs had at least one reconviction for any crime with the mean time to reoffense being 60.95 months. However, only 9 JSOs in their sample had been reconvicted for a sexual reoffense. Borduin, Henggeler, Blaske, and Stein (1990) also found that there is a significantly greater chance that JSOs will engage in a general offense versus a sexual offense after treatment.

In contrast, however, nonsexual recidivism rates, or offenses that are criminal versus sexual, have been shown to be quite high for this population. Nonsexual recidivism rates, for periods up to 10 years, range from 34.8% to 90% (Becker & Hunter, 1997; Hagan & Gust-Brey, 1999; Kahn & Chambers, 1991; Langstrom & Grann, 2000; Smith & Monastersky, 1986). Thus, although current evidence suggests that most JSOs do not go on to repeat sexual offenses, many remain active in perpetrating some form of juvenile offense. Therefore, the question remains whether treatment of JSOs produces generalized positive outcomes.

Positive outcomes, particularly when experienced by at-risk youth, are often associated with resiliency. Resiliency is conceptualized as being demonstrated by at-risk youth who overcome adversity, develop competence, and persevere despite significant hardship. In this article, research on both the juvenile sex offender and resiliency will be reviewed. First, characteristics of JSOs and recidivism risk factors identified by existing research will be explored. Next, factors associated with resiliency will be discussed. Finally, a critical discussion of the literature and implications for future treatment and research will be provided. Specifically, implications for considering resiliency in the treatment and research of JSOs will be addressed.

FACTORS INFLUENCING RECIDIVISM

Despite a clear demonstration of differences in recidivism, the majority of research does not allow for a clear identification of factors that predict sexual versus nonsexual recidivism. In general, prominent characteristics and risk factors associated with JSO recidivism discussed in the literature include the following: (a) failure to achieve treatment success or complete treatment, (b) a family history of dysfunction, (c) prior abuse or mistreatment, (d) delinquent peer relations and behaviors, (e) characteristics of the JSO offenses, (f) deviant arousal and/or sexual maladjustment, and (g) mental health diagnosis and defenses.

Lack of Treatment Completion

Failure to complete treatment is one of the most salient risk factors for reoffending behaviors (Studer & Reddon, 1998). The variable of treatment completion has been predictive for both adult sex offender and JSO populations. In their meta-analysis, Hanson and Bussiere (1998) found that one of the strongest predictors of sexual reoffending among adult and juvenile sex offenders was failure to complete treatment (with the other being sexual deviance). Sipe, Jensen, and Everett (1998) studied 124 former non-violent JSOs who completed treatment and found that only 9.7% were arrested as adults, with follow-up being 11 to 14 years. Further, in their 10-year longitudinal study of adolescent rapists, Hagan and Gust-Brey (1999) found that only 8 of 50 individuals completing a sex offender treatment program had perpetrated another sexual assault. Analyzing recidivism among a sample of 96 JSOs, Prentky, Harris, Frizzell, and Righthand (2000) found a 4% sexual recidivism rate for those completing treatment. Other studies confirm that JSOs who successfully complete treatment have low (generally under 10%) sexual recidi- vism rates (Bremer, 1992; Kahn & Chambers, 1991) and that sexual recidivism is significantly associated with failure to complete treatment (Rasmussen, 1999). Outcome studies in both the adult and JSO research support the completion of sexual offender treatment programs as one of the most predictive factors for decreasing sexual recidivism.

Family History and Dysfunction

Family dysfunction is a known risk factor associated with juvenile sex offending (Bourke & Donohue, 1996; see Righthand & Welch, this issue), and research is beginning to show that family dysfunction also affects recidivism risk. Many JSOs appear to fail in treatment programs not because of underlying pathology, but because they seem to lack motivation and proper familial support and supervision (Borduin et al., 1990). Rasmussen (1999) found that divorce/separation of parents was a statistically significant variable in nonsexual recidivism, while parental absence resulting from the death of a parent or parents who never married was not statistically significant. Mathews, Hunter, and Vuz (1997) showed that female JSOs had higher rates of sexual reoffending when family psychopathology and dysfunction were more extensive and severe. Given that a high percentage of JSOs live in single-parent homes (Rasmussen, 1999), the role of family disruption such as divorce may be an important risk factor for recidivism.

Prior Abuse and/or Mistreatment

The relationship between early maltreatment and later sexual acting out is undoubtedly complex, and the reason why some mistreated youths later perpetrate and others do not has yet to be explicated fully (Hunter & Becker, 1994;

for further discussion of the connection between early maltreatment and sexual offending, see Knight & Sims-Knight, this issue). More complex is the relationship between mistreatment and recidivism. Research shows that abuse and mistreatment are useful in predicting juveniles who will offend sexually (Kahn & Lafond, 1988: Mathews et al., 1997; Rasmussen, 1999). However, this risk factor has a weak association with recidivism.

Kahn and Chambers (1991) found that a sexual abuse history and/or siblings with a sexual abuse history were significant variables in predicting non-sexual recidivism, but not sexual recidivism. Smith and Monastersky (1986) reported that the absence of physical or sexual abuse in the families of their sample was characteristic of JSOs who did not reoffend. In a study comparing 156 JSOs who had not been abused and 134 JSOs who had been abused, Cooper, Murphy, and Haynes (1996) found that abused JSOs had an earlier onset of offending, a greater number of victims, were more likely to abuse both male and female victims, demonstrated more psychopathology, and had a higher level of interpersonal problems.

However, Rasmussen (1999) found that a history of sexual abuse was only weakly related to sexual recidivism in her sample of 170 JSOs. Langstrom and Grann (2000) showed that historical factors including adverse upbringing and sexual abuse were not predictive of relapse into sexual criminality. Further, a recent meta-analysis did not find a relationship between prior sexual victimization and later recidivism in sex offenders (Hanson & Bussiere, 1998). Thus, when examined in isolation, abuse history does not appear useful in predicting juvenile sexual recidivism.

Delinquent Behaviors and Peer Groups

Involvement with delinquent peers has been shown to allow for correct classification of juveniles who reoffend (Prentky et al., 2000). Moreover, delinquent behaviors and prior juvenile offenses have been associated with nonsexual recidivism (Kahn & Chambers, 1991; Rasmussen, 1999). For example, truancy has been linked to sexual recidivism (Shram, Milloy, & Rowe, 1991, as cited in Hunter & Becker, 1994) and to non-sexual recidivism (Kahn & Chambers, 1991). School behavior problems also significantly relate to nonsexual recidivism (Kahn & Chambers, 1991). Furthermore, Rasmussen (1999) found that almost one-half of her sample of 170 JSOs had a history of delinquent offenses, and greater than one-half reoffended during the observation period by committing new nonsexual offenses.

Characteristics of JSO Offenses

Research suggests that certain characteristics of JSO offenses such as age at the time of the referral offense, victim demographics, sexual acts committed, victim blame, and methods used to recruit victims can be predictive of sexual recidivism. The ages most indicative of recidivism in JSOs have been conflictual in existing research. Research has found both younger JSOs (Hanson & Bussiere, 1998; Kahn & Chambers, 1991) and older JSOs (Kraemer & Salisbury, 1998; Smith & Monastersky, 1986) are at risk for recidivism, either through known rates of reoffending or treatment failure. With ambiguous research findings, clinicians must rely on other characteristics of the JSO offense(s) when assessing risk of recidivism.

Sexual offenses committed by JSOs may be instigated by a variety of methods that are considered when predicting recidivism rates. JSOs who use verbal threats in the commission of their offenses reoffended sexually at higher rates than those who did not threaten their victims (Kahn & Chambers, 1991). Further, use of death threats or weapons during a sex offense has been predictive of nonsexual recidivism (Zolondek, Abel, Northey, & Jordan, 2001). However, Smith and Monastersky (1986) found an inverse relationship between seriousness of the referral offense and recidivism. These researchers also found that JSOs who victimized same age or older peers who were strangers had higher sexual recidivism rates.

Gender of JSO victims has not consistently been shown to be predictive of recidivism. Both perpetration against males (Langstrom & Grann, 2000; Smith & Monastersky, 1986) and females (Rasmussen, 1999) have been linked to JSO recidivism. Finally, a consistent predictor of future offending has been the number of victims. Specifically, JSOs who have multiple female or a larger number of total victims are more likely to commit additional sexual offenses (Langstrom & Grann, 2000; Rasmussen, 1999).

Deviant Arousal and Sexual Knowledge

In existing research, the role of deviant sexual arousal, sexual drive, and sexual preoccupation as risk factors for JSO recidivism is unclear (Prentky et al., 2000). Hanson and Bussiere (1998) found sexual deviance as one of the risk factors strongly associated with recidivism in their adolescent and adult populations. Therapist-identified deviant arousal patterns also appear suggestive of sexual recidivism, although not statistically significantly so (Kahn & Chambers, 1991). Also, JSOs with high rates of sexual maladjustment are more likely to be expelled from treatment (Hunter & Figueredo, 1999). Thus, because failure to complete treatment is a risk factor for recidivism, high rates of sexual maladjustment may be indirectly associated with recidivism.

Mental Health Problems

The relationship between JSO mental health symptomatology and recidivism is complex. The reasons why some mental health diagnoses and symptoms are predictive of recidivism and others are not remain unclear in existing research. For example, the ability of JSOs to identify strengths and positive personal attributes has actually been associated with higher nonsexual recidivism (Smith & Monastersky, 1986). Contrary to what might be expected, healthier (i.e., not depressed or defensive) JSOs have been found to be more likely to reoffend sexually (Smith & Monastersky, 1986). This is somewhat surprising given the prevalence of depression and defensiveness in JSOs (Becker, Kaplan, Tenke, & Tartaglini, 1991; Kavoussi, Kaplan, & Becker, 1988) and the previously described low rates of sexual recidivism. Researchers in the same study also found that less well-adjusted JSOs had a reduced likelihood of reoffending nonsexually (Smith & Monastersky, 1986).

Diagnoses of personality disorders such as Antisocial Personality Disorder and psychopathy have also been effective in predicting JSO recidivism (Hanson & Bussiere, 1998; Jacobs, Kennedy, & Meyer, 1997; Langstrom & Grann, 2000). In contrast, there is little support that substance abuse, which is common among JSOs, is a predictor for JSO recidivism (Zolondek et al., 2001). Research has generally found that substance abuse is not predictive of relapse into sexual criminality, but is predictive of nonsexual recidivism (Hanson & Bussiere, 1998).

RESILIENCY

Evaluating recidivism of JSOs has largely been a means of predicting the utility and success of various treatments (Camp & Thyer, 1993). It is obvious from the previous description of research that certain characteristics of JSOs are useful in predicting recidivism. What is missing from existing research is attention to factors that can predict successes of JSOs, or factors associated with resilience. Resilience is conceptualized in this article as existing on the opposite end of a continuum from risk. Specifically, resilience is viewed as a construct related to positive outcomes, whereas risks are related to negative outcomes. While it may be safe to assume that most individuals will achieve positive outcomes in some aspect of their lives at some point, demonstration of resilience is unique because it involves achieving positive outcomes while exposed to significant risk factors expected to result in an adverse outcome.

Many have found consistent protective factors that distinguish high-risk children who become resilient adults from their high-risk peers who succumb to the circumstances of their youth (Doll & Lyon, 1998). This consistency suggests that there may be common developmental pathways toward patterns of adult maladaption and common factors by which these pathways may be diverted (Masten & Coatsworth, 1998). These common factors are considered to be both intrinsic and extrinsic components of an individual's experience, and are associated with overcoming adverse circumstance. Furthermore, resilience has been viewed as an interaction of genetic, biological, psychological, and sociological factors in the context of environmental support (Henry, 1999). It is important to note that there is limited empirical literature focused on resiliency in the JSO population.

Resiliency Defined

Resilience is generally defined as "a central notion of successfully coping with or overcoming risk and adversity or the development of competence in the face of severe stress and hardship" (Doll & Lyon, 1998, p. 349). Resilience requires existence of a significant risk or threat to the individual and a high quality of adaptation or development despite the risk (Masten & Coatsworth, 1998).

There are three types of resilience described in the literature (Masten, Best, & Garmezy, 1990). The first type is achieving a good outcome despite a high-risk status. Individuals demonstrating resiliency via this process are characterized as achieving more positive outcomes than expected given their life circumstances. The second type consists of sustaining competence under threat. These individuals demonstrate resiliency by enduring hardship and functioning as though their environment did not threaten them. The final resilience experience is described as recovery from trauma. Individuals demonstrating resiliency through this process are characterized by the ability to encounter events that are considered traumatic, such as a sexual assault, and managing to function as well as or better than their competence level/abilities before the trauma. It should be noted that resilience waxes and wanes (Cicchetti & Garmezy, 1993; Wolff, 1995) but can have a cumulative impact on an individual's well being (Masten & Coatsworth, 1998).

Internal Factors Associated with Resiliency

Evidence suggests that youth have a large capacity to regulate and adapt to life circumstances (Eisenberg et al., 1998), and it is the responsibility of professionals to be cognizant of and seek out these qualities in order to promote resilience. Several variable have been identified as dispositional or personality features of the resilient person: (a) above average cognitive abilities and coping strategies, (b) high self-esteem and self-efficacy, (c) self-regulation or control, (d) internal locus of control, (e) faith, and (f) the biological hardiness of the individual (Heller, Larrieu, D-Imperio, & Boris 1999; Valentine & Feinauer, 1993; Walsh, 1996). A brief exploration of each variable follows.

Intellectual and cognitive abilities. Many have argued that better intellectual abilities lead to more effective coping strategies (Heller et al., 1999; Jew, Green, & Kroger, 1999; Masten et al., 1990; Masten & Coatsworth, 1998; Wolff, 1995). For example, Heller and colleagues (1999) found that greater intellectual abilities may lead to effective coping strategies in children exposed to abuse or neglect. Further, Himelein and McElrath (1996) found a greater tendency to engage in four types of cognitive strategies predictive of resilience in a non-clinical sample of child sexual abuse survivors (i.e., disclosing and discussing sexual abuse, minimization, positive reframing, and refusing to dwell on negative experiences). Moreover, resilient children appear to be resourceful and effective problem solvers (Masten et al., 1990). Researchers suggest that the cognitive coping strategies and reappraisal skills of resilient individuals appear to be associated with psychological well-being (Himelein & McElrath, 1996).

Intellectual abilities of resilient youth also have been shown to facilitate positive life experiences. For example, language competence and verbal abilities in precocious youngsters have been associated with greater abilities to engage in interactions with others, providing the engaging youngsters with many positive life experiences (Dalzell, 1998). Most JSOs are verbally coercive (Kahn & Chambers, 1991), which may suggest that they are able to successfully use verbal persuasion skills. Further, research has shown that even in the face of adverse circumstance during the first years of life, cognitive abilities can improve (Kagan, 1975).

However, some have argued that more developed intellectual abilities can actually serve as a risk factor (Luthar, 1991), presumably because higher intelligence allows for an increased sensitivity to environmental stressors and situations. Despite the potential risk that heightened awareness of reality could present, above average intellectual abilities likely can buffer negative life events. Because cognitive abilities develop and increase with age, the capacity for resilience may also develop or be taught.

Self-esteem and self-efficacy. The ability of at-risk youth to intellectually engage others and extract positive experiences from interactions facilitates the discovery of competence and positive self-worth in the individual. Researchers have found that high self-esteem–the ability to think well of oneself–is predictive of competence in children (Seifer, Sameroff, Baldwin, & Baldwin, 1992). Moreover, Dumont and Provost (1999) found that well-adjusted and resilient groups of individuals exhibit higher self-esteem than vulnerable adolescents. These researchers also found that those with high self-esteem were more likely to use effective problem-solving strategies and be more involved in their environment.

Self-efficacy, like self-esteem, concerns individuals' self-concepts and their feelings about their environment, their competence in handling life's obstacles, and their perceptions of control in determining outcomes (Winfield, 1991). The capacity to understand one's self in relation to long-term family stressors can enhance self-regard and feelings of competence (Rak & Patterson, 1996; Valentine & Feinauer, 1993). Thus, research appears to support the existence of more positive self-evaluations (i.e., high self-esteem) and more positive views of one's abilities (i.e., high self-efficacy) among resilient youth.

Self-regulation. Consistently, research has linked pro-social, adaptive behaviors as stemming from self-regulation and disruptive behaviors as stemming from a lack of self-regulation (Freitas & Downey, 1998). Resilient individuals are those who come to regulate their emotional reactivity in social or non-social contexts and react relatively positively to stressful events (Eisenberg et al., 1998). Self-control involves monitoring one's susceptibility or vulnerability to the environment (Cicchetti & Garmezy, 1993). Resilient individuals have been suggested to regulate vulnerability by controlling and modifying their emotions, behaviors, and attention to life stressors (Eisenberg et al., 1998). Further, Doll and Lyon (1998) suggested that the subjective meaning an individual attaches to life circumstances has the potential to alter the experience of "risk," leading to a variety of different and potentially positive outcomes.

Internal locus of control. Through self-regulation, individuals can develop the belief that they can influence their own life course. In other words, they may be people who demonstrate an internal locus of control. Resilient individuals often acquire the belief that their lives have meaning and that they have control over their own fates (Egeland, Carlson, & Sroufe, 1993). For example, Jew and colleagues (1999) found that individuals scoring higher on a resiliency scale had higher internal locus of control orientation. In contrast, external locus of control has been associated with increased vulnerability to stress in both boys and girls (Weist, Freedman, Paskewitz, Proescher, & Flaherty, 1995). Also, Valentine and Feinauer (1993) found internal locus of control to be an important theme related to resilience in their qualitative research examining positive outcomes of 22 women sexually abused as children.

Applying this research to youth, resilient youth may be those who are likely to take control of their responses to events, internalize positive outcomes, and externalize negative situations and outcomes. An inner-directed locus of control seems to emanate from internal values and beliefs rather than from expectations and directions of others (Valentine & Feinauer, 1993). The assertion could be made, then, that resilience is part of a plan or strategy (Felten, 2000), developed with an internal locus of control.

Faith. Religion, faith, and/or spirituality may influence appraisals of stressful situations and coping behaviors of individuals (Masten et al., 1990). For example, Henry (1999) found that the majority of adolescents in her qualitative study had religious beliefs about a higher power that watched over and protected them. Spirituality also was believed to serve as a protective factor for female survivors of sexual abuse in Valentine and Feinauer's (1993) qualitative study of 22 women. Those researchers found that spirituality promoted a sense of purpose, elevated self-esteem, and provided an external support system for interaction.

Biological hardiness. Resilient youth often have been described as having a personality structure characterized by biological hardiness, or a survival instinct (Walsh, 1996). Further, inherent differences in resilience, such as age, gender, and personality, often have been noted in existing research. For instance, research has shown that vulnerability and resistance to stressful experiences may shift as a function of ongoing developmental changes (Masten et al., 1990). Masten and colleagues found that both very young infants and older children have shown less distress in response to separations and strange situations. Moreover, factors that support resilience in girls may be different from those that support resilience in boys (Heller et al., 1999). Patterns of age and sex differences in studies of adaptation to stress are similar to patterns of psychopathology observed across the literature (Masten et al., 1990). Finally, personal dispositions may be indicative of resilience. In a landmark longitudinal study of resilience by Werner and Smith (1982), physical health and temperament were found to contribute to resilience, particularly in young children. Individual traits of independence and autonomy also serve as protective factors for individuals, particularly for children raised in abusive homes (Henry, 1999; Wolin & Wolin, 1993). These individuals learn to maintain safe boundaries and to distinguish between safe and dangerous relationships (Henry, 1999).

Summary. In summary, it is important to acknowledge the characteristics an individual brings to his or her environment. Considering aspects of resiliency inherent in individuals allows for an appreciation of uniqueness and perseverance. However, by focusing on the traits of an individual in isolation, we limit our consideration of resilience. The environmental context in which intrapersonal variables are supported and fostered warrants consideration.

External Factors Associated with Resiliency

Resilience to adversity depends as much upon the characteristics of the contexts in which youth develop as upon characteristics of the youth themselves (Doll & Lyon, 1998). Unless multiple domains of development are assessed, only a partial picture of adaptation can be formulated (Cicchetti & Garmezy, 1993). To complete the picture of resilience and attend to relevant developmental contexts, youth interactions with the family environment, parents and family members, the school environment, peers, and the community environment are considered and discussed below.

Socioeconomic status. Childhood poverty has been described as the most consistent predictor of dysfunction in adulthood (Doll & Lyon, 1998). Families growing up in poverty with a low socioeconomic status (SES) should produce vulnerable children. However, this often is not the case. For example, Long and Vaillant (1984) found that poverty was not necessarily predictive of adverse outcomes in their longitudinal study of 456 inner-city men. In their review of the literature, Engle, Castle, and Menon (1996) found that low-income mothers are often capable of utilizing agencies and community resources to meet their family needs (e.g., churches, neighborhood support groups, and neighborhood bartering systems). Mothers able to meet family needs also report higher confidence and self-efficacy, suggesting a sense of agency that may extend into mother-child relationships and the family environment. This research suggests that family interventions in the face of economic hardship could increase resilience in youth.

Family environment. Beyond financial and economic situations, the relationship that a child has with members of his or her family also appears to affect resiliency. For example, Elder, Nguyen, and Caspi (1985) found that fathers showing more affection toward their daughters appeared to ameliorate the risk of their daughters developing negative behaviors. Also, researchers have suggested that normalizing the environment within families may foster resilience (Henry, 1999; Wolff, 1995). Finally, existing research makes it evident that a sensitive, consistent, and safe care-giving environment is an important protective factor for maltreated youth (Heller et al., 1999).

Caregivers. Across accounts, the most important and consistent protective factor for youth at risk for the development of negative behavioral and emotional outcomes is that of adults caring for them during or after major stressors (Elder et al., 1985; Masten et al., 1990). Parents and other caregivers function as the first environmental protective agents of development. Under normative conditions, their relationships appear to foster several protective psychological processes (Masten et al., 1990). Effective parents also may generate or increase not only intellectual abilities, but self-efficacy and self-esteem as well.

In another longitudinal study, Seifer and colleagues (1992) found that high-risk but resilient youth were distinguished from non-resilient youth by effective parental teaching, limited parental criticism, and low rates of maternal depression. From existing research, the importance of a warm, consistent attachment system to the well-being and resilience of children is apparent (Masten & Coatsworth, 1998).

Family relationships. Relationships within a family, even when not with parents, can serve the function of providing warm, loving environments (Werner & Smith, 1992). For example, Barnes (1999) found that in addition to parental relationships, good sibling relationships and social support from adults outside the family facilitated positive adjustment in children after divorce. Further, in a study of intergenerational abuse, mothers who were able to abstain from abusing their own children, thus ending the cycle of abuse, reported that a salient protective factor was foster parents or a relative providing them with emotional support (Egeland, Jacobvitz, & Sroufe, 1988). Positive familial support appears to protect at-risk youth from negative outcomes, perhaps because early experience is critical in shaping the way later experience is organized (Egeland et al., 1993).

Peer groups. Positive peer groups and competence in building positive friendships not only promote social skills of at-risk youth, but also provide an enriching social context for personal development. Jew and colleagues (1999) found high self-perceived competence in friendships among resilient youth. This finding suggests that youth who utilize their abilities to interact with others, thus building support systems, are more resilient. Further, friendships support individuals in times of hardship, providing sustained relationships for resilient youth (Valentine & Feinauer, 1993).

Community support. Other extra-familial sources of support can provide important buffering roles (Engle et al., 1996; Seifer et al., 1992). For example, the resilient women in Valentine and Feinauer's (1993) study reported that school and college played a crucial role in their lives, serving as a refuge from a painful environment. Engagement in school and community activities also predicted resilience in 75 at-risk men in Long and Vaillant's (1984) longitudinal study. Further, community relations were found protective in the research review of Doll and Lyon (1998). Church relations can provide opportunities for friendship, role models, mentors, and confidants (Valentine & Feinauer, 1993). Protection through these interactions could be attributed to the increased social support (Walsh, 1996). School and community interactions may also help at-risk youth by increasing prosocial skills, which has been shown to be a protective factor for youth (Luthar, 1991).

Summary. Existing theoretical and empirical literature suggests that resilience in the face of adversity is fostered when individuals possess specific abilities and are exposed to particular environmental circumstances that serve to protect against threats to development (Masten & Coatsworth, 1998). Thus, a given heritable trait or exposure to environmental experiences is moderated by a host of associated risk and protective factors, eventually leading to a variety of phenotypic expressions (Heller et al., 1999). From discussed characteristics of JSOs and JSOs who reoffend, it is apparent that creating the context so that these individuals are more likely to succeed and be resilient is necessary. By capitalizing on existing strengths and systems, namely the treatment context, it is theorized that JSO risk for recidivism can be counteracted. That is, JSOs can develop resilience and competence in their lives, too.

RESILIENCY ADDRESSED IN JSO TREATMENT

Despite the tendency of research to ignore the concept of resilience in discussion of goals, locations, interventions, and modalities of JSO treatments, JSOs appear to demonstrate resiliency through low rates of sexual recidivism and other delinquent behaviors. Further, review of existing clinical and empirical literature on the treatment of JSOs suggests that interventions are designed to foster resiliency, although authors do not discuss approaches using this terminology. It is important to note that there is limited empirical literature focused on resilience in the JSO population, so only general factors related to resilience may be reviewed. These extrapolations from existing resilience literature should be viewed cautiously.

Internal Factors

Many internal factors associated with resiliency are addressed in existing JSO treatment. Although increasing self-esteem, self-regulation, cognitive abilities, and developing an internal locus of control are not stated as explicit goals for JSO treatment, interventions described in the literature appear to focus on these factors. For example, increasing positive self-evaluation (i.e., self esteem) is addressed in both individual and group therapies (Kahn & LaFond, 1988; Lombardo & DiGiorgio-Miller, 1988; Mathews et al., 1997). Also, developing a stronger ability to self-regulate and a development of an internal locus of control are addressed in cognitive-behavioral techniques that target a JSO's control over impulsive behavior, anger, and deviant arousal (Becker, Kaplan, & Kavoussi, 1988; Bourke & Donohue, 1996; Hunter & Becker, 1994).

Attempts to promote attitudes of openness and accountability that are common among JSO treatment (Hunter & Figueredo, 1999) also may promote resiliency. Specifically, encouraging JSOs to honestly relate to others may increase their ability to be honest with themselves and recognize treatment needs more readily. Monitoring and capitalizing on instances when JSOs take responsibility for their own actions can be one way to strengthen a cognitive style of openness and honesty (Hunter & Figueredo).

In addition to addressing sexual offending behavior, JSO treatments are geared toward addressing the overall mental health of JSOs (Becker, 1990). Mental health issues addressed range from substance abuse (Ertl & McNamara, 1997) to cognitive distortions (Becker, 1990). By incorporating broader mental health issues, treatment may affect overall functioning of JSOs. Specifically, treatments may be beginning to consider how to promote resilience in JSOs through improving functioning in multiple areas versus only eliminating offending behaviors. Doing so creates a situation in which the JSO may be better equipped psychologically to cope with adverse/stressful environments.

External Factors

External factors associated with resiliency are also indirectly addressed in existing treatments. Family therapy and multi-systemic therapy both attend to the caregiver and family characteristics that may maintain offending behavior (Borduin et al., 1990; Ertl & McNamara, 1997). Furthermore, assessments tend to include family interviews (Sciarra, 1999; Veneziano & Veneziano, 2002), which allow treatment providers to assess levels of family dysfunction and develop interventions accordingly. Empathy training also allows JSOs to consider the impact of their offending behaviors beyond the immediate consequences of getting caught (Ertl & McNamara, 1997). For example, JSOs are taught to consider the impact of their actions on the victim, the victim's family, and their own family. Further, group therapy and psycho- educational techniques provide JSOs with an opportunity to develop skills that promote prosocial peer development.

Many treatments promote resilience through external factors by including schools, families, communities, and groups in interventions. Incorporating individuals beyond the JSO's existing support structures presumably would have the benefit of producing treatment gains across settings. For example, by including school personnel in treatment, JSOs can not only begin to experience academic successes, but also can begin to develop problem solving and intellectual skills that can be utilized in discharge planning. Specifically, JSOs can begin to practice skills useful in developing strategies to prevent recidivism and to cope with difficult situations. Thus, integrating different aspects of the community allows JSOs to extend their skills and develop larger support groups.

Summary

In summary, while JSO treatment programs do not target resilience directly as a goal of treatment, currently used intervention techniques and modalities do provide an opportunity to develop resilience. The implications of existing research suggest that incorporating resilience into JSO treatment may improve rehabilitative efforts of treatment providers (Dewhurst & Nielsen, 1999). This is especially salient given that the one efficacy study of JSO treatment to date has involved incorporating into treatment important strategies to promote resiliency and has demonstrated effectiveness in reducing recidivism rates (Borduin et al., 1990). Incorporating resilience into existing treatment designs by enhancing internal and external factors associated with resilience will benefit all parties involved in JSO treatments.

DISCUSSION AND FUTURE DIRECTIONS

The research literature on characteristics of JSOs who reoffend, factors associated with resiliency, and characteristics of JSO treatments were reviewed in this article. Concerns have been raised about the paucity of empirical studies, problems in definition, and the scientific quality of existing research (Camp & Thyer, 1993; Swenson, Henggeler, & Schoenwald, 1998). These concerns are largely due to high rates of attrition (Hunter & Figueredo, 1999), low base rates of juvenile sex offending in the general population (Kahn & Chambers, 1991), and the infancy of juvenile sex offending as a recognized criminal offense (Zolondek et al., 2001).

While researchers may have little control over extraneous variables mentioned above, they do have the ability to assess successes of JSOs; that is, it is possible to assess outcomes suggestive of resilience as opposed to focusing almost exclusively on recidivism. Despite the abilities of treatment providers and researchers to learn about past successes and areas of competence in JSOs, it is unclear whether these persons do so. To date, there is only one published article, a literature review, which suggests including the concept of resilience in treatment of sex offenders (Dewhurst & Nielsen, 1990).

Studying resilience in JSOs is complicated because resilience has not been consistently defined in the literature. Presumably this is the case because the construct is both difficult to quantify and not well understood. Literature on resiliency in general has few standards to guide the operational definitions of the construct. Furthermore, there are few agreed upon standards regarding research methodology and data analysis techniques when studying resilience (Heller et al., 1999). While there have been longitudinal studies on the topic (Werner & Smith, 1982), there are few empirical studies/measures that evaluate resilience (Jew et al., 1999).

Resilience literature includes studies of overcoming a variety of risk factors and situations. While this research has not directly examined resilience in youth who sexually offend, it provides a wide knowledge base for inference. That is, this literature has examined both internal and external factors associated with resilience that can be compared to characteristics of JSOs. Comparing resilience factors with characteristics of JSOs who reoffend and JSOs who do not reoffend may prove more useful. Utilizing the concept of resiliency within JSO treatment allows treatment providers and JSOs to identify healthy solutions to emotional and situational problems (Dewhurst & Nielsen, 1999), and may prevent recidivism.

While research on JSOs has examined risk factors for negative outcomes, there have been no attempts to identify the protective, resilience factors of JSOs. Practitioners working with this population could save time by utilizing existing areas of competence and mastery in treatment of JSOs. Individuals who experience success in at least one area of their life may well be demonstrating the capacity for success in other areas. JSOs are a heterogeneous group, but research has already shown that they exhibit success through low rates of substance use, infrequent gang membership, low rates of truancy, and demonstration of acceptable social skills (Kaufman, Hilliker, & Daleiden, 1996; Zolondek et al., 2001). Incorporating approaches that promote resiliency may result in more frequent and significant positive outcomes for JSOs.

Research has demonstrated that JSOs and delinquent peers are similar in areas of deficit or psychopathology (e.g., Blaske, Borduin, Henggeler, & Mann, 1989; Ford & Linney, 1995; Hastings, Anderson, & Hemphill, 1997) and that both groups are different from normal peers (e.g., Hastings et al., 1997; Valliant & Bergeron, 1997). However, presuming that these patterns would exist when examining resiliency may be problematic, and thus comparisons of internal and external factors associated with resiliency (i.e., a strength-based approach) appear needed.

Given the nonexistence of current literature on the topic, the methodologically simple approach of obtaining a sample of JSOs and a similar group of other non-offending adolescents and comparing scores on a measure of resilience would serve as a first step to further this line of research. To that end, Efta-Breitbach and Freeman (2003) recently compared the scores of 28 JSOs and 29 normal peers on the Behavioral and Emotional Rating Scale (BERS), a measure specifically designed to investigate strengths (Epstein & Sharma, 1998). Results showed that JSOs had lower resilience scores in the domains of overall resilience, interpersonal strength, family involvement, intrapersonal strength, and affective strength. No differences were found with regards to school functioning. These initial results suggest that JSOs are different than non-offending, non-delinquent peers in many areas of strength.

In addition to evaluating similarities and differences in patterns of strength among JSOs as compared to other adolescent populations, research assessing JSOs' resilience factors prior to entering treatment, and when completing (or dropping out of) treatment would be useful in determining if existing treatments are specifically promoting resilience. Again, relatively simplistic methodological approaches (e.g., pre-post comparisons with a control group) could be used to evaluate how interventions affect resiliency. Finally, outcome studies comparing different modalities of treatments and resilience levels at completion of treatment are warranted. This research would help providers select the most appropriate treatments to promote positive outcomes. Of course, these last two areas of proposed research are predicated on the increase of systematic evaluation of treatment for JSOs in general, which in and of itself is lacking (Veneziano & Veneziano, 2002).

In conclusion, JSOs represent a population in particular need of research and services. Professionals treating JSOs have experienced success in decreasing sexual offending behaviors (Becker & Hunter, 1997; Hagan & Gust-Brey, 1999; Langstrom & Grann, 2000). However, little attention has been paid to assessing whether more generalized positive outcomes are demonstrated, which would suggest promotion of resilience. In fact, the findings that JSOs often have high nonsexual offending recidivism rates argues that current intervention attempts may not be well suited to foster resiliency. The field is plagued not only by an absence of empirical research to support existing treatment methodologies, but also by a quest for knowledge complicated by the legal rights and complexities associated with juvenile offenders and their justice system.

Existing research has not adequately addressed positive outcomes or resilience in JSOs. The introduction of a resiliency-based approach to sexual offender treatment has the potential of shifting the perspective of JSO treatment providers away from the "deficit" mentality that often underpins their thinking about this population (Dewhurst & Nielsen, 1999). Positive strengths and positive traits that coexist with the offending behavior are often ignored or if acknowledged, not addressed in treatment because they are not directly related to risk factors that predict recidivism (Dewhurst &

Nielsen, 1999). It is difficult for people to progress in treatment and maintain change if they are only avoiding negative behaviors. For change to be
maintained and generalized, JSOs need to move toward goals and replace
offense behaviors with positive behaviors. While some current treatment
interventions and goals are consistent with fostering resilience in JSO
youth, many are not. JSO treatments need to integrate more of the existing
positive behaviors and outlooks in current treatments to build resilience.
Promoting resilience and competence in the development of at-risk youth,
including JSOs, is a fundamental aspect of decreasing dire circumstance in
their futures.

REFERENCES

Able, G.G., Becker, J.V., Mittelman, M., Cunningham-Rathner, J., Rouleau, J.L., &
Murphy, W.D. (1987). Self-reported sex crimes of nonincarcerated paraphiliacs.
Journal of Interpersonal Violence, 2, 3-25.

Able, G.G., Mittleman, M.S., & Becker, J.V. (1985). Sexual offenders: Results of assessment and recommendations for treatment in clinical criminology. In M.H.
Ben-Aron, S.J. Hucker, & C.D. Webster (Eds.), *The assessment and treatment of
criminal behavior* (pp. 191-205). Toronto: M&M Graphic.

Barnes, G.G. (1999). Divorce transitions: Identifying risk and promoting resilience for
children and their parental relationships. *Journal of Marital and Family Therapy, 25*,
425-441.

Becker, J.V. (1990). Treating adolescent sexual offenders. *Professional Psychology:
Research and Practice, 21*, 362-365.

Becker, J.V., & Hunter, J.A. (1997). Understanding and treating child and adolescent
sexual offenders. *Advances in Clinical Child Psychology, 19*, 177-197.

Becker, J.V., Kaplan, M.S., & Kavoussi, R. (1988). Measuring the effectiveness of
treatment for the aggressive adolescent sexual offender. *Annals of the New York
Academy of Science, 528*, 215-222.

Becker, J.V., Kaplan, M.S., Tenke, C.E., & Tartaglini, A. (1991). The incidence of depressive symptomatology in juvenile sex offenders with a history of abuse. *Child
Abuse & Neglect, 15*, 531-536.

Blaske, D.M., Borduin, C.M., Henggeler, S.W., & Mann, B.J. (1989). Individual, family, and peer characteristics of adolescent sex offenders and assaultive offenders.
Developmental Psychology, 25, 846-855.

Borduin, C.M., Henggeler, S.W., Blaske, D.M., & Stein, R.J. (1990). Multisystemic
treatment of adolescent sexual offenders. *International Journal of Offender Therapy
and Comparative Criminology, 34*, 105-113.

Bourke, M.L., & Donohue, B. (1996). Assessment and treatment of juvenile sex offenders: An empirical review. *Journal of Child Sexual Abuse, 5*, 47-70.

Bremer, J.F. (1992). Serious juvenile sex offenders: Treatment and long-term follow-up. *Psychiatric Annals, 22*, 326-332.

Brown, F., Flanagan, T., & McLeod, M. (Eds.). (1984). *Sourcebook of criminal justice statistics.* Washington, DC: Bureau of Justice Statistics.

Camp, B.H., & Thyer, B.A. (1993). Treatment of adolescent sex offenders: A review of empirical research. *The Journal of Applied Social Sciences, 17,* 191-206.

Cicchetti, D., & Garmezy, N. (1993). Prospects and promises in the study of resilience. *Development and Psychopathology, 5,* 497-502.

Cooper, C.L., Murphy, W.D., & Haynes, M.R. (1996). Characteristics of abused and nonabused adolescent sexual offenders. *Sexual Abuse: A Journal of Research and Treatment, 8,* 105-119.

Dalzell, H.J. (1998). Giftedness: Infancy to adolescence–a developmental perspective. *Roeper Review, 20,* 259-265.

Dewhurst, A.M., & Nielsen, K.M. (1999). A resiliency-based approach to working with sexual offenders. *Sexual Addiction & Compulsivity: The Journal of Treatment and Prevention, 6,* 271-279.

Doll, B., & Lyon, M.A. (1998). Risk and resilience: Implications for the delivery of educational and mental health services in schools. *School Psychology Review, 27,* 348-364.

Dumont, M., & Provost, M.A. (1999). Resilience in adolescents: Protective role of social support, coping strategies, self-esteem, and social activities on experience of stress and depression. *Journal of Youth and Adolescence, 28,* 343-363.

Efta-Breitbach, J., & Freeman, K.A. (2003). *Assessing resilience among juvenile sex offenders and non-offending peers.* Unpublished manuscript.

Egeland, B., Carlson, E., & Sroufe, L.A. (1993). Resilience as process. *Development and Psychopathology, 5,* 715-528.

Egeland, B., Jacobvitz, P., & Sroufe, L.A. (1988). Breaking the cycle of abuse. *Child Development, 59,* 1080-1088.

Eisenberg, N., Guthrie, I.K., Fabes, R.A., Reiser, M., Murphy, B.C., Holgren, R., Maszk, P., & Losoya, S. (1998). The relations of regulation and emotionality to resiliency and competent social functioning in elementary school children. *Child Development, 68,* 295-311.

Elder, G.H., Nguyen, T.V., & Caspi, A. (1985). Linking family hardship to children's lives. *Child Development, 56,* 361-375.

Engle, P.L., Castle, S., & Menon, P. (1996). Child development: Vulnerability and resilience. *Social Science & Medicine, 43,* 621-635.

Epstein, M.H., & Sharma, J.M. (1998). *Behavioral and Emotional Rating Scale-Manual.* Austin, Texas: Pro-Ed, Incorporated.

Ertl, M.A., & McNamara, J.R. (1997). Treatment of juvenile sex offenders: A review of the literature. *Child and Adolescent Social Work Journal, 14,* 199-221.

Felten, B.S. (2000). Resilience in a multicultural sample of community-dwelling women older than age 85. *Clinical Nursing Research, 9,* 102-124.

Ford, M.E., & Linney, J.A. (1995). Comparative analysis of juvenile sexual offenders, violent nonsexual offenders, and status offenders. *Journal of Interpersonal Violence, 10,* 56-70.

Freitas, A.L., & Downey, G. (1998). Resilience: A dynamic perspective. *International Journal Behavioral Development, 22,* 263-285.

Hagan, M.P., & Gust-Brey, K. L. (1999). A ten-year longitudinal study of adolescent rapists upon return to the community. *International Journal of Offender Therapy and Comparative Criminology, 43*, 448-458.

Hanson, R.K., & Bussiere, M.T. (1998). Predicting relapse: A meta-analysis of sexual offender recidivism studies. *Journal of Consulting and Clinical Psychology, 66*, 348-362.

Hastings, T., Anderson, S.J., & Hemphill, P. (1997). Comparisons of daily stress, coping, problem behavior, and cognitive distortions in adolescent sexual offenders and conduct-disordered youth. *Sexual Abuse: Journal of Research & Treatment, 9*, 29-42.

Heller, S.S., Larrieu, J.A., D-Imperio, R., & Boris, N.W. (1999). Research on resilience to child maltreatment: Empirical considerations. *Child Abuse & Neglect, 23*, 321-338.

Henry, D.L. (1999). Resilience in maltreated children: Implications for special needs adoption. *Child Welfare, 78*, 519-541.

Himelein, M.J., & McElrath, J.V. (1996). Resilient child sexual abuse survivors: Cognitive coping and illusion. *Child Abuse & Neglect, 20*, 747-758.

Hunter, J.A., & Becker J.V. (1994). The role of deviant sexual arousal in juvenile sexual offending: Etiology, evaluation, and treatment. *Criminal Justice and Behavior, 21*, 132-149.

Hunter, J.A., & Figueredo, A.J. (1999). Factors associated with treatment compliance in a population of juvenile sexual offenders. *Sexual Abuse: A Journal of Research and Treatment, 11*, 49-67.

Jacobs, W.L., Wallace, K.A., & Meyer, J.B. (1997). Juvenile delinquents: A between-group comparison study of sexual and nonsexual offenders. *Sexual Abuse: A Journal of Research and Treatment, 9*, 201-217.

Jew, C.L., Green, K.E., & Kroger, J. (1999). Development and validation of a measure of resiliency. *Measurement & Evaluation in Counseling & Development, 32*, 75-91.

Kagan, J. (1975). Resilience in cognitive development. *Ethos, 3*, 231-247.

Kahn, T.J., & Chambers, H.J. (1991). Assessing reoffense risk with juvenile sexual offenders. *Child Welfare, 70*, 333-345.

Kahn, T.J., & Lafond, M.A. (1988). Treatment of the adolescent sexual offender. *Child and Adolescent Social Work, 5*, 135-148.

Kaufman, K.L., Hilliker, D.R., & Daleiden, E.L. (1996). Subgroup difference in the modus operandi of adolescent sexual offenders. *Child Maltreatment, 1*, 17-24.

Kavoussi, R.J., Kaplan, M., & Becker, J.V. (1988). Psychiatric diagnosis in adolescent sex offenders. *Journal of the American Academy of Child and Adolescent Psychiatry, 27*, 214-243.

Knight, R.A., & Sims-Knight, J.E. (2004). Testing an etiological model for male juvenile sexual offending against females. *Journal of Child Sexual Abuse, 13*(3/4), pp. 33-56.

Kraemer, B.D., & Salisbury, S.B. (1998). Pretreatment variables associated with treatment failure in a residential juvenile sex-offender program. *Criminal Justice & Behavior, 25*, 190-203.

Langstrom, N., & Grann, M. (2000). Risk for criminal recidivism among young sex offenders. *Journal of Interpersonal Violence*, *15*, 855-871.

Lombardo, R., & DiGiorgio-Miller, J. (1988). Concepts and techniques in working with juvenile sex offenders. *Journal of Offender Counseling, Services & Rehabilitation*, *13*, 39-53.

Long, J.V.F., & Vaillant, G.E. (1984). Natural history of male psychological health, XI: Escape from the underclass. *American Journal of Psychiatry*, *141*, 341-346.

Luthar, S.S. (1991). Vulnerability and resilience: A study of high-risk adolescents. *Child Development*, *62*, 600-616.

Masten, A.S., Best, K.M., & Garmezy, N. (1990). Resilience and development: Contributions from the study of children who overcome adversity. *Development and Psychopathology*, *2*, 425-444.

Masten, A.S., & Coatsworth, J.D. (1998). The development of competence in favorable and unfavorable environments: Lessons from research on successful children. *American Psychologist*, *53*, 205-220.

Mathews, R., Hunter, J.A., & Vuz, J. (1997). Juvenile female sexual offenders: Clinical characteristics and treatment issues. *Sexual Abuse: A Journal of Research and Treatment*, *9*, 187-199.

Office of Juvenile Justice and Delinquency. (1999, September 30). *OJJDP statistical briefing Book*. Retrieved from http://www.ojjdp.ncjrs.org/ojstatbb/qa136.html

Prentky, R., Harris, B., Frizzell, K., & Righthand, S. (2000). An actuarial procedure for assessing risk with juvenile sex offenders. *Sexual Abuse: A Journal of Research and Treatment*, *12*, 71-93.

Rak, C.F., & Patterson, L.F. (1996). Promoting resilience in at-risk children. *Journal of Counseling & Development*, *74*, 368-374.

Rasmussen, L. A. (1999). Factors related to recidivism among juvenile sexual offenders. *Sexual Abuse: A Journal of Research and Treatment*, *11*, 69-86.

Righthand, S., & Welch, C. (2004). Characteristics of youth who sexually offend. *Journal of Child Sexual Abuse*, *13*(3/4), pp. 15-32.

Sciarra, D. T. (1999). Assessment and treatment of adolescent sex offenders: A review from a cross-cultural perspective. *Journal of Offender Rehabilitation*, *28*, 103-118.

Seifer, R., Sameroff, A.J., Baldwin, C.P., & Baldwin, A. (1992). Child and family factors that ameliorate risk between 4 and 13 years of age. *Journal of the American Academy of Child and Adolescent Psychiatry*, *31*, 893-903.

Sipe, R., Jensen, E.L., & Everett, R.S. (1998). Adolescent sexual offenders grown up: Recidivism in young adulthood. *Criminal Justice and Behavior*, *25*, 109-124.

Smith, W.R., & Monastersky, C. (1986). Assessing juvenile sexual offenders' risk for reoffending. *Criminal Justice and Behavior*, *13*, 115-140.

Studer, L.H., & Reddon, J.R. (1998). Treatment may change risk prediction for sexual offenders. *Sexual Abuse: Journal of Research & Treatment*, *10*, 175-181.

Swenson, C.C., Henggeler, S.W., & Schoenwald, S.K. (1998). Changing the social ecologies of adolescent sexual offenders: Implications of the success of multisystemic therapy in treating serious antisocial behavior in adolescents. *Child Maltreatment*, *3*, 330-339.

Valentine, L., & Feinauer, L. L. (1993). Resilience factors associated with female survivors of childhood sexual abuse. *The American Journal of Family Therapy*, *21*, 216-224.

Valliant, P.M., & Bergeron, T. (1997). Personality and criminal profile of adolescent sexual offenders, general offenders in comparison to nonoffenders. *Psychological Reports*, *81*, 483-489.

Veneziano, C., & Veneziano, L. (2002). Adolescent sex offenders: A review of the literature. *Trauma Violence & Abuse*, *3*, 247-260.

Walsh, F. (1996). The concept of family resilience: Crisis and challenge. *Family Process*, *35*, 261-281.

Weist, M.D., Freedman, A.H., Paskewitz, D.A., Proescher, E.J., & Flaherty, L.T. (1995). Urban youth under stress: Empirical identification of protective factors. *Journal of Youth and Adolescence*, *24*, 705-721.

Werner, E.E., & Smith, R.S. (1982). *Vulnerable but invincible*. New York: McGraw-Hill Book Company.

Winfield, L.F. (1991). Resilience, schooling, and development in African-American youth. *Education & Urban Society*, *24*, 5-15.

Wolff, S. (1995). The concept of resilience. *Australian and New Zealand Journal of Psychiatry*, *29*, 565-574.

Wolin, S.J., & Wolin, S. (1993). *The resilient self*. New York: Villard Books.

Zolondek, S., Abel, G.G., Northey, W.F., & Jordan, A.D. (2001). The self-reported behaviors of juvenile sexual offenders. *Journal of Interpersonal Violence*, *16*, 73-85.

Treatment Effectiveness
for Male Adolescent Sexual Offenders:
A Meta-Analysis and Review

Donald F. Walker
Shannon K. McGovern
Evelyn L. Poey
Kathryn E. Otis

SUMMARY. Research concerning the treatment of sexual offenders has generally focused on the treatment of adult offenders. The effectiveness of treatments for male adolescent sexual offenders ($N = 644$) was assessed in a meta-analysis of 10 studies. Overall, the results were surprisingly encouraging, suggesting that treatments for male adolescent sexual offenders appear generally effective ($r = .37$). Studies which used self-report measures of outcome obtained a 6% higher effect size than studies which used measures of arousal in response to deviant stimuli, and a 22% higher effect size than studies using actual recidivism rates. A descriptive review of the set of 10 studies indicates that studies utilizing cognitive-behavioral therapy approaches were the most effective. *[Article copies available for a fee from The Haworth Document Delivery Service: 1-800-HAWORTH. E-mail*

Address correspondence to: Donald F. Walker, MA, 789 North Orange Grove Boulevard, Pasadena, CA 91103 (E-mail: dfwalker@hotmail.com).

[Haworth co-indexing entry note]: "Treatment Effectiveness for Male Adolescent Sexual Offenders: A Meta-Analysis and Review." Walker, Donald F. et al. Co-published simultaneously in *Journal of Child Sexual Abuse* (The Haworth Maltreatment and Trauma Press, an imprint of The Haworth Press, Inc.) Vol. 13, No. 3/4, 2004, pp. 281-293; and: *Identifying and Treating Youth Who Sexually Offend: Current Approaches, Techniques, and Research* (ed: Robert Geffner et al.) The Haworth Maltreatment and Trauma Press, an imprint of The Haworth Press, Inc., 2004, pp. 281-293. Single or multiple copies of this article are available for a fee from The Haworth Document Delivery Service [1-800-HAWORTH, 9:00 a.m. - 5:00 p.m. (EST). E-mail address: docdelivery@haworthpress.com].

Digital Object Identifier: 10.1300/J070v13n03_14

address: <docdelivery@haworthpress. com> Website: <http://www.Haworth Press.com>

KEYWORDS. Adolescent, male, sex offenders, treatment effectiveness, meta-analysis

Research indicates that approximately 20% of rapes and 30% to 50% of child molestations are committed by adolescent sexual offenders (Morenz & Becker, 1995), and that as many as 50% of adult sexual offenders committed their first sexual offense in adolescence (Davis & Leitenberg, 1987). Although the effectiveness of treatments for adult sexual offenders has been hotly debated (e.g., Furby, Weinrott, & Blackshaw, 1989; Hall, 1995; Marshall, 1993; Marshall & Pithers, 1994; Quinsey, Rice, Harris, & Lalumiere, 1993), this concern has generally not extended to the treatment of adolescent sexual offenders. This suggests the need for further study of treatment approaches for adolescent sexual offenders (Barbaree, Marshall, & Hudson, 1993).

Since Barbaree and associates' (1993) call for additional work concerning male adolescent sexual offenders, two review articles and additional treatment studies have been done in the area, suggesting that it is now appropriate to perform a meta-analysis of the accumulated research. The purpose of this study is to provide a meta-analysis and review of treatments for male adolescent sexual offenders. What follows is a review of the treatment outcome literature for male adolescent sexual offenders, followed by a meta-analysis of the effectiveness of treatment for adolescent sexual offenders, and a descriptive review of treatment effectiveness for male adolescent sexual offenders by type of treatment modality.

TREATMENT APPROACHES
FOR MALE ADOLESCENT SEXUAL OFFENDERS

Morenz and Becker (1995) provided the most recent review of treatment approaches for adolescent sexual offenders. They noted that the most common treatment modalities consisted of cognitive-behavioral therapy, individual and family therapy, psychoeducational interventions, relapse prevention, and biological treatment. Cognitive-behavioral approaches are quite common and typically include (a) confrontation of the offense, (b) the development of empathy for the victim, (c) the use of the offender's own experience of being sexually victimized, (d) anger and stress management, (e) social skills training, (f) relapse prevention, and (g) treatment of substance abuse (for a detailed description of a cognitive-behavioral treatment model, see Kolko, Noel, Thomas, & Torres, this issue). Relapse prevention attempts to make adolescent offenders aware of the multiple factors that may lead to reoffending and help the adolescent manage each of the factors. Psychoeducational interventions typically address such topics as sexual knowledge, problem solving, and moral judgment. Biological treatment is far less frequent in the United States due to its controversial nature and includes castration, cyproterone acetate, medroxyprogesterone acetate, and stereotaxic neurosurgery (Camp & Thyer, 1993).

MEASURING TREATMENT EFFECTIVENESS

An important theoretical distinction is necessary between treatment effectiveness and treatment efficacy. Treatment efficacy is demonstrated when studies utilize random clinical trials in which participants are randomly assigned to either a treatment or comparison group (Chambless & Hollon, 1998). This provides a controlled manipulation in which it is reasonable to conclude that the effects are due to treatment rather than to confounding factors not under the control of the experimenter. There are relatively few studies of treatment efficacy available in the treatment literature for male adolescent sexual offenders. Treatment effectiveness, conversely, refers to whether or not a treatment can be demonstrated to work in clinical practice (Chambless & Hollon, 1998). Research designs attempting to demonstrate treatment effectiveness can include experimental designs with control groups, as well as nonexperimental and quasi-experimental research designs.

Treatment effectiveness with male adolescent sexual offenders has been measured through three ways: (a) recidivism rates, (b) self-report measures, and (c) the measurement of the adolescent offender's arousal while exposed to sexual stimuli such as audio or videotapes. Camp and Thyer (1993) reviewed these three methods of assessing treatment effectiveness and concluded that the use of recidivism rates continued to be the most popular method. This is regardless of the fact that recidivism rates may be unreliable due to (a) follow-up periods that are too short, (b) empirical evidence suggesting that recidivism rates for adolescent sexual offenders are extremely low (e.g., Davis & Leitenberg, 1987), and (c) methodological problems inherent in using recidivism rates as a scale, including problems of different definitions of recidivism across studies and in accurately recording recidivism. Camp and Thyer noted that self-report measures were used less frequently due to the fear of methodological problems and the questionable validity of self-report measures with this population. Finally, Camp and Thyer questioned the reliability of the measurement of arousal and the degree to which it may be susceptible to faking. Hence, further evaluation of treatment effectiveness needs to check the similarity of results across these methods of evaluating outcomes.

Addressing the adolescent offender treatment literature more broadly, Mulvey, Arthur, and Reppucci (1993) argued that a major methodological barrier to assessing the effectiveness of treatment for adolescent offenders is the "lack of specification of the theoretical bases or mediating processes that tie specific strategies to expected decreases in delinquent behavior" (p. 135). Such variables could include type of treatment and therapist qualifications in the delivery of treatment.

This study sought to add to the treatment literature for adolescent sexual offenders in several ways. First, recent reviews provided by Camp and Thyer (1993) and Morenz and Becker (1995) have identified common treatment modalities used in the treatment of adolescent sexual offenders and difficulties associated with measuring treatment outcomes. Our meta-analysis sought to extend those reviews by first quantitatively determining the effectiveness of treatment for adolescent sexual offenders by computing an overall weighted, averaged r across all studies. Second, we attempted to compare the degree to which the effectiveness of treatment was dependent upon the type of measure being used to assess outcome (i.e., recidivism, self-report, or measurement of arousal to deviant sexual stimuli). Finally, we sought to descriptively review variables (such as type of treatment and therapist qualifications in the delivery of treatment) that affected the outcome of treatment.

METHOD

Study Selection

Studies were selected for the meta-analysis using (a) major reviews of the literature provided by Camp and Thyer (1993) and Morenz and Becker (1995), (b) literature searches in both the PsychInfo and Dissertation Abstracts International databases using the search terms "adolescent sexual offenders" and "treatments for adolescent sexual offenders," (c) Internet searches using the phrase "treatments for adolescent sexual offenders," (d) electronic mail sent to organizations and individuals identified via the Internet search who appeared to possibly have unpublished reports on treatments for adolescent sexual offenders, and (e) electronic mail and phone calls both to authors who had previously published work in the area and to editors of relevant journals who might have articles not yet published. Unpublished studies such as dissertations and unpublished reports were solicited because it has been suggested that most published studies yield significant results and higher effect sizes more often than unpublished studies. Rosenthal (1979) calls this the "file drawer problem" and warns that meta-analyses that do not include unpublished studies may produce larger overall effect sizes than the entire body of literature would suggest.

On the basis of these searches, 12 studies were identified. Of the 12 studies, 2 used a dependent measure of outcome which did not involve (a) recidivism, (b) self-report measures of deviant sexual attitudes and behaviors, or (c) level of arousal in relation to deviant sexual stimuli. These studies were excluded, leaving 10 studies. Three studies used measures of recidivism as their dependent measure, four studies used paper and pencil tests of deviant sexual attitudes and behaviors, and three studies used level of arousal in response to deviant sexual stimuli as their dependent measure. Of these 10 studies, 7 were published journal articles and 3 were unpublished dissertations.

Coding of Studies

The 10 studies that contained outcome measures of interest were coded for the meta-analysis using several categories suggested by Rosenthal (1991). These categories included (a) type of treatment as labeled by the author(s), (b) therapist qualifications, (c) mortality rate within the treatment group, (d) mortality rate within the control group, (e) type of publication (published article vs. unpublished dissertation), and (f) outcome measure (recidivism, self-report, or level of arousal).

Calculations

An overall weighted averaged *r* for the 10 studies was computed as an effect size for treatment, as recommended by Rosenthal (1991). In this procedure, the individual correlation in a given study is multiplied times the number of participants in the study. This is done for each study, and then summed. The sum is then divided by the total number of participants in all studies to provide the overall averaged correlation.

Studies that reported indices other than *r* were transformed into *r*'s using formulas provided by Rosenthal (1991). Chi-square values were converted to correlations by dividing the chi-square by the total number of participants in the study and then taking the square root of that number. *F* values were converted to correlations by dividing the *F* value by the *F* value plus the degrees of freedom error and then taking the square root of that number.

Separate overall weighted, averaged *r*'s were also calculated for the three studies that used recidivism as an outcome measure, the four studies that used self-report measures, and the three studies that used a measure of arousal in relation to deviant sexual stimuli. These were weighted by the number of participants in each individual study being included in the computation of the overall weighted averaged *r*.

Estimates of observed variance, sampling error variance, and population variance were also calculated. Observed variance is the sum of the weighted squared difference between the observed correlation in each study and the overall averaged correlation. Sampling error refers to the difference between the value of a sample statistic and the value of a corresponding population parameter (Jaccard & Becker, 1990). Population variance was calculated by subtracting the sampling error variance from the observed error variance. Finally, the number of studies averaging null results that were needed to bring the overall *p* level to .05 was calculated using a formula from Rosenthal (1991). In this formula, the *Z* value for *p* = .05 is 1.645, which is equal to the number of studies combined (in this instance, 10) times the mean *Z* obtained for the 10 studies, divided by the square root of the number of studies (10) plus *X*, the number being solved for.

RESULTS

To determine the overall effectiveness of treatments for adolescent sexual offenders across all 10 studies, the overall weighted averaged *r* was computed (*r* = .37). Next, estimates of observed error (.05), sampling error (.01), and population variance (.04) were calculated. Then, a series of small meta-analyses were conducted by calculating separate overall weighted averaged *r*'s for the set of three studies which used future sexual recidivism as an outcome measure (*r* = .26), the set of four studies which used self-report measures as an outcome measure (*r* = .48), and the set of three studies which used level of arousal in relation to deviant sexual stimuli (*r* = .42). Finally, the number of studies with null results required to bring the overall *p* level to .05 was calculated. Rosenthal's (1991) formula indicated that 139 studies with null results would be required to bring these results to a *p* level of .05.

A description of the 10 studies that were included in the meta-analysis is presented in Table 1. An inspection of Table 1 indicates that three of the four studies which had effect sizes higher than .50 contained treatment packages that were either cognitive-behavioral or multi-systemic therapy.

The impact upon treatment effect size by therapist qualifications was the other relationship of interest to us. An inspection of Table 1 indicates that 5 of the 10 studies did not report the qualifications of the therapists in their study. Of the remaining five, licensed psychologists (only one in this category, and it had a mix of master's level practitioners) or doctoral level students were used in four of the studies, yielding r's in the range of .39 to .77. The remaining study (Brannon & Troyer, 1991) utilized bachelor's level therapists, and obtained an effect size of .14. The odds of these results occurring due to chance are .2.

An attempt was made to determine whether the mortality of the treatment or control group impacted the effect size obtained in the study. This analysis was not possible, due to the fact that five studies (50%) did not report the mortality of the treatment group in the study, and eight studies (80%) did not have a control group as part of the study.

A final descriptive analysis attempted to compare the effect sizes obtained in journals versus those obtained in dissertations. This was not possible, due to the fact that two of the three dissertations used cognitive-behavioral treatment methods, and, as noted earlier, cognitive-behavioral treatments yielded the largest effect sizes of any treatment modality.

DISCUSSION

The central purpose of this study was to determine the effectiveness of treatments for male adolescent sexual offenders via meta-analysis. Somewhat surprisingly, the results obtained in this meta-analysis suggested that treatments appear effective (overall weighted averaged $r = .37$). Indeed, even the poorest result with the least impacted dependent variable (recidivism) compares quite favorably (overall weighted averaged $r = .26$) with those obtained by Hall's (1995) meta-analysis of 12 studies of treatments for primarily adult sexual offenders, in which recidivism rates were used exclusively as an outcome measure and an overall effect size of .12 was obtained. Also somewhat surprisingly, a strikingly small amount of variance due to error (.01) was obtained, which suggests that the results were largely due to treatment effects.

As noted earlier, larger overall weighted averaged r's were obtained in separate meta-analyses for those studies which used self-report ($r = .48$) and level of arousal in response to deviant sexual stimuli ($r = .42$), than for those studies which used a measure of sexual offense recidivism ($r = .26$). As suggested earlier, the use of recidivism rates in any study of treatment effectiveness for adolescent sexual offenders is problematic, due to difficulties with follow-up periods that may not reflect the actual amount of recidivism, and with inaccurate reporting

TABLE 1. Description of the 10 Studies Included in the Meta-Analysis

Study	N	Type of Tx	Therapist	MT	MC	Pub	r	DV
Haines, Herrman, Baker, & Graber (1986)	9	Psycho Ed	Psychologist, MSW	-	-	Journal	.65	SR
Borduin, Henggler, Blake, & Stein (1990)	16	MST	PhD Students	37.5%	37.5%	Journal	.54	R
Brannon & Troyer (1991)	53	Residential	BA Level	-	NA	Journal	.14	R
Bromberg (1991)	199	Eclectic	-	-	NA	Diss	.48	SR
Kahn & Chambers (1991)	221	Eclectic	-	-	NA	Journal	.27	R
Hunter & Goodwin (1992)	27	ST	-	-	NA	Journal	.42	P
Kaplan, Morales, & Becker (1993)	15	CBT	-	62%	NA	Journal	.66	P
Knox (1994)	25	CBT	PhD Students	0	NA	Diss	.39	SR
Piliero (1994)	10	CBT	PhD Students	0	40%	Diss	.77	SR
Weinrott, Riggan, & Frothingham (1997)	69	VS	-	26%	NA	Journal	.37	P

Note. MT = mortality of treatment condition; MC = mortality of control group; Pub = publication type; r = Pearson's product moment correlation; DV = type of dependent variable; MST = multisystemic therapy; CBT = cognitive behavioral therapy; PsychoEd = psychoeducational therapy; ST = satiation therapy; VS = vicarious sensitization; - = not reported in the study; NA = not available as part of the study due to not including it in the study; Diss = dissertation; R = sexual recidivism; SR = self-report; P = penile plethysmograph. In studies that did not utilize a control group, pre and post measures for the single group were the independent variables correlated with outcome.

procedures (Camp & Thyer, 1993). These difficulties account for the differences in effect size that are obtained when using different outcome measures.

It should be noted, however, that both the overall averaged *r* calculated for recidivism and the overall averaged *r* across all 10 studies were at least twice as high as the effect size of .12 obtained in Hall's (1995) meta-analysis, which was comprised mainly of adult sex offender samples. As Camp and Thyer (1993) noted that methodological difficulties arise in this population regardless of the type of outcome measure being used, one recommendation for the assessment of therapy outcome with this population is to use all three methods of measuring outcome if possible. If more immediate results are desired and the collection of long-term recidivism data is not possible, both the measurement of arousal in relation to deviant sexual stimuli and the administration of self-report measures can be used in conjunction with each other, and can be administered in a relatively short amount of time.

Studies using cognitive-behavioral treatments (CBT) had the largest effect sizes. Given the generally positive results for this treatment modality, therapists treating male adolescent sexual offenders are encouraged to use cognitive-behavioral approaches. Becker and Murphy (1998) described a typical CBT approach to the treatment of adolescent sexual offenders. They noted that treatment typically focuses on reducing denial and cognitive distortions that adolescent sex offenders use to justify their offenses, and on identifying internal and external precursors to offending. Cognitive-behavioral techniques are also used to identify and reduce deviant sexual arousal and behavior. Social skills (such as assertiveness), problem solving, and anger management, are taught. Finally, empathy training is provided, with the rationale that the ability to experience empathy for a victim will help avoid future sexual offenses.

Given the effectiveness of CBT, it is suggested that future studies begin to test the effectiveness of cognitive-behavioral therapy against that of multisystemic therapy (MST, Henggeler, Schoenwald, & Pickrel, 1995), the other therapeutic modality that appeared promising in this study (e.g., Borduin, Henggler, Blake, & Stein, 1990). Such studies would allow the utilization of experimental designs with randomized clinical trials that are necessary to demonstrate the efficacy of treatment. Such studies would also provide additional information about the effectiveness of MST with adolescent sexual offenders. This information is needed given the general effectiveness of MST with violent juvenile offenders and other adolescent nonsexual offender populations.

In addition, as Becker and Johnson (2001) noted, it is important that researchers begin to evaluate the effectiveness of treatment with different categories of adolescent sexual offenders. Such research could be undertaken using a taxonomic classification system of sexual offenders that has been developed (e.g., Knight & Prentky, 1993; Prentky & Knight, 1991), but not utilized in studies of treatment effectiveness with adolescent sexual offenders.

Previous reviews of psychotherapy in general have indicated that clients of more qualified therapists have better outcomes in therapy (Stein & Lambert, 1995), and that the quality of the therapeutic relationship is the most significant predictor of positive change (Whiston & Sexton, 1993). The results of our descriptive review indicated that studies using more qualified therapists had better outcomes. One implication of these results for therapeutic practice is that agencies should utilize more qualified and experienced therapists. Training sites using student therapists would serve male adolescent sexual offender clients better by using therapists at a higher level such as internship rather than a lower level such as practicum. Such sites would also best serve their clientele and the public by providing interns with experienced postdoctoral supervisors rather than unlicensed doctoral personnel or postdoctoral supervisors who have just obtained their license. Additional supervision need not be limited to pre-doctoral therapists, however. As Mothersole (2000) noted, the idea that supervision is for junior staff only and that experienced clinicians cannot benefit from it is a myth.

Limitations of the Current Study

Methodologically, a large number of studies did not report mortality rates for the treatment group, and did not have either a control group or other comparison group that received a different form of treatment. This made it impossible to document the treatment efficacy of the treatments in the studies. As Henggeler, Smith, and Schoenwald (1994) noted in their review of adolescent offender research issues, research must show that treatment has an effect beyond what could be explained by other confounding factors such as cohort effects or other interventions. Such a task is difficult to complete without a comparison group receiving another treatment. Until more studies are conducted in which a control group is provided, the degree to which the overall effect size ($r = .37$) obtained here is due strictly to treatment effects must be interpreted cautiously.

However, an estimate of sampling error was computed precisely for the purpose of providing an index of how much the results were due to factors other than treatment. The index obtained as an estimate of sampling error was extremely low (.01), and strengthens the amount of confidence that can be placed in the results. In addition, the purpose of this study was to quantitatively determine the treatment effectiveness, not treatment efficacy, of treatments for adolescent sexual offenders at this time. As observed earlier, treatment effectiveness can be demonstrated with non-experimental and quasi-experimental studies such as were included in this meta-analysis. Further research is necessary using randomized clinical trials before these treatments can be considered efficacious (Chambless & Hollon, 1998).

This study was also limited by the relatively small number of studies *(N = 10)* available to perform the meta-analysis. Although the number of studies available for meta-analysis was small, this number was comparable to the number of studies meta-analysis was performed on in Hall's (1995) study of primarily adult sexual offenders. In addition to computing an effect size for the effectiveness of treatment, an index of the number of studies that would be required to make the obtained results null was also computed. The number of studies required to obtain null results according to this index was 139. This also strengthens the degree to which confidence can be placed in the results obtained here.

An argument could be made that combining the eight studies that did not have control groups with the two studies that did have control groups is an inappropriate use of meta-analysis. Rosenthal (1991) refers to this criticism of meta-analytic studies as that of the problem of heterogeneity of method. Following Glass (1978), Rosenthal refers to this also as the "apples and oranges issue," and suggests that they are good things to mix when attempting to generalize to fruit. In this meta-analysis, both studies that failed to include a comparison group and the two studies that did include comparison groups provided indexes of the overall effectiveness of treatment, allowing a generalization to a common index of effectiveness across those studies.

This study sought to determine how effective treatments are for male adolescent sexual offenders. Overall, the results obtained in this meta-analysis and review are surprisingly encouraging. While the number of studies is low at this time, the importance of reducing sexual aggression is so important that any guidance from these studies is needed. As practitioners continue to develop treatments to intervene in this critical period in the development of a male adolescent sexual offender, the profession can look forward to new advances in treatment, and ultimately, prevention.

REFERENCES

Barbaree, H. E., Marshall, W. L., & Hudson, D. (1993). *The juvenile sex offender.* New York: Guilford Press.

Becker, J. V., & Johnson, B. R. (2001). Treating juvenile sex offenders. In J. Ashford & B. Sales (Eds.), *Treating adult and juvenile sex offenders with special needs* (pp. 273-289). Washington, DC American Psychological Association.

Becker, J. V., & Murphy, W. D. (1998). What we know and do not know about assessing and treating sex offenders. *Psychology, Public Policy, and the Law, 4,* 116-137.

Borduin, C. M., Henggler, S. W., Blake, D. M., & Stein, R. J. (1990). Multisystemic treatment of adolescent sexual offenders. *International Journal of Offender Therapy and Comparative Criminology, 34,* 105-113.

Brannon, J. M., & Troyer, R. (1991). Peer group counseling: A normalized residential alternative to the specialized treatment of adolescent sex offenders. *International Journal of Offender Therapy and Comparative Criminology, 35,* 225-234.

Bromberg, C. K. (1991). *Pretreatment status, treatment intensity, and treatment outcome in male adolescent sex offenders.* Unpublished doctoral dissertation, California School of Professional Psychology.

Camp, B. H., & Thyer, B. A. (1993). Treatment of adolescent sex offenders: A review of empirical research. *The Journal of Applied Social Sciences, 17,* 191-206.

Chambless, D., & Hollon, S. D. (1998). Defining empirically supported therapies. *Journal of Consulting and Clinical Psychology, 66,* 7-18.

Davis, G. E., & Leitenberg, H. (1987). Adolescent sex offenders. *Psychological Bulletin, 101,* 417-427.

Furby, L., Weinrott, M. R., & Blackshaw, L. (1989). Sexual offender recidivism: A review. *Psychological Bulletin, 105,* 3-30.

Glass, G. V. (1978). In defense of generalization. *The Behavioral and Brain Sciences, 3,* 394-395.

Hains, A. A., Herrman, L. P., Baker, K. L., & Graber, S. (1986). The development of a psycho-educational group program for adolescent sex offenders. *Journal of Offender Counseling, Services, and Rehabilitation, 11,* 63-76.

Hall, G. C. N. (1995). Sexual offender recidivism revisited: A meta-analysis of recent treatment studies. *Journal of Consulting and Clinical Psychology, 63,* 802-809.

Henggeler, S. W., Schoenwald, S. K., & Pickrel, S. G. (1995). Multisystemic therapy: Bridging the gap between university and community-based treatment. *Journal of Consulting and Clinical Psychology, 63,* 709-717.

Henggeler, S. W., Smith, B. H., & Schoenwald, S. K. (1994). Key theoretical and methodological issues in conducting treatment research in the juvenile justice system. *Journal of Clinical Child Psychology, 23,* 143-150.

Hunter, J. A., & Goodwin, D. W. (1992). The clinical utility of satiation therapy with juvenile sex offenders: Variations and efficacy. *Annals of Sex Research, 5,* 71-80.

Jaccard, J., & Becker, M. A. (1990). *Statistics for the behavioral sciences* (2nd ed.). Belmont, CA: Brooks/Cole Publishing.

Kahn, T. J., & Chambers, H. J. (1991). Assessing reoffense risk with juvenile sexual offenders. *Child Welfare, 70,* 331-345.

Kaplan, M. S., Morales, M., & Becker, J. V. (1993). The impact of verbal satiation on adolescent sex offenders: A preliminary report. *Journal of Child Sexual Abuse, 2,* 81-88.

Knight, R. A., & Prentky, R. A. (1993). Exploring characteristics for classifying juvenile sex offenders. In H.E. Barbaree, W.L. Marshall, & D. Hudson (Eds.), *The juvenile sex offender* (pp. 45-83). New York: Guilford Press.

Knox, S. (1994). *Effectiveness of cognitive behavioral therapy: Evaluating self-instructional training with adolescent sex offenders.* Unpublished doctoral dissertation, University of Texas at Austin.

Kolko, D.J., Noel, C., Thomas, G., & Torres, E. (2004). Cognitive-behavioral treatment for adolescents who sexually offend and their families: Individual and family applications in a collaborative outpatient program. *Journal of Child Sexual Abuse, 13*(3/4), pp.157-192.

Marshall, W. L. (1993). The treatment of sex offenders: What does the outcome data tell us? A reply to Quinsey et al. *Journal of Interpersonal Violence, 8,* 524-530.

Marshall, W. L., & Pithers, W. D. (1994). A reconsideration of treatment outcome with sex offenders. *Criminal Justice and Behavior, 21,* 10-27.

Morenz, B., & Becker, J. (1995). The treatment of youthful sexual offenders. *Applied and Preventive Psychology, 4,* 247-256.

Mothersole, G. (2000). Clinical supervision and forensic work. *The Journal of Sexual Aggression, 5,* 45-58.

Mulvey, E. P., Arthur, M. W., & Reppucci, N. D. (1993). The prevention and treatment of juvenile delinquency: A review of the research. *Clinical Psychology Review, 13,* 133-167.

Piliero, C. A. (1994). *Cognitive restructuring and the mental states of adolescent sex offenders: A quasi-experimental study of the effects of three interventions.* Unpublished doctoral dissertation, University of Pennsylvania.

Prentky, R. A., & Knight, R. A. (1991). Identifying critical dimensions for distinguishing among rapists. *Journal of Consulting and Clinical Psychology, 59,* 643-661.

Quinsey, V. L., Rice, M. E., Harris, G. T., & Lalumiere, M. L. (1993). Assessing treatment efficacy in outcome studies of sex offenders. *Journal of Interpersonal Violence, 8,* 512-523.

Rosenthal, R. (1979). The file drawer problem and tolerance for null results. *Psychological Bulletin, 86,* 638-641.

Rosenthal, R. (1991). *Meta-analytic procedures for social science research* (revised ed.). Newbury Park, CA: Sage Publications.

Stein, D. M., & Lambert, M. J. (1995). Graduate training in psychotherapy: Are therapy outcomes enhanced? *Journal of Consulting and Clinical Psychology, 63,* 182-196.

Weinrott, M. R., Riggan, M., & Frothingham, S. (1997). Reducing deviant arousal in juvenile sex offenders using vicarious sensitization. *Journal of Interpersonal Violence, 12,* 704-728.

Whiston, S. C., & Sexton, T. L. (1993). An overview of psychotherapy outcome research: Implications for practice. *Professional Psychology: Research and Practice, 24,* 43-51.

An Investigation
of Successfully Treated
Adolescent Sex Offenders

Kristina Crumpton Franey
Donald J. Viglione
Peter Wayson
Clark Clipson
Robert Brager

SUMMARY. Little is known about the characteristics of adolescent sex offenders who do not reoffend. Most studies emphasize reoffense rates, recidivism and those who reoffend. Moreover, these studies provide quantitative summaries without describing the individual, his behavior, and challenges after treatment. The present study seeks to provide novel information about the life experiences of adolescent sex offenders who have not reoffended after reentering society. Through a structured questionnaire and an in-depth qualitative interview, the adolescents ($N = 7$) provided information regarding their

---

Address correspondence to: Kristina Crumpton Franey, PsyD, Forensic Psych Consultants, 614 5th Avenue Suite A, San Diego, CA 92101 (E-mail: kfraney@earthlink.net).

[Haworth co-indexing entry note]: "An Investigation of Successfully Treated Adolescent Sex Offenders." Franey, Kristina Crumpton et al. Co-published simultaneously in *Journal of Child Sexual Abuse* (The Haworth Maltreatment and Trauma Press, an imprint of The Haworth Press, Inc.) Vol. 13, No. 3/4, 2004, pp. 295-317; and: *Identifying and Treating Youth Who Sexually Offend: Current Approaches, Techniques, and Research* (ed: Robert Geffner et al.) The Haworth Maltreatment and Trauma Press, an imprint of The Haworth Press, Inc., 2004, pp. 295-317. Single or multiple copies of this article are available for a fee from The Haworth Document Delivery Service [1-800-HAWORTH, 9:00 a.m. - 5:00 p.m. (EST). E-mail address: docdelivery@haworthpress.com].

http://www.haworthpress.com/web/JCSA
10.1300/J070v13n03_15

life experiences after treatment with an emphasis on the challenges they face in society. *[Article copies available for a fee from The Haworth Document Delivery Service: 1-800- HAWORTH. E-mail address: <docdelivery@ haworthpress.com> Website: <http://www.HaworthPress.com> © 2004 by The Haworth Press, Inc. All rights reserved.]*

KEYWORDS. Sex offender, adolescent, recidivism, qualitative, success

Until recently, the phenomenon of adolescent sexual offending has been largely ignored (Becker & Hunter, 1997). For instance, prior to 1970, only nine major papers were published on adolescent sex offenders. During the past 20 years researchers and clinicians have devoted much more attention to this problem with over 100 major papers published by 1993 (Barbaree, Hudson, & Seto, 1993).

What is missing in the literature is an understanding of what happens to male adolescent sex offenders once they leave treatment. Researchers have focused on recidivism and predictors of reoffense without investigating those adolescent offenders who have successfully reintegrated into society. It would seem that studying what we have done right and what has helped these offenders might allow us to evaluate and to enhance treatment models.

Whereas many studies provide quantitative summaries of adolescent sex offenders' characteristics and reoffense rates, few studies have described their lives and experiences. Although reviewing re-arrest statistics and recidivism rates are vital for assessing dangerousness and treatment efficacy, interviewing the adolescents directly may deepen our understanding of their lives after treatment as well as why they reoffend (Grubin & Wingate, 1996).

Only one study has adopted this idiographic, qualitative approach in researching adolescent sex offenders. Bremer (1992) conducted an idiographic study of adolescent sex offenders after treatment. She explored the experiences of 193 adolescent sex offenders from a residential treatment program. The length of stay varied from 30 days to 30 months, with an average stay of 7-12 months. Bremer completed a record review of the participants' juvenile criminal records. Also, each participant completed a questionnaire either by telephone or by mailing. This questionnaire addressed sexual offending since leaving the program as well as aspects of the treatment program that the participants felt were particularly helpful.

Six percent of the participants were convicted of subsequent sexual offenses after leaving treatment. Of note, 11% of the population admitted to sexually reoffending but were not convicted, indicating that criminal records underreported the actual rate of reoffense. Unfortunately, the author did not assess rates of nonsexual reoffending behavior. In response to a question that asked what they found most helpful, the majority of participants felt that the caring relationship with the therapists and the participants' abilities to express emotions aided them in changing their offensive behavior. Other helpful components included "learning the meaning of or how to have a relationship" and "learning to identify or express feelings appropriately" (p. 230). Bremer calls for more qualitative studies to assist in gaining a more complete understanding of the adolescent sex offender.

We present a qualitative, idiographic study addressing experiences of "successful" adolescent offenders who do not reoffend when they reenter society. The study focuses on the challenges they face when returning to society and on their attributions for success. Through both a structured and an in-depth qualitative interview, it is hoped that themes will emerge which represent their experiences and any elements associated with their success. This study will not assess the effectiveness of the specific treatment program nor is it a study on recidivism. It is an exploratory study that hopes to provide the literature with an in-depth understanding of who these young offenders are as human beings.

That is not to say that their experiences in treatment will not be addressed. On the contrary, important information about the treatment program will be asked. We will explore how participation in the treatment program has impacted the lives of these adolescents who have abstained from reoffending. Other questions include, from the participant's point of view, what aspects of treatment were most beneficial? What aspect of treatment provided them with the skills needed to successfully re-enter society? What difficulties in the world do they encounter due to labeling effects? How do they overcome such difficulties and continue to abstain from offending? By listening to their individual stories, it is the expectation that we can develop an understanding of their life experiences after treatment, and therefore offer insight that could be used to enhance relapse prevention and devise better treatment programs to address the reintegration process into society.

By utilizing an idiographic, qualitative approach to access the thoughts and experiences of this successful group, we hope to communicate important knowledge about this overlooked subpopulation.

METHOD

This study took place in three stages: (a) a record review, (b) a questionnaire, and (c) an in-depth qualitative interview. It is an ancillary study of longitudinal research conducted at a day treatment program for adolescent sex offenders in conjunction with the California School of Professional Psychology at San Diego. The treatment program is a county funded, 2-year treatment program for male adolescent offenders between the ages of 12 and 17 years. The adolescents are usually court mandated into the program. The first phase of the longitudinal study involved collecting psychological assessment and demographic data on participants at intake, 18 months, and discharge from the program. A wide cross section of the program members participated in this study. At the last assessment of data, the participants ($N = 101$) had an average of four reported victims, with the number of victims ranging from 1 to 20.

Record Review

The sample population ($N = 101$) was used for the record review phase of the current study. A record review was completed on all participants who had left the program at least 1 year prior to the start of the current study ($N = 51$). A court order was obtained to gain access to both their juvenile court and probation records. An additional security clearance was obtained to gain access to the Department of Justice database to widen the search of adult criminal records, supplementing a search of the San Diego County adult criminal record database. Finally, a review of the participants' clinical records and previously collected assessment data was completed.

The record reviews served to narrow down the participant pool. Initially, 51 participants were eligible for the study. Twenty were then excluded because of a new crime (3 sexual crimes, 17 nonsexual crimes), and 11 others had been terminated from the treatment program. From the remaining 20 potential participants, 13 could be located; however, 4 refused to participate and 4 were under the age of 18, leaving 7 to be interviewed for the study.

The second and third phases to this study (questionnaire and interview) drew participants from the record reviews. Stringent inclusion criteria were implemented for the final phases, such that only successful participants would be included. For the purposes of this study, "success" was defined as a participant who graduated from the treatment program and abstained from reoffending, both sexually and non-sexually according to a criminal record review. Any subject who had reoffended since leaving was excluded from the final phases of the research. Likewise, due to research ethical concerns, anyone who was under the age of 18 regardless of their "success" was not included in the study. In all, 16 people met the inclusion criteria, and 7 eventually participated.

Participants

The participants of the questionnaire and interview phase of the study ($N =$ 7) were male adolescents who agreed to participate in the longitudinal study described above, and had been away from the treatment program for a minimum of 1 year (average time since graduation = 36 months). The participants ranged in age from 18 to 23. Four of the 7 participants were Caucasian, and 3 were Hispanic. Five of the 7 participants remained in the home during their time in treatment, with 2 requiring placements in a group home.

Participant recruitment. A letter first alerted the potential participants and their families that a researcher would be contacting them via telephone to ask them to participate in interviews regarding their life after treatment. This letter served to prepare the participants for the telephone call and to encourage their continued participation in the research project. If the participant was a ward of the state, his caseworker or parole officer was contacted to obtain current information for the participant.

Participants who met the inclusion criteria were then recruited by telephone and asked if they would like to participate in an in-person interview. The participants were informed that the interview would consist of both a semi-structured and an open-ended interview between 2- to 2-1/2 hours. The participants were reimbursed for travel expense and earned two movie-passes for their participation.

Number of participants. The number of participants ($N = 7$) was determined when a point of saturation was met. This method of setting an N states that interviews are conducted until such a time that newly gathered data becomes redundant (Maykut & Morehouse, 1994). Saturation was determined when subsequent subjects provided no new themes or information. Therefore, data analysis was completed after each interview.

Questionnaire

The instrument utilized in this study was an 82-question demographic interview developed by this researcher. It is based on work by Dwyer (1997) and Viglione, Brager, Flitton, Crumpton, and Moore (2000). While Dwyer's (1997) study addresses adult reoffending behavior after treatment, it is one of only two studies that this author has found that includes actual contact with the offenders. Dwyer's questionnaire was revised and combined with a questionnaire previously developed by Drs. Viglione and Brager. The questionnaire addressed major components of adolescent development (e.g., family support, education, peer relationships, romantic relationships, occupation) as well as mental health, criminal behaviors, and substance abuse. The answers to the questionnaire provided initial data on all of the participants. Additionally, the replies to the questionnaire were utilized in developing the open-ended, qualitative interview schedule.

Interview

The participants completed an in-depth qualitative interview. The goal of the interview was to obtain a thorough understanding of the participants as individuals. The interview was based upon the findings from the questionnaire as well as areas of difficulty that are often addressed in the literature regarding re-entering society. An initial interview schedule was developed which addressed domains that the primary researcher hypothesized were important elements of the participant's challenges since reentering society. The main domains addressed included peer relationships, romantic relationships, familial relationships, educational difficulties, occupational difficulties, use of relapse prevention techniques, self-esteem, prior sexual history, prior criminal history, mental health issues, substance abuse, and treatment program-specific questions (e.g., what was helpful about treatment). The qualitative data was analyzed in hopes of understanding common experiences shared by all of the participants.

Procedure

Definitions of reoffense and success incorporated both sexual and non-sexual offenses, arrests, convictions, and losses of liberty. Reoffense was defined as self-reported or reported incidence of sexual crimes (voyeurism, frotteurism, child molestation, or rape) or any nonsexual criminal behavior (e.g., burglary, shoplifting, drug possession, or assault). It should be noted that the very limited definition of success utilized in this research is intended to be an operational definition and does not represent the concept of overall adaptation to life.

Following the record reviews, data collection took place through in-person questionnaires and interviews. The data were encoded with the participants' assigned subject numbers. Factual information gathered during the interview or questionnaire (e.g., number of victims) was then compared to the participants' legal and clinical files for verification.

The quantitative questionnaire was read to each participant, and his answers were recorded on the form. Once the questionnaire was complete, participants were asked to complete an in-depth, open-ended interview with the primary researcher. New consent and assent forms were signed prior to the interviews taking place. The participants were given a Subject's Bill of Rights, which explained that they were free to stop the interview at any time. They were also provided with names and telephone numbers of a treatment program therapist in case they had any questions or felt they needed support following the interview.

All interviews took place at the program offices and were audio taped. In an effort to ensure accurate transcripts of the interview, a professional transcriptionist was hired to type all interviews. This transcriptionist was bonded, and she signed a confidentiality agreement form prior to receiving the tapes.

Qualitative Data Analysis

The analysis of the qualitative interview data followed the emergent design as described by Maykut and Morehouse (1994). Before the first interview, initial themes were identified based on the literature. In turn, these were amended based on the results of the first interview. After each interview, new themes were identified and revisited with participants who had already completed their interviews. In other words, any new themes or experiences that the participants disclosed were added to the interview schedule. Likewise, those experiences that were initially included in the interview schedule but did not emerge in the interviews were noted and eliminated. When saturation was reached (when redundant themes were emerging), the interviews were discontinued. The initial participants were then contacted to assess the new themes that emerged during later data analysis.

RESULTS

Description of the "Successful" Graduates

Demographic and mental health information collected via questionnaire and interview for each of the 7 participants is summarized in Table 1, followed by a discussion of the findings.

Educational history. Despite their history of learning disabilities and educational challenges, 6 of the 7 participants completed high school. The seventh participant stated plans to earn a GED certificate. During the interviews, when describing their schooling, most participants reported, "School was difficult," explaining, "I'm not very good in school. Sometimes, I just don't like to apply myself in school." Others reported having difficulty "getting my work done" and that school "kind of got boring after awhile." Five of the 7 participants had decided to continue their education at the junior college level.

Table 1. Description of the Participants' Demographic and Mental Health Issues

Participant number and name[a]	Ethnicity	Age	Years past discharge	KBIT VIQ	KBIT–Matrices	KBIT–Composite	Education Challenges	DSM-IV Diagnoses	Out of Home Placement and Hospitalizations	Family Structure
1–Matthew	Hispanic	21	4	86	100	92	Special ed. speech, reading, math, behavior (bx)	Schizoaffective Disorder, r/o PTSD, LD NOS, Paraphilia NOS, hearing loss	Multiple group homes, inpatient, outpatient and day treatment (tx)	Father out of home, witnessed domestic violence (dv)
2–Pat	Caucasian	18	2	78	92	83	Special ed.; retained in 2nd grade, learning disability memory & reading	Paraphilia NOS, r/o PTSD, Depressive disorder NOS, LD NOS, auditory processing	Mother jailed twice, placed with family members, outpatient tx	Father out of home, death of stepfather, witnessed dv, mother out of home
3–Michael	Hispanic	18	2	91	96	93	Special education, did not complete high school	Paraphilia NOS	Group home placement	Witnessed dv
4–Christopher	Caucasian	21	5	93	101	97	Hyperactive, incomplete work, low grades	Paraphilia NOS, Impulse Control d.o. NOS, ADHD, left heel cord shorter than right, r/o hearing impairment	No placement, outpatient tx, history of depression	Corporal punishment, intact family
5–Nicholas	Caucasian	20	4	116	128	125	No special ed.	Paraphilia NOS, Dysthymia, asthma, history of bypass surgery	No placements, outpatient tx	Father chronically depressed, sisters required out of home placement
6–Timothy	Caucasian	19	3	87	86	85	No special ed.	Paraphilia NOS, asthma	No placement, outpatient tx	Parents divorced, witnessed dv
7–Lucas	Hispanic	19	1	75	46	57	Special ed., writing and bx problems	R/o Dysthymia, r/o Communication d.o., r/o LD	Outpatient tx, gang activity	Witnessed dv

Note. [a]Participants are numbered in order of interview completion; all names have been changed to protect the identity of the participants.

Concomitant mental health diagnoses. Four of the 7 participants were dealing with depressive or anxiety-based disorders (such as Posttraumatic Stress Disorder) upon entering treatment. Three experienced suicidal ideation during this time. During their interviews, they explained, "I wanted to commit suicide . . . I climbed up on the ledge and I was like, 'what should I do?'" After getting caught for offending, one participant explained, " I felt like I wasn't human . . . I seemed like nothing, nobody." One participant described having continued moments of suicidal ideation. When asked what keeps him from making an attempt, he explained, "If I were to kill myself, or if I were to die in a car accident, how are people going to think of me?" Of note, at the time of the interview, only 1 of the 7 participants admitted to suicidal ideation. This participant signed a no-harm contract and was given resources for local therapists as well as the crisis line.

Three of the 7 participants required medication for depressive symptoms during their involvement with treatment. However, at the time of this study, only 1 participant was still on medication. This participant, who has been diagnosed with a psychotic disorder, has also required hospitalization since leaving treatment, and is currently involved in therapy. One additional participant sought therapy after leaving treatment, participating in family therapy.

Family structure and dysfunction. All of the participants reported difficulty in family relationships. Three of the participants were raised without a father in the home. Even those with fathers in the home reported challenging relationships with their fathers. Statements during their interviews such as, "He has a drinking problem," "He had a nervous breakdown . . . he stays in his room," and "He would come into my life for like a month or whatever and then he'd leave" illustrate these challenges. The participants' relationships with their mothers were also challenging. During the interview, statements such as, "She treats me like a mental patient instead of like her son," "My mom wasn't there most of the time," and "She did drugs for 21 years" describes the participants' relationships with their mothers. Similarly, clinical files denote that 5 of the 7 participants reported being exposed to domestic violence during their childhood. It is clear that most of the participants grew up in chaotic homes.

However, looking back to their time in treatment, most of the participants described their families as being active in their treatment program. When asked during the interview, "How was your family supportive of your treatment?" some described how their families attended the multi-family groups each week ("my dad and mom were like one of the leaders in the program"). Others stated, "They fought for me to get in here (treatment vs. juvenile detention)," and "They never left me alone." Unfortunately, this was not the experience of all of the participants. Some stated, "him (father) coming to anything was practically a miracle," "(my) family still thinks of me like an unstable person," and "they were very numb."

Now that most of the participants have moved away from home, they described their relationships with their families as greatly improved. Statements such as, "(we are) closer than ever," and "I see my father more as a friend now, more as a someone I look to for guidance than a father" reflect this change in perspective. However, some were still struggling to find peace within their families. The participants stated, "We still argue sometimes," "I don't care about them that much," and "I just kind of realized that I've got to kind of step away from them . . . I don't want to live like that."

Abuse histories. As is consistent with the literature, 6 of the 7 participants reported being victims of physical abuse. Most of the participants described physical abuse as a means of discipline. For instance, "If we didn't do our homework right, we'd get like hit with a belt," and "I was brought up with the belt." One participant associated his physical abuse with his later offending behavior, "Somebody was hurting you, and you didn't know what to do with all that anger and hurt . . . I had to get out somehow, but I hurt someone else."

In this study, 4 of the 7 were victims of sexual abuse. They expressed confusion and long lasting negative effects of their own sexual abuse: "I thought it was just a game my cousin was playing," and "I have flashbacks from when I was 1 and 2 but I still remember."

Prior legal involvement. None of the participants in this study had a formal criminal record at the time of intake into the program. This includes the sexual offense that resulted in their referral to treatment. One of the 7 participants had an extensive history of legal involvement prior to attending treatment, which included being cited for gang involvement and truancy. However, despite their criminal behavior, no formal charges could be found during the record review. Most likely participants' criminal records were sealed or they were informally adjudicated and therefore no record exists (B. Stevens, personal communication, May 9, 2002).

Index sexual offense. The index offenses are summarized in Table 2. A review of clinical records indicated that the 7 participants offended against an average of two victims per participant (range = 1-4 victims). However, as is consistent with Bremer's (1992) findings, the self-report number of victims was higher than reported in their clinical and legal files, with an average of three victims per participant (range = 1-8).

COMMON THEMES AND TRENDS

By implementing the constant comparative method (Maykut & Morehouse, 1994) certain themes and common experiences emerged from the data gathered during the interview. As a new category emerged (spirituality), it was

TABLE 2. Summary of Sexual Offense Histories

Participant Number[a]	Number of documented victims	Number of self-reported victims	Gender of victims	Ages range of victims	Relation to victims	Offenses	Level of Coercion and Severity
1–Matthew	2	1	Female	Age 5	Stranger	Fondled, masturbated victims	Denies
2–Pat	2	2	Males	Ages 6-7 yr.	1 Friend, 1 Stranger	Exposed self, fondled, frotteurism, oral copulation	Used guilt to coerce
3–Michael	3	2	2 Males, 1 Female	Males–11-12 yr. Female–17 yr.	All family members	Showed porn., exposed self, had victim orally copulate him	Promised special rewards, hit victims, restrained victim
4–Christopher	1	1	Female	Age 5	Friend	Frotteurism, exposed self, fondling, oral copulation, digital and penile penetration	Told her he loves her, promised her rewards, used a threatening tone, hit her, restrained her, threatened to tell, admits to hurting her
5–Nicholas	4	8	2 Males, 6 Females	Males–6-7 yr. Females–1-51 yr.	3 Family member 3 Extra family members, 2 Strangers	Showed porn., exposed self, fondled, had victim masturbate him, digital penetration	Denies
6–Timothy	1	1	Female	From age 5-14	Family member	Showed porn., fondling, exposed self, oral copulation, penile penetration	Promised would do favors for victim
7–Lucas	1	8	1 Male, 7 Females	Male age 8, females age 15-30	Male–family member, Females strangers	Females–sexual harassment; male–exposed self, fondling, anal penetration	Promised special rewards, used guilt statements, used a threatening tone with victim, admits to hurting victim

Note. [a]Participant names have been changed to protect the identity of the participants.

305

added to the interview schedule and addressed in each subsequent interview. Attempts were made to contact the first participant after his interview to address the new domain that was not in place during his interview, but he was not available for further interviews. No additional categories emerged during the interviews. Following is a description of the primary categories or themes that emerged during the data analysis.

An Understanding of the Sexual Offenses Committed

When asked to provide a detailed description of their sexual offenses, all 7 participants showed visible discomfort. However, once they began discussing the offenses, each answered in a detailed and almost detached manner. Most of the participants graphically described the specific offensive behavior. Some explained that during their treatment they were taught to be thorough and explicit when discussing their offenses. When asked to describe antecedents to their behaviors (e.g., "What was going on for you at that time in your life?"), all of the participants provided what appeared to be insightful, well thought out answers. Table 3 summarizes their statements.

The Participants' Views of the Treatment Program

Each participant was asked to describe his experience of the program. Six of the 7 participants stated they believe they needed the program, and that they found it to be very helpful. They described how the program, "changed my life," "woke me up," and "opened my eyes." The participant who did not believe he needed the program stated, "You had to say some things so you can get out," and "I don't agree with the theories that go on here." He did not identify his behavior as abusive, and to this day believes he engaged in mutual sex

Table 3. Self-Reported Antecedents to Sexual Offenses

Offense Antecedents	Example Statements
Low Self-Esteem/Self Hatred	"I felt alone. I felt like I didn't have anybody" "I thought everybody hated me" "I couldn't stand myself"
Confusion/Curiosity	"I think a lot of my offenses were out of curiosity and inappropriate boundaries" "Being confused . . . not knowing right from wrong at that time" "In our lives, for whatever reason, it was natural"
Re-Enactment/Revenge	"I treated her like I was paying her back for everything that happened" "In our tradition, the oldest one is the person who tells the younger ones what to do" "We were both molested"

play with his sibling. He did however have a suggestion of adding a spiritual component to the program, which will be discussed in a later section.

The participants were asked, "What about treatment did you find to be most helpful?" Whereas 1 participant mentioned, "nothing," the remaining 6 gave answers with three main themes, which represent key elements to the program: (a) peer support, (b) structure, and (c) therapeutic relationships. Statements that support these three themes are presented in Table 4.

Many of the participants reported that they had also learned techniques at the program that they find themselves still utilizing. These skills include relapse prevention plans, such as recognizing high-risk situations and removing themselves from these situations, anger management skills, and recognizing triggers that lead to their offending. Others gave more generalized answers, such as "looking at the big picture," "think before I act," and "empathy."

The final questions regarding the program addressed how the participants would change the program. The answers given regarding changing the program can be placed into two main categories: (a) emphasizing accountability and (b) adding skill building. The participants indicated that learning to hold themselves accountable for their decisions was most helpful. Some indicated that they continue to utilize this skill. Yet they also described times during treatment when they felt sorry for themselves, or seemed to forget why they were in the program. They suggested that staff "Keep the focus on the reasons we're here" and to give "reminder of the reasons why they were there, it's not for them, it's for the ones they offended."

Additional recommendations for changes to the program included having a chaplain on call for spiritual crises, increasing the amount of exercise the juveniles receive, and adding a unit on life skills to the group component. As one person explained, he was released from the program and sent to the "real world," but he did not know how to interview for a job, write a resume, balance a checkbook, or maintain a healthy relationship. He felt that the two years

TABLE 4. Elements of Treatment Participants Found Most Helpful

Treatment	Statements
Peer Support	"We looked out for each other" "We were always a family" "More of a brotherhood kind of community" "We finally connected . . . bonding"
Structure	"limits" "boundaries . . . structure . . . be accountable" "like a boot camp . . . lock down" "The in your face stuff was cool" "I need to stay focused and stay responsible"

of treatment was so focused on his offense, that the other areas of his life were overlooked. He stated that success was a struggle because he was lacking family support and had to teach himself how to navigate adult tasks.

Adjusting to Life After Treatment

The next part of the interview focused on the participants' lives after their time in treatment. This included exploring their readjustment into society, their identity, and any challenges they faced following treatment. It became clear that one of the obstacles they would have to face upon returning to society was deciding whom they would tell about their treatment, and what would be said.

Who they tell, who they don't. Three of the participants were able to complete their high school education during their treatment. The program has an agreement with a local high school, which enables the participants to graduate from that particular high school even though their course work is completed in treatment. These three did not have to face the challenge of returning to their original school and peer groups after a 2-year absence. While one stated, "I never got to enjoy high school," the other two saw graduating from high school through the program as a blessing. They stated, "I wanted to keep that separation. I protected myself; I had to," and "It would have been pretty awkard to re-transition."

Two participants returned to their original schools, while the remaining two were able to attend a new school. Those that went to new schools still ran into old friends. When asked how they handled the situation, all stated they told lies about why they left their old school. These lies included, "I told them I blew up at a teacher," "I was going through things with the family," and "I told them . . . because of my grades or something." Yet some describe how peers found out about their sexual offenses. They said, "They totally teased me about it" and "It was pretty embarrassing, you know pretty awkward."

Similarly, many of the participants had to decide which of their friends they would tell about their offenses. This was especially difficult for those who were placed in group-homes as a result of the offense. Many of the participants made friends with fellow clients, but all stated they ended those friendships after leaving treatment. One described this need for new friends as, "I didn't want to deal with the past anymore; it was time to move on." Those who told friends outside of the program stated they were pretty honest regarding what they told them, "I just told them straight up."

In contrast to being open with their friends, the participants did not always inform those with whom they have had romantic relationships about their pasts. One participant who had been living with his girlfriend for 2 years and plans to marry her within the next year stated, "No, I believe that when I graduated I said to myself this part is behind me. Knowing her past, I don't want to reveal it to her." Others decided to be forthcoming about their pasts. They explained, "I had to be straight up with her," and "I told her if we were going to have a relationship, I'm going to at least be honest with her."

Identity and Spirituality

A primary task of adolescence is the development of an identity separate from one's parents. When a significant event such as committing a sexual offense occurs during adolescence, it would seem that this event would alter the course of the adolescent's development. Therefore, two primary questions were posed to the participants regarding their self-identity: "What was it like the first time you were called a sex offender?" and "Will you always be a sex offender?"

First time called an offender. As is common with sex offender treatment programs, the participants were required to admit to their sexual offenses in great detail. This detailed description has multiple purposes, including breaking down denial, tracking faulty cognitions, and identifying triggers to the behavior, and it is often utilized in offense-specific treatment programs (R. Brager, personal communication, January 24, 2002). The participants of this study provided a glimpse into their memories of what it was like the first time they were called a sex offender. It seems that the participants experienced apprehension, guilt, and confusion. Table 5 summarizes their responses.

Putting the past behind them. The majority of participants made comments about their desire to "move on" and "put it behind me." When asked to elaborate, many of the participants explained that it was too painful to dwell on their past offenses. They have to strike a delicate balance between honoring their victims and

TABLE 5. Participants' Reactions When First Called a Sex Offender

Emotional Responses	Statements
Apprehension/Fear/Confusion	"I was really scared" "It was kind of crazy, you know, being a child molester and being a child at the same time. It was confusing" "Where am I going to go in life with all of these labels that are in my records?"
Guilt/Remorse/Sadness	"My heart had dropped" "I felt kind of dirty and bad" "Am I a horrible person?"
Awareness	"I just realized I raped this little girl, I took her innocence away" "It kind of hits home" "I took it to heart"

moving forward with their lives. One of the participants explained that becoming a successful, productive member of society is one way to honor his victim.

Current identity. One might assume that following 2 years of sexual offending treatment, the 7 participants would be permanently identified by their crimes. This hypothesis corresponds with a 12-step model, in which one admits that once an addict, always an addict. Therefore, the question, "Will you always be an offender?" was based upon this model of treatment. However, this was not the case. None of the 7 participants identified themselves as being at risk to reoffend. The participants still struggle with the label and strive to move forward with their lives. Their responses to this question, as outlined in Table 6, illustrate this point.

Spirituality. An unanticipated aspect to the participants' self-identity was their spirituality. This topic was not included in the original interview schedule. The second participant interviewed brought this up as an important part of his life. As is expected in the emergent design, this theme was then added to all remaining interviews. Unfortunately, the first participant was no longer available for a follow-up interview, so his answer is not reflected here. This is the only new theme that emerged in the data analysis.

The remaining 7 participants responded to the question, "Please tell me about your spiritual beliefs as they apply to your recovery." There were responses that reflected anger at God. For instance, one young man stated, "God didn't help her when I raped her. God wasn't there," while another stated he had lost his faith in God at that time. Yet others were able to find comfort in their belief that God was able to forgive them for their offenses. One participant explained, "It definitely has a lot of bearing on my life–it helps me to forgive myself if I know God can forgive me" while others explained that God's forgiveness allows them to release the guilt associated with their crimes.

Many stated that God or the church acts as a centering agent in their lives, bringing them a sense of peace. As one explained, "It gives us time to think and contemplate what we're doing and whether or not we're going the right

TABLE 6. Participants' Responses to "Will You Always Be an Offender?"

Responses	Statements
Struggling to accept the past	"I just hate myself for it sometimes" "Just trying to cope with what I've done and who I am as a person" "No, but in my soul I am"
Moving forward	"You should never look back . . . pushing on, pushing forward. It's just like you have to leave the past in the past" "That was just a label. That label comes off when you forgive yourself . . . you saw what you did wrong and you make a difference" "I don't think I ever was an offender"

way." He went on to explain that his religion helps him to be "more down-to-earth" and more honest, which in turn makes him more apt to reach out to help others. Still others expressed a belief that God has a plan for their future. As another participant explained, "God's going to put me in a place where He's going to want me to preach His word. God has a plan for me; no matter what I do, He has a plan."

The Future as Seen by the Participants

Challenges and future concerns. The 7 participants of this study completed the program and have not reoffended criminally or sexually according to their criminal records. They have begun the process of reintegration into society and have generally succeeded. Yet each faces the normal challenges of a person in their early 20s (e.g., career, education, success) as well as unique challenges based on their offending behaviors and past criminal histories. They expressed concerns regarding raising their own children. As one explained, "What if I offend my own kids? What if I have a kid and my wife won't let me hold him because of the past?"

Future dreams and goals. The participants readily shared their future dreams and goals during the interview. Like many 20-year-olds, the participants held dreams of a good career, family, and a home "with a white picket fence." They dream about financial security and future education. Yet most of the participants expressed rather mature goals given their young ages. These goals focused on the desire to better themselves and to never stop evolving. They made statements such as, "for me to be someone," "to walk the talk," "to always change, always work on myself, being aware of who I am, where I'm going and just never stop changing" and "to focus, practice, and just go for it." One participant sees himself living one day at a time and chooses to not focus on the future. He explained, "I'm not in prison where I could have been, so I'm living my dream." Perhaps most inspirational was a participant's dream to return to the program to work with current clients. He explained he wants to "come back here, look at everybody and say hey, I made it!"

Why Successful and Advice to Current Clients

Most were surprised to learn that they fit the definition of "successful." When asked to explain, "To what do you attribute your success?" many had difficulty answering the question. After much deliberation, the participants were able to quantify the reasons for their success. Their answers can be classified into three categories: (a) family support, (b) therapeutic support, and (c) mindset. The statements supporting these categories can be found in Table 7.

The participants had similar advice to give to current participants. They emphasized the need to believe in one's self, remain focused, and to remain hopeful. As mentioned earlier, 6 of the 7 participants found the program to have a positive impact on their lives. They wanted to share their messages of hope with the current clients. Their messages are summarized in Table 8.

DISCUSSION

The aim of this study was to describe the life experiences of adolescent sex offenders who had successfully completed a 2-year day treatment program for moderate level offenders and who had not reoffended afterwards. The challenges faced by the participants of this study are consistent with challenges often discussed in the literature when describing adolescent sex offenders. The literature often depicts adolescent offenders as having a history of educational problems (Awad & Saunders 1989; Awad, Saunders, & Levene, 1984; Fehrenbach, Smith, Monastersky, & Deisher, 1986), poor peer relations (Awad & Saunders, 1989;

TABLE 7. Participants' Attributions of Success

Responses	Statements
Family Support	"They were really there for you all the time" "It was really good to have my family supporting me" "Knowing they care for you"
Therapeutic Support	"Because they put up with me, the real me" "(They) were always there for me when I had a hard time"
Planning	"Live one day at a time" "Think ahead" "Realize everything before I act" "To prove to myself that I know I can do it" "Just like planning for everything"

TABLE 8. Messages for Current and Future Clients

Responses	Statements
Believe in Yourself & Stay Determined	"You just can't give up" "You've just got to realize you can change, you can become a better person"
Dedication	"Mean what you are saying–care about what you are doing" "Put everything on the line and go for it" "Tell everything. Tell the truth no matter what"

Blaske, Borduin, Hengeler, & Mann, 1989; Fehrenbach et al., 1986; Weinrott, 1996), familial instability (Awad, Saunders et al., 1984; Ford & Linney, 1995), and histories of their own abuse (Freeman-Longo, 1986; Knight & Prentky, 1993; Van Ness, 1984). The literature previously covered also suggests that adolescent sex offenders are at risk for nonsexual offending (Becker, Kaplan, Cunningham-Rathner, & Kavoussi, 1986; Ford & Linney, 1995; Weinrott 1996). Most of the participants in this study fit this description.

Life Experiences of Successful Adolescent Sex Offenders

During the interviews, each of the 7 participants discussed their lives prior to treatment. Each came from chaotic homes; 5 came from homes where domestic violence took place. Six of the boys were themselves victims of physical abuse. There were discussions of learning disabilities, repeating grades, and having difficulties with peers.

Likewise, when discussing their lives immediately prior to and during their offenses, the participants each identified feelings of confusion, self-hatred, loneliness, and anger. The life stories of these participants do not excuse their behaviors. Yet as one listens to their descriptions of sadness and hopelessness, a new level of empathy for the offender emerges.

The participants expressed feelings of guilt, shame, embarrassment, and sadness when recalling their offenses. Most of the participants spoke of the desire to "move on," and to leave the label "sex offender" behind them. Moreover, the participants were visibly uncomfortable during their interviews. They made comments about wanting to cancel their appointments and their hesitancy to return the researcher's telephone calls. Many described how difficult it was for them to return to the treatment office, and the memories this brought up for them. Coupled with those participants who had qualified for the study but either declined or refused to accept phone calls from someone calling with the program, it is clear that asking participants to revisit their past was more distressing than was assumed.

Yet most were enthusiastic in their descriptions of why they needed to attend the program and of the elements that they found most helpful. They suggested peer support, structure, and therapeutic relationships were very important to them. This supports Bremer's (1992) findings in which her participants mentioned therapeutic support and the ability and opportunity to express themselves as vital components to their treatment. The added elements of peer support and structure may enhance Bremer's findings or may be unique to this treatment program. This should be explored further in future research.

Additionally, the participants identified the concept of accountability as the most important element of treatment that they utilize currently. The participants each explained that the treatment program emphasizes the need to hold oneself accountable for one's actions. Many feel they are more responsible and mature than same aged peers because of the treatment they completed. Other important elements identified include open communication and active listening skills.

One unanticipated suggestion for changes to treatment programs was adding a component of spirituality. As each consecutive participant was asked about his beliefs, it became clear that some form of spirituality is important to this group of participants. The belief in God's ability to forgive appears to play a crucial role in their healing process. This should be investigated in future research.

The participants made comments about "moving on" but never forgetting. Finding this balance in their lives appears to be an important element in their success. It allows them to integrate their past identities with their adult identities. As one participant explained, it is a matter of survival. Given the recent influx of media coverage, registration programs, and three-strike laws surrounding sex offenders, his insight is accurate. Letting the world know you were/are a sex offender is not a wise choice. Disclosing one's "secrets" would require a certain level of self-confidence and courage in the face of possible rejection by another person. This likely explains why only one of the four participants who are engaged has told his significant other about his past.

Nonetheless, the participants' desire to integrate their past behaviors into their adult identity is a sign of positive adult identity development. To dwell on the past and never forgive oneself would be damaging, as was exhibited by one participant's occasional suicidal ideation. To choose to be successful and a productive member of society out of respect for one's victim is a healthy and positive manner of integrating the past with the future. Many of the participants suggested that treatment programs address this challenge before the adolescents are sent into the adult world.

Lessons Learned from Successfully Treated Adolescent Sex Offenders

Enhancing treatment programs. This study started with a limited definition of success–that is, graduating from the treatment program and not committing new sexual or nonsexual crimes since leaving treatment. However the self-reported life experiences of these "success" stories illustrates how tenuous this success truly is. The participants continue to face similar global social challenges (e.g., peer relations, familial discord, poor social skills) that may have contributed to their offending in the first place. Yet many of the specialized treatment programs that help adolescent sex offenders to stop offending often do not address these underlying difficulties.

It is unknown how many treatment programs include modules in relationship skills, money management, and life skills, yet that is what "successful" sex offenders suggest be added to treatment. It is clear that the scope of treatment must move beyond offense-specific behaviors. By listening to the participants, and learning the challenges they face upon reentering society, clinicians and researchers can learn how to enhance existing treatment programs.

The role of qualitative methods in studying adolescent offenders. This is the third study this researcher knows of in which the participants were actually interviewed after treatment. So often, follow-up studies end after a record review. Bremer (1992) and Dwyer (1997) were pioneers in utilizing qualitative methods with sex offenders. This study took their method a step further. Rather than focusing solely on treatment factors that the participants found helpful, this study sought to truly understand their experiences both in treatment and after returning to society. It is hoped that clinicians reading this study will gain a personal perspective on what their sexual offending client is facing after leaving treatment.

As is mentioned throughout this paper, qualitative research methods allowed access to data that is normally overlooked–the participants' own experiences. This study could have stopped at the second phase, with a record review and reporting of reoffense rates of the 51 clients who left the treatment program.

The qualitative research design utilized in this study provided a venue for the adolescent offenders to be the experts. By presenting the goal of the interview to the participants, that is, to understand what has happened to them since leaving treatment and to allow us to learn from their success, the participants became valuable teachers. Although many stated they do not feel like "success stories," they were happy to provide the program and its clients advice to remain successful. They were able to articulate the challenges they faced growing up, as well as their own thoughts as to why they sexually offended others. The participants also sent messages to treatment facilities, reminding the facilities that a more global treatment approach would better serve offenders like themselves. A study confined to record review would have missed this invaluable information.

Yet this study is not without its limitations. For instance, given the small number of participants, a pilot study was not possible. By utilizing a pilot study to test the coding system developed, additional themes may have emerged or been able to be eliminated prior to interviewing the participants. Likewise, it does not provide statistically significant elements related to "success" after treatment. Finally, given the limited amount of time between graduation and this study, it is possible that the participants in this study may not meet the definition of success in the future. A longitudinal study of these 7 participants would address this question. However, it is hoped that this study lays the groundwork for future exploration, including the different experiences of those who were unsuccessful and possible mitigating factors that determine whether an adolescent offender will be successful or go on to reoffend after leaving treatment.

REFERENCES

Awad, G., & Saunders, E. (1989). Adolescent child molesters: Clinical observations. *Child Psychology and Human Development, 19*, 195-206.

Awad, G., Saunders, E., & Levene, J. (1984). A clinical study of male adolescent sexual offenders. *International Journal of Offender Therapy and Comparative Criminology, 28*, 105-116.

Barbaree, H. E., Hudson, S., & Seto, M. C. (1993). Sexual assault in society: The role of the juvenile offender. In H. E. Babaree, W. L. Marshall, & S. Hudson (Eds.), *The juvenile sex offender* (Vol. 1, pp. 1-24). New York: Guilford Press.

Becker, J. P., Kaplan, M. P. D., Cunningham-Rathner, J., & Kavoussi, R. J. M. (1986). Characteristics of adolescent incest sexual perpetrators: Preliminary findings. *Journal of Family Violence, 1*(1), 85-97.

Becker, J. V., & Hunter Jr., J. A. (Eds.). (1997). *Understanding and treating child and adolescent sexual offenders* (Vol. 19). New York: Plenum Press.

Blaske, D. M., Borduin, C. M., Hengeler, S. W., & Mann, B. J. (1989). Individual, family and peer characteristics of adolescent sex offenders and assaultive offenders. *Developmental Psychology, 25*, 846-855.

Bremer, J. (1992). Serious juvenile sex offenders: Treatment and long-term follow-up. *Psychiatric Annals, 22*(6), 326-332.

Dwyer, S. M. (1997). Treatment outcome study: Seventeen years after sexual offender treatment. *Sexual Abuse: A Journal of Research and Treatment, 9*(2), 149-161.

Fehrenbach, P. A., Smith, W., Monastersky, C., & Deisher, R. W. (1986). Adolescent sexual offenders: Offender and offense characteristics. *American Journal of Orthopsychiatry, 36*(2), 225-223.

Ford, M. E., & Linnery, J. A. (1995). Comparative analysis of juvenile sexual offenders, violent non-sexual offenders, and status offenders. *Journal of Interpersonal Violence, 10*(1), 56-70.

Freeman-Longo, R. E. (1986). The impact of sexual victimization on males: A brief communication. *Child Abuse and Neglect, 10*, 411-414.

Grubin, D., & Wingate, S. (1996). Sexual offence recidivism: Prediction versus understanding. *Criminal Behaviour and Mental Health, 6*, 349-356.

Knight, R. A., & Prentky, R. A. (1993). Exploring characteristics for classifying juvenile sex offenders. In H. E. Babaree, W. L. Marshall, & S. Hudson (Eds.), *The juvenile sex offender* (Vol. 1, pp. 45-83). New York: The Guilford Press.

Maykut, P., & Morehouse, R. (1994). *Beginning qualitative research. A philosophic and practical guide*. Philadelphia: The Falmer Press.

Van Ness, S. R. (1984). Rape as instrumental violence: A study of youth offenders. *Journal of Offender Counseling, Services, and Rehabilitation, 9*, 161-170.

Viglione, D. J., Brager, R., Flitton, A., Crumpton, K., & Moore, T. (2000, March). *Rorschach and other assessment data from adolescent sex offenders in treatment.* Paper presented at the Annual Meeting of the Society for Personality Assessment, Albuquerque, New Mexico.

Weinrott, M. R. (1996). *Juvenile sexual aggression: A critical review* (Center Paper 005 F-1450). Boulder, CO: Institute of Behavioral Science, Regents of the University of Colorado.

Index

BOOK ORDER FORM!

Order a copy of this book with this form or online at:
http://www.haworthpress.com/store/product.asp?sku=5497

Identifying and Treating Youth Who Sexually Offend
Current Approaches, Techniques, and Research

____ in softbound at $39.95 ISBN: 0-7890-2787-9.
____ in hardbound at $59.95 ISBN: 0-7890-2786-0.

COST OF BOOKS _____	❑**BILL ME LATER:**
	Bill-me option is good on US/Canada/ Mexico orders only; not good to jobbers, wholesalers, or subscription agencies.
POSTAGE & HANDLING _____	
US: $4.00 for first book & $1.50 for each additional book	❑ **Signature** _____
Outside US: $5.00 for first book & $2.00 for each additional book.	❑ **Payment Enclosed: $** _____
SUBTOTAL _____	❑ **PLEASE CHARGE TO MY CREDIT CARD:**
In Canada: add 7% GST. _____	❑ Visa ❑ MasterCard ❑ AmEx ❑ Discover
STATE TAX _____	❑ Diner's Club ❑ Eurocard ❑ JCB
CA, IL, IN, MN, NJ, NY, OH, PA & SD residents please add appropriate local sales tax.	**Account #** _____
FINAL TOTAL _____	**Exp Date** _____
If paying in Canadian funds, convert using the current exchange rate, UNESCO coupons welcome.	**Signature** _____
	(Prices in US dollars and subject to change without notice.)

PLEASE PRINT ALL INFORMATION OR ATTACH YOUR BUSINESS CARD

Name

Address

City   State/Province   Zip/Postal Code

Country

Tel   Fax

E-Mail

May we use your e-mail address for confirmations and other types of information? ❑Yes ❑No We appreciate receiving your e-mail address. Haworth would like to e-mail special discount offers to you, as a preferred customer.
We will never share, rent, or exchange your e-mail address. We regard such actions as an invasion of your privacy.

Order from your **local bookstore** or directly from
The Haworth Press, Inc. 10 Alice Street, Binghamton, New York 13904-1580 • USA
Call our toll-free number (1-800-429-6784) / Outside US/Canada: (607) 722-5857
Fax: 1-800-895-0582 / Outside US/Canada: (607) 771-0012
E-mail your order to us: orders@haworthpress.com

For orders outside US and Canada, you may wish to order through your local
sales representative, distributor, or bookseller.
For information, see http://haworthpress.com/distributors

(Discounts are available for individual orders in US and Canada only, not booksellers/distributors.)

Please photocopy this form for your personal use.
www.HaworthPress.com

BOF05